A Practical Approach to Neurophysiologic Intraoperative Monitoring

A Practical Approach to Neurophysiologic Intraoperative Monitoring

Edited by

Aatif M. Husain, MD
Department of Medicine (Neurology)
Duke University Medical Center
Durham, North Carolina

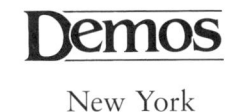

Demos
New York

Acquisitions Editor: R. Craig Percy
Cover Designer: Aimee Davis
Indexer: Joann Woy
Compositor: TypeWriting
Printer: Edwards Brothers Incorporated

Visit our website at www.demosmedpub.com

© 2008 Demos Medical Publishing, LLC. All rights reserved. This book is protected by copyright. No part of it may be reproduced, stored in a retrieval system, or transmitted in any form or by any means, electronic, mechanical, photocopying, recording, or otherwise, without the prior written permission of the publisher.

Library of Congress Cataloging-in-Publication Data

A practical approach to neurophysiologic intraoperative monitoring / edited by Aatif M. Husain.
    p. ; cm.
  Includes bibliographical references and index.
  ISBN-13: 978-1-933864-09-9 (pbk. : alk. paper)
  ISBN-10: 1-933864-09-5 (pbk. : alk. paper)
  1. Neurophysiologic monitoring. I. Husain, Aatif M.
  [DNLM: 1. Monitoring, Intraoperative—methods. 2. Evoked Potentials—physiology. 3. Intraoperative Complications—prevention & control. 4. Trauma, Nervous System—prevention & control. WO 181 P895 2008]
  RD52.N48P73 2008
  617.4'8—dc22
                                                                    2008000450

Medicine is an ever-changing science undergoing continual development. Research and clinical experience are continually expanding our knowledge, in particular our knowledge of proper treatment and drug therapy. The authors, editors, and publisher have made every effort to ensure that all information in this book is in accordance with the state of knowledge at the time of production of the book.

Nevertheless, this does not imply or express any guarantee or responsibility on the part of the authors, editors, or publisher with respect to any dosage instructions and forms of application stated in the book. Every reader should examine carefully the package inserts accompanying each drug and check with a his physician or specialist whether the dosage schedules mentioned therein or the contraindications stated by the manufacturer differ from the statements made in this book. Such examination is particularly important with drugs that are either rarely used or have been newly released on the market. Every dosage schedule or every form of application used is entirely at the reader's own risk and responsibility. The editors and publisher welcome any reader to report to the publisher any discrepancies or inaccuracies noticed.

Made in the United States of America
09 10 5 4 3 2

This book is dedicated with love and respect to my parents,
Mairaj and Suraiya Husain,
who have given me the foundations to do what I have done,
what I am doing, and what I will ever do.

Contents

Foreword .... *ix*
Preface .... *xiii*
Contributors .... *xv*

I Basic Principles

1. Introduction to the Operating Room 3
   Kristine H. Ashton, Dharmen Shah, and Aatif M. Husain

2. Basic Neurophysiologic Intraoperative Monitoring Techniques 21
   Robert E. Minahan and Allen S. Mandir

3. Remote Monitoring 45
   Ronald G. Emerson

4. Anesthetic Considerations 55
   Michael L. James

5. Billing, Ethical, and Legal Issues 67
   Marc R. Nuwer

6. A Buyer's Guide to Monitoring Equipment 73
   Greg Niznik

II Clinical Methods

7. Vertebral Column Surgery 95
   David B. MacDonald, Mohammad Al-Enazi, and Zayed Al-Zayed

8. Spinal Cord Surgery 117
   Thoru Yamada, Marjorie Tucker, and Aatif M. Husain

9. Lumbosacral Surgery 139
   Neil R. Holland

10. Tethered Cord Surgery 155
    Aatif M. Husain and Kristine H. Ashton

11. Selective Dorsal Rhizotomy 169
    Daniel L. Menkes, Chi-Keung Kong, and D. Benjamin Kabakoff

12. Peripheral Nerve Surgery 181
    Brian A. Crum, Jeffrey A. Strommen, and James A. Abbott

13. Cerebellopotine Angle Surgery: Microvascular Decompression 195
    Cormac A. O' Donovan and Scott Kuhn

14. Cerebellopotine Angle Surgery: Tumor 213
    Dileep R. Nair and James R. Brooks

15. Thoracic Aortic Surgery 227
    Aatif M. Husain, Kristine H. Ashton, and G. Chad Hughes

16. Carotid Surgery 261
    Jehuda P. Sepkuty and Sergio Gutierrez

17. Epilepsy Surgery 283
    William O. Tatum, IV, Fernando L. Vale, and Kumar U. Anthony

    Index *303*

Foreword

Neurophysiologic intraoperative monitoring (NIOM) is undertaken in an effort to reduce neurological morbidity associated with some types of surgeries. Postoperative outcomes of some orthopedic, neurosurgical, and otologic surgeries reveal a significant incidence of adverse outcomes with intraoperatively acquired neurologic lesions. Presumably there is a time in the development of many lesions when the pathologic process leading to a lesion is reversible. Initially it seemed reasonable that although the patient cannot be directly examined during the surgical procedure, that demonstration of changes in electrophysiology might give warnings that pathophysiologic changes were taking place. If the changes were corrected, the surgically induced lesion could be avoided. These assumptions proved to be true, and various animal studies revealed that neural damage was accompanied by changes of evoked response amplitude, latency, or both and/or changes of evoked and spontaneous electromyographic (EMG) activity. Nonpathologic factors, such as temperature and anesthetic type and depth, cause changes in activity, which may be misinterpreted as an impending neural lesion. Unfortunately such changes may also be due to purely technical factors. When changes are seen, the monitoring technologist should begin a search for technical causes and simultaneously inform the monitoring neurophysiologist and surgeon of the changes.

Initially, the technology provided only limited capacity for remote monitoring, requiring the neurophysiologist to be present in the operating room, at least during critical periods of surgery when a neural lesion was likely to occur.

Our medicolegal experiences have led us to examine many surgical records in which there was an adverse outcome. Too often the operating surgeon was not informed promptly, usually because response amplitude diminished progressively until it was not clear whether a response was present or not. The surgeon should be aware that false positives are common. He or she should be aware that not all neurophysiologic changes are the result of surgical manipulations. We advised technologists that the surgeon should be informed *immediately* of the difficulty and the possibility or even likelihood that the cause was purely technical. Then as now, rapid troubleshooting is imperative. It is the surgeon, not the technologist, who knows the anatomy of the current surgery. Thus a change in cortical and/or subcortical responses in spinal surgery may be of little concern if the surgeon is taking a bone graft and has not been near the spine for many minutes.

The avoidance of some anesthetic agents as well as the study and documentation of the relative resistance of far-field subcortical responses to anesthetic changes, commonly altering near-field cortical responses, greatly enhanced the utility of evoked potentials (EP) in the operating room setting. Early in the application of NIOM, with the exception of direct cord stimulation, the study of EMG (both spontaneous and evoked responses) was in its infancy. Now, motor responses from stimulation techniques, including transcranial electrical and magnetic stimulation, are no longer investigative but are routine in many centers.

The technical aspects of electroencephalography (EEG), EP, and NIOM are now largely resolved. Guidelines were published by the American EEG Society in 1986, 1988, 1994, and 2006, which represented consensus knowledge and approaches to these techniques.

In the mid-1990s we were introduced to a new postdoctoral fellow in clinical neurophysiology. Aatif Husain was one of the first to take a combined EEG/Epilepsy/EMG fellowship at Duke University Medical Center. To us he expressed a keen interest in NIOM, and he was one of the few fellows to respond to our invitations to come to the operating room for an orientation to NIOM. He would arrive in the operating room at 6:00 A.M. to watch the technical staff prepare patients for monitoring. In a short time he was asking probing questions and assisting in "setting up" the patients for surgery. With his training in EMG, it was not long before Aatif was making suggestions as how to better monitor EMG activity when the surgeon deemed such monitoring to be appropriate. Those who have experienced the operating room environment know well the potential pitfalls related to interfacing with operating room staff. When the monitoring team sets up a new monitoring service and intrudes with additional personnel and equipment, they are not always welcomed with open arms. As in the early days of EEG, technologists and interpreters of EP and NIOM were either self-taught or the product of "on-the-job training" in centers where such diagnostic procedures were done. We were training residents, fellows, and technologists informally, usually structured by the number of trainees present. In a short time we found requests for technologist and interpreter training to be almost overwhelming. Space and the time demands of Duke University Medical Center allowed us to offer only extended weekend courses. We realized the inadequacy of such training, but too little training was considered preferable to no training. Interpreter classes on EP in general and NIOM in particular could be larger than technologist classes, in part because lab time was not offered. We felt that technologists required a lab exposure, and thus their classes were limited to 20 attendees. Dr. Husain attended many of these technician training sessions, realizing that technologist training was both important and necessary. Subsequently, Dr. Husain championed the long Duke tradition of emphasizing intensive training for technologists, and he has actively supported the American Society of Electroneurodiagnostic Technologists (ASET) courses and the American Board of Registration in Electroencephalographic and Evoked Potential Technology (ABRET) by serving initially as an invited examiner and later as an elected board member.

Course offerings in these topics were and are now available at numerous medical centers and national technologist and physician societies have incorporated EP and NIOM into their course offerings at their annual meetings. For physicians, the American Board of Clinical Neurophysiology (ABCN) developed a special NIOM certification examination and the American Board of Psychiatry and Neurology (ABPN) developed the Subspecialty Examination in Clinical Neurophysiology, which incorporated NIOM questions. Early on there was a continuing need to educate surgeons and anesthesiologists on strategies for enhancing NIOM techniques, because cooperation between the surgical and monitoring teams is essential. Dr. Husain's text will no doubt serve well to promote such cooperation. On the technologist front, ABRET offered the first examination of Certification in Neurophysiologic Intraoperative Monitoring (CNIM) in 1996.

Since that time, Aatif's career in clinical neurophysiology has progressed impressively; his publications alone attest to his broad interest in the field. Aatif directs Duke's NIOM program. We have retired from the active practice of medicine and left clinical neurophysiology and NIOM to younger eyes and minds.

On all these levels, from local teaching to national society offerings to national board examinations, Dr. Husain has contributed his time and expertise to the benefit of trainees at all experience levels. We feel that we must all be trainees; otherwise we close our minds to new information. We share Dr. Husain's enthusiasm for the field and this text. No text can solve all of the training issues of such a broad audience, but this work is clearly an important step forward. We are honored to have been asked to write this foreword and to have participated in the formative period of this fascinating field.

C. William Erwin, MD
Professor Emeritus
Duke University Medical Center
Past President ABRET and ACNS
Past Chairman, ABCN

Andrea C. Erwin, R EP T, CNIM
Past Manager
Clinical Neurophysiology Laboratories
Duke University Medical Center
Past ABRET Section Chair
EP Examining Committee

Preface

Seldom has a field in medicine grown as rapidly as neurophysiologic intraoperative monitoring (NIOM). Twenty-five years ago, few people had heard of NIOM. About 20 years ago, the initial seminal papers appeared, documenting the utility of somatosensory and brainstem auditory evoked potential monitoring in reducing the morbidity of scoliosis and brainstem surgery. Fifteen years ago, NIOM was available only in large, academic hospitals, often with equipment cobbled together by experienced neurophysiologists. As recently as 10 years ago, there were few educational offerings where one could learn more about NIOM.

The last decade has seen remarkable advances in NIOM. Not only have new modalities, such as motor evoked potentials, become available, but the equipment used for monitoring has improved considerably. Advances in telecommunications have enabled remote real-time review of NIOM data by neurophysiologists. Educational programs and courses in NIOM are much more common and are offered during meetings of many neurophysiology societies. Trained technologists have done much to further advance the field. Research has documented the utility of many types of NIOM in reducing the morbidity not only in orthopedic surgery and neurosurgery but also otolaryngologic, vascular, and cardiothoracic surgery. Surgeons, anesthesiologists, neurologists, and other healthcare professionals now accept the value of NIOM in making many types of surgeries safer.

Although most large academic and many community hospitals now offer NIOM services, there remains a shortage of qualified neurophysiologists and technologists to meet the demand. Education in NIOM is seldom available in traditional residency, fellowship, or other training programs. Technologists also learn on the job and often have no formal curriculum to follow. Textbooks on the subject are few and often limited in scope to neurosurgical and orthopedic procedures. Learning about medicolegal issues surrounding NIOM is even more difficult.

With this book I hope to bridge some of the gaps on NIOM education and clinical practice. It is divided in two main sections. In the first section, "Basic Principles," the reader will learn the basics of NIOM. This includes not only the modalities used in monitoring, but also topics not usually discussed. The novice will find an introduction to the operating room, where basics about sterile technique and the various machines that might be encountered are discussed. Chapters on remote monitoring, billing, and ethical issues will help those trying to set up laboratories. All will benefit from the buyer's guide to NIOM machines. The second part of the book, "Clinical Methods," reviews the use of NIOM in various types of surgeries. The chapters present the basics of anatomy, physiology, and surgery of the various procedures so that the reader will better understand what happens during these procedures. Details of the monitoring modalities and their interpretive criteria are then presented. Whenever possible, data supporting the use of NIOM in the particular type of surgery is also presented. A unique feature of every chapter is that it is written not only by an experienced neurophysiologist but also a senior technologist who has contributed to a technical section. This section reviews practical information about the logistics of monitoring a particular type of surgery, and it will be especially useful for technologists.

Many different professionals will find this book useful. Neurophysiology trainees and technologists will benefit in reading it in its entirety. Experienced neurophysiologists will find it useful every day in clinical practice, as information about many different types of surgery and monitoring is easily accessible. Surgeons and anesthesiologists will find useful information that will help them understand what the NIOM team does. Laboratory managers will find material that will help them set up laboratory procedures and protocols.

There are many individuals that have contributed to this book and must be recognized. Foremost, I am extremely grateful to my colleagues who contributed to this text. They have helped create a truly unique book. R. Craig Percy and his colleagues at Demos Medical Publishing have been incredibly supportive of this project and must be recognized and appreciated for their foresight in seeing the need for such a book. A special note of thanks is due to the many technologists, neurophysiologists, and surgeons at Duke University Medical Center who have taught me extensively. Special mention is due to Dr. C. William Erwin and Andrea Erwin, my mentors, without whom I would not have been introduced to NIOM. Of course, none of this would be possible without our patients, who have done the most to advance this field. Finally, I am indebted to my wife, Sarwat, and children, Aamer and Aayaz, for enduring my absenteeism for the many, many nights and weekends I worked on this book.

Aatif M. Husain

Contributors

James A. Abbott, R ED T
Department of Neurology
Mayo Clinic College of Medicine
Rochester, Minnesota
Chapter 12: Peripheral Nerve Surgery

Kumar U. Anthony, R EEG/EP T, CNIM, R PSG T
Department of Neurology
Tampa General Hospital
Tampa, Florida
Chapter 17: Epilepsy Surgery

Kristine H. Ashton, R EEG T, CNIM
Department of Medicine (Neurology)
Duke University Medical Center
Durham, North Carolina
Chapter 1: Introduction to the Operating Room
Chapter 10: Tethered Cord Surgery
Chapter 15: Thoracic Aortic Surgery

James R. Brooks, R PSG T, CNIM
Epilepsy Center
The Neurological Institute
Cleveland Clinic
Cleveland, Ohio
Chapter 14: Cerebellopontine Angle Surgery: Tumor

Brian A. Crum, MD
Department of Neurology
Mayo Clinic College of Medicine
Rochester, Minnesota
Chapter 12: Peripheral Nerve Surgery

Ronald G. Emerson, MD
Department of Neurology
The Neurological Institute
Columbia University College of Physicians and Surgeons
New York, New York
Chapter 3: Remote Monitoring

Mohammad Al-Enazi
Department of Neurosciences
King Faisal Specialist Hospital & Research Centre
Riyadh, Saudi Arabia
Chapter 7: Verterbral Column Surgery

Sergio Gutierrez, MD
Department of Neurology
Johns Hopkins University and Hospital
Baltimore, Maryland
Chapter 16: Carotid Surgery

Neil R. Holland, MB BS
Neurology Specialists of Monmouth County
West Long Branch, New Jersey
Department of Neurology
Drexel University College of Medicine
Philadelphia, Pennsylvania
Chapter 9: Lumbosacral Surgery

G. Chad Hughes, MD
Department of Surgery (Thoracic and Cardiovascular)
Duke University Medical Center
Durham, North Carolina
Chapter 15: Thoracic Aortic Surgery

Contributors

Aatif M. Husain, MD
Department of Medicine (Neurology)
Duke University Medical Center
Neurodiagnostic Center
Veterans Affairs Medical Center
Durham, North Carolina
Chapter 1: Introduction to the Operating Room
Chapter 8: Spinal Cord Surgery
Chapter 10: Tethered Cord Surgery
Chapter 15: Thoracic Aortic Surgery

Michael L. James, MD
Departments of Anesthesiology and Medicine (Neurology)
Duke University Medical Center
Durham, North Carolina
Chapter 4: Anesthetic Considerations

D. Benjamin Kabakoff, R EEG T, CNIM, R PSG T
Department of Clinical Neurophysiology
Baptist Memorial Hospital
Memphis, Tennessee
Chapter 11: Selective Dorsal Rhizotomy

Chi-Keung Kong, MBChB, FHKAM (Paed)
Department of Paediatrics
The Chinese University of Hong Kong,
Hong Kong, People's Republic of China
Chapter 11: Selective Dorsal Rhizotomy

Scott Kuhn, BS, CNIM
Department of Diagnostic Neurology
Wake Forest University Baptist Medical Center
Winston-Salem, North Carolina
Chapter 13: Cerebellopontine Angle Surgery: Microvascular Decompression

David B. MacDonald, MD, FRCP(C), ABCN
Department of Neurosciences
King Faisal Specialist Hospital & Research Centre
Riyadh, Saudi Arabia
Chapter 7: Verterbral Column Surgery

Allen S. Mandir, MD, PhD
Department of Neurology
Georgetown University
Washington, DC
Chapter 2: Basic Neurophysiologic Intraoperative Monitoring Techniques

Daniel L. Menkes, MD
Department of Neurology
University of Tennessee Health Sciences Center at Memphis
Department of Clinical Neurophysiology
Baptist Memorial Hospital
Memphis, Tennessee
Chapter 11: Selective Dorsal Rhizotomy

Robert E. Minahan, MD
Department of Neurology
Georgetown University
Washington, DC
Chapter 2: Basic Neurophysiologic Intraoperative Monitoring Techniques

Dileep R. Nair, MD
Epilepsy Center
The Neurological Institute
Cleveland Clinic
Cleveland, Ohio
Chapter 14: Cerebellopontine Angle Surgery: Tumor

Greg Niznik, MSc, CNIM, DABNM
Allied Neurodiagnostics
Atlanta, Georgia
Chapter 6: A Buyer's Guide to Monitoring Equipment

Marc R. Nuwer, MD, PhD
Department of Neurology
UCLA School of Medicine
Department of Clinical Neurophysiology
UCLA Medical Center
Los Angeles, California
Chapter 5: Billing, Ethical, and Legal Issues

Cormac A. O'Donovan, MD
Department of Neurology
Wake Forest University Baptist Medical Center
Winston-Salem, North Carolina
Chapter 13: Cerebellopontine Angle Surgery: Microvascular Decompression

Jehuda P. Sepkuty, MD
Epilepsy Center/Clinical Neurophysiology
Swedish Neuroscience Institute
Seattle, Washington
Johns Hopkins University and Hospital
Baltimore, Maryland
Chapter 16: Carotid Surgery

Dharmen Shah, MD
Department of Medicine (Neurology)
Duke University Medical Center
Durham, North Carolina
Chapter 1: Introduction to the Operating Room

Jeffrey A. Strommen, MD
Department of Physical Medicine and Rehabilitation
Mayo Clinic College of Medicine
Rochester, Minnesota
Chapter 12: Peripheral Nerve Surgery

William O. Tatum, IV, DO
Department of Neurology
Tampa General Hospital and University of South Florida
Tampa, Florida
Chapter 17: Epilepsy Surgery

Marjorie Tucker, CNIM, R EEG/EP T, R NCS T
Department of Neurology
Roy J. and Lucille A. Carver College of Medicine
University of Iowa Hospital and Clinics
Iowa City, Iowa
Chapter 8: Spinal Cord Surgery

Fernando L. Vale, MD
Department of Neurosurgery
Tampa General Hospital and University of South Florida
Tampa, Florida
Chapter 17: Epilepsy Surgery

Thoru Yamada, MD
Department of Neurology
Roy J. and Lucille A. Carver College of Medicine
University of Iowa Hospital and Clinics
Iowa City, Iowa
Chapter 8: Spinal Cord Surgery

Zayed Al-Zayed, MD, FRCS
Department of Orthopedics
King Faisal Specialist Hospital & Research Centre
Riyadh, Saudi Arabia
Chapter 7: Verterbral Column Surgery

A Practical Approach to Neurophysiologic Intraoperative Monitoring

1 Basic Principles

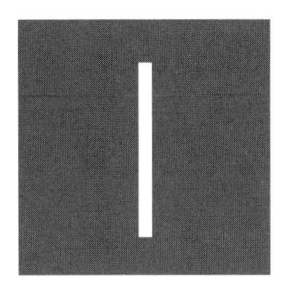

1 Introduction to the Operating Room

Kristine H. Ashton
Dharmen Shah
Aatif M. Husain

The operating room can be an intimidating environment for most nonsurgical healthcare personnel. Lack of operating room knowledge, unfamiliarity with aseptic techniques and sterile field, and minimal surgical training contribute to the anxiety. This basic knowledge is critical for neurophysiologic intraoperative monitoring (NIOM) staff, since it helps them to understand the roles of various personnel and how their jobs dovetail with those of others. Familiarity with the personnel, instrumentation, and environment of the operating room can help make NIOM successful. This chapter serves as an introduction to the operating room, discussing aseptic technique, personnel, equipment likely to be encountered, and the basics of preparation, safety, and cleanup related to NIOM.

ASEPTIC TECHNIQUE

"Aseptic technique" refers to practices used to minimize the patient's exposure of pathogens, usually one undergoing a surgical procedure. This technique involves not only cleaning surgical instruments so that they are free of pathogens but also routines followed by surgeons and operating room personnel to minimize the spread of microorganisms. In this section, sterilization techniques are discussed first, followed by a review of how surgeons and other staff should be attired.

Sterilization Methods

Sterilization is a process by which objects are cleansed of living organisms, including spores. It is important to differentiate sterilization from disinfection. Disinfection reduces the number of viable organisms, whereas sterilization kills all organisms. Common disinfectants include alcohol and phenolic compounds. However, sterilization—not disinfection—is necessary in the operating room.

Three methods of sterilization are available: thermal, chemical, and radiation. Each method uses different devices to measure and ensure the integrity of the sterilization. Knowing about methods of sterilization is important for NIOM staff, as instruments needing to be sterilized must be packed according to the method that will be used to sterilize them.

Thermal Sterilization

Heat is a reliable method of sterilization. Moisture, in the form of steam, combined with heat hastens the process. This process causes denaturation and coagulation of enzymes and protein systems of microorganisms. All living organisms are killed with steam at a temperature of 115°C (240°F) for 15 minutes (1). Higher temperatures require less time. The exact temperature and time needed to thermally sterilize an object depends on its size and what else is placed in the sterilization chamber.

Steam sterilizers are often referred to as autoclaves. Three types of steam pressure sterilizers are commonly used: prevacuum sterilizers, gravity displacement sterilizers, and flash/high-speed pressure sterilizers. As name indicates, the prevacuum sterilizer vacuums air for several minutes prior to entry of the steam into the chamber. Because of the vacuum created, as soon as steam enters the chamber it penetrates to the center of packages placed in the chamber. A temperature between 132° and 141°C (270° and 285°F) at 27 lb/in^2 for 15 to 30 minutes is needed for sterilization in prevacuum sterilizers (1).

A gravity displacement sterilizer has two openings. Steam enters the chamber through one opening, displacing heavy air out of the chamber from the other opening. Once the heavy air is removed from the chamber, the second opening is closed. The steam penetrating objects within the chamber kills the organisms. Gravity displacement sterilizers require a temperature of 121° to 123°C (250° to 254°F) at 15 lb/in^2 for 15 minutes to complete sterilization (1).

A flash/high-speed pressure sterilizer uses either a prevacuum or gravity displacement cycle. If a prevacuum cycle is used, the temperature requirement is 132° to 134°C (270° to 275°F) at 27 lb/in^2 for 3 minutes to kill microorganisms on a nonporous object. For porous objects, the time must be extended to 4 minutes. If the gravity displacement cycle is used, the time should be extended to at least 10 minutes (1). Flash/high-speed sterilization should be used only in emergencies and not to compensate for a shortage of supplies.

Electrodes, stimulators, and other objects used in NIOM that require sterilization should be thermally sterilized. Flash/high-speed pressure sterilization should be used only in emergencies, as when a one-of-a-kind instrument is inadvertently contaminated, such as by dropping on the floor.

The advantages of thermal sterilization are that it is fast, easy, inexpensive, and safe. It disadvantages include the need for cleaning the objects prior to sterilization, ensuring the steam contact with items in the chamber, and different standards regarding exposure time and temperature according to object size.

Chemical Sterilization

Multiple different chemicals have been utilized for chemical sterilization; however, only those listed by the U.S. Environmental Protection Agency (EPA) as chemical sterilants should be used as such. This list includes ethylene oxide gas, hydrogen peroxide, formaldehyde, and formaldehyde gas. Most of these chemical agents interfere with the metabolism of the organism, leading to cell death and ensuring sterility. Chemical sterilization is most commonly used for items that can easily erode and have low melting points, such as plastic. It is extensively used by commercial companies to prolong the shelf life of their products. In general, items that can be sterilized with steam should not be sterilized with chemical agents. Electrodes and other objects used by the NIOM team needing sterilization should not be chemically sterilized.

Radiation Sterilization

Ionizing radiation is mostly used for commercial sterilization. It kills microorganisms by forcefully dislodging electrons from ions and disrupting their deoxyribonucleic acid (DNA). The free electrons from gamma rays penetrate objects to be sterilized; efficacy depends on the electrons penetrating the entire object. Thus thick and dense objects may not get properly sterilized. However, high heat is not involved, so heat-sensitive objects can be sterilized in this manner. Gamma radiation is very expensive, and exposure of healthcare personnel to the radiation must be closely monitored (2). Radiation sterilization is seldom needed by NIOM personnel.

Operating Room Attire

Since human skin is harbors living organisms, operating room attire has been created to provide an effective barrier against the spread of these organisms to the patient. To maintain the integrity of the sterile environment of the operating room, street clothes are not allowed into the restricted area, and operating room attire should not be worn outside the operating room. Different clothing requirements exist for those individuals who are scrubbed for a procedure and for those not scrubbed.

Individuals who are not scrubbed for the actual surgery have four required components of their attire: body cover, head cover, shoe covers, and mask. Body covers are available in either two-piece pantsuits or one-piece overalls. If a two-piece suit is worn, the shirt should be tucked inside the pants' drawstring to avoid contact with the sterile field. The required head and shoe covers are usually made of special paper and should be replaced each time the individual exits and enters the restricted area. Two types of face masks are available, conical and cup-shaped. The application of the mask is also critical for its effective use. The upper strings should always be tied at the back of the head, while the lower strings are tied behind the neck. Multiple different personal protective devices are also available—such as aprons, eyewear, nonsterile glove, etc.—however, their use is not mandatory. NIOM personnel must wear the prescribed attire when they are in the operating room.

Personnel who are operating or otherwise scrubbed in for the surgery must undergo three processes to become sterile: scrubbing, gowning, and gloving. Scrubbing the hands and arms with special soaps removes many organisms. Operating rooms may have requirements for how long or how many brush strokes are necessary for adequate scrubbing. After drying with a sterile towel, a sterile gown is immediately put on. Details about gowning and gloving are not be discussed further, as NIOM personnel will generally do not need to be scrubbed. Such details can be found elsewhere in operating room texts (1,3).

Sterile Field

Knowledge of the sterile field is critical as a small mistake can result in a significant disruption to the operating room environment. The sterile field includes the patient and his or her periphery, personnel wearing sterile attire, furniture covered with sterile drapes, and items within the sterile field. The integrity of the sterile field must be maintained by allowing only sterile items to enter or touch it. If there is a question regarding an item's sterility, it should be considered nonsterile.

Sterile gowns worn by the surgeon and the staff assisting him or her are considered sterile in front of the chest, at and above the level of the sterile field but not below it. Also, the area 2 inches above the elbows to the cuffs is considered sterile. The back of the gown is considered nonsterile, as it is not under close observation. Persons wearing sterile attire should keep their hands at or above waist level or at the level of the sterile field. All surgical team members should maintain the same height in relation to other surgical team member to protect the integrity of the sterile field. A drastic change in the position of one surgical team member, such as the sitting position, will require a change in position of all other members of the surgical team as well (3).

Sterile tables are considered sterile only on the top areas. Drapes extending below the operating tables are considered nonsterile. The NIOM personnel must secure all electrical cords with nonperforating clips to prevent them from sliding onto the sterile areas. Sterile items on the table are continuously observed and maintained by the main scrub nurse. The circulating nurse (discussed later) is responsible for getting instruments and supplies that are not on the sterile tray of instruments. He or she will then hand the instrument to the scrub nurse or place them in the sterile field, maintaining integrity of the object and the sterile field. If the item is wrapped in a peel package, the edges of the package should be rolled over the presenter's hands and the inner sterile contents presented to the scrub nurse. This must be done in a manner that avoids contamination of the object, the scrub nurse, and the sterile field. Nonsterile persons should never reach over the sterile field to transfer the sterile items. On the other hand, a sterile person should never reach over a nonsterile area (1,3).

The NIOM staff must be able to follow the sterile technique and learn to transfer objects such as electrodes and stimulators in a sterile manner. If they are unable or not sure how to do so, they should consider using the circulating nurse to transfer their supplies to the operating table. Like all other personnel in the operating room, the NIOM staff also have a responsibility of helping keep the sterile field intact and alerting the appropriate personnel (scrub or circulating nurse) if a breach occurs.

PERSONNEL

Many different people are likely to be encountered by the NIOM team in the operating room. It is useful to know who these people are, what responsibilities they have, and how they can affect NIOM.

Surgical Team

In addition to the attending surgeon, other members of the surgical team may be present in the operating room. Several of these may scrub in the case and assist the surgeon. The NIOM staff must know who is in charge of the case, as this person must be kept abreast of any changes or other issues with NIOM.

Attending Surgeon

The surgical team consists first of an attending surgeon, the physician ultimately responsible for the patient and everything that occurs during the surgery. The attending surgeon decides which patients should undergo NIOM and, in conjunction with the neurophysiologist, decides what type of NIOM to use. Changes in NIOM during surgery must be communicated to the attending surgeon so that appropriate corrective action can be taken if possible. Additionally, any issues with setup of a case should be referred to the attending surgeon so that he or she is aware and can address them if necessary. The attending surgeon is usually not in a position to serve as the interpreter of NIOM data.

Surgical Resident

One or more surgical residents (surgeons in training) may be training with the attending surgeon and assist with the case. Senior residents may open and close the case independently. Depending on their skill level, chief residents may perform most of a surgery independently. When the attending surgeon is not in the room, the senior resident is in charge. In such a situation, responsibilities noted above for the attending surgeon are assumed by the resident in charge. Changes in NIOM data must then be communicated to this resident.

Medical Students

At some centers, particularly teaching hospitals, medical students may be present and perform certain duties, such as inserting Foley catheters. With the surgeon's permission, they may scrub in on the case. They generally are not present in the surgery by themselves. Whereas informing medical students about NIOM may be educational for them, it is not a substitute for informing the surgeon in charge. Medical students should not be relied upon to convey NIOM information to the attending surgeon.

Physician Assistants (PAs) and Nurse Practitioners (NPs)

PAs and NPs work in large and small hospitals and may scrub in to assist the attending surgeon when necessary. In these situations, PAs and NPs play a role similar to that of a surgical resident. However, they will seldom perform large parts of the surgery independently. If the PA or NP is the only member of the surgical team present in the room, he or she must be kept informed of NIOM changes; if the attending surgeon is present, he or she must be informed.

Anesthesia Team

The anesthesia team typically consists of an attending physician and technician who float between several operating rooms and an anesthesia resident or clinical registered nurse anesthetist (CRNA) who is dedicated to one operating room. The monitoring technologist should communicate with the anesthesia team about the best time to apply electrodes and other requirements for NIOM.

Attending Anesthesiologist

The attending anesthesiologist is the physician in charge of all aspects of the patient's anesthesia. Often he or she is responsible for overseeing the anesthetic care of patients in multiple rooms. Although the attending anesthesiologist will not be physically present in the operating room for the duration of the surgery, an anesthesia resident or CRNA will be present at all times. The attending anesthesiologist will usually interview the patient in the preoperative holding area prior to surgery. The NIOM team should communicate any special requirements, such as total intravenous anesthesia (TIVA), with the attending anesthesiologist. When changes in NIOM data occur, in addition to the surgeon being informed, the anesthesiologist should also be kept aware in case changes in anesthesia are needed.

Anesthesia Resident

The anesthesia resident is an anesthesiologist in training and is responsible for the patient's immediate care; he or she remains in the operating room with the patient at all times. The monitoring technologist will frequently encounter the resident in the operating room very early in the morning while both are setting up equipment to begin a case. It is courteous to begin communications regarding anesthetic requirements at this time, since the anesthesia team may need to gather different drugs than anticipated. Additionally, they may require additional infusion pumps and some extra time to program these. During the surgery, if NIOM changes are noted, along with the surgeon, the anesthesia resident should be kept apprised of these if the attending anesthesiologist is not in the room.

Clinical Registered Nurse Anesthetist

A CRNA is an anesthesia team member who has completed a master's degree program in nurse anesthesia. This person functions in much the same way as the anesthesia resident and is present with the patient during the entire surgery.

Anesthesia Technician

Anesthesia technicians assist the team in setting up the case in a variety of ways. They gather equipment, set up infusion pumps, prepare electrocardiogram leads and blood pressure cuffs, gather intravenous supplies, and do any other job that can help the anesthesia team get a case started. Throughout the case, the technician takes samples to the lab, gets blood, operates machines such as the cell saver, and again carries out other duties as needed.

Nursing Team

The nursing team usually consists of two nurses who are assigned to the operating room for all of the cases scheduled in that room for the day. They are almost always registered nurses (RNs) and may have a number of other degrees/certifications.

Circulating Nurse

The circulating nurse, also known as the circulator, is responsible for keeping track of personnel in the room, retrieving items required during surgery, maintaining documentation, answering the phone, and doing any other task that need to be done by someone who is not sterile. It is important for the monitoring technologist to check in with the circulating nurse at the start of the case. A cooperative relationship about the location of equipment, access to the patient, and draping of electrodes is essential to successful monitoring of a case.

Scrub Nurse

The scrub nurse scrubs in prior to the case in order to set up the instruments. He or she remains sterile throughout the case and passes instruments to the surgeons. If the monitoring technologist has any sterile probes, stimulators, electrodes, or cables for the surgeon to use, these are passed in a sterile fashion to the scrub nurse.

Room Attendant

The room attendant brings large equipment such as beds or microscopes into the room. He or she also helps to turn and position the patient. The circulating nurse will often call on the room attendant to locate odds and ends, such as extension cords or hair clippers. Attendants are usually assigned to several operating rooms and run between rooms, helping out wherever they can. An experienced room attendant can be an invaluable resource to the monitoring technologist, since he or she often arrives early in the morning to set up rooms, knows how the rooms are arranged and where best to place the NIOM equipment, knows where to find supplies, and knows a variety of personnel who may be of help.

Allied Health Personnel

Depending on the type of surgery, a variety of allied health personnel may be called in to help or may be present in the room throughout the surgery.

Radiology Technician

The radiology technician is one of the allied health professionals whom the monitoring tech will encounter often in the operating room. The radiology technician is usually operating one of two types of equipment, either a traditional x-ray or a C-arm machine. It is important for the monitoring technologist to establish communication with the radiology technician about the location of any wires or cords on the patient or bed so that the movement of the radiology machines does not disrupt NIOM.

Perfusionist

A perfusionist is present in cardiothoracic surgeries and operates the cardiopulmonary bypass (CPB) machine. The monitoring technologist should be aware that the perfusionist can deliver anesthetic agents through the CPB machine. Consequently, in these cases, not only the anesthesia team but also the perfusionist must be asked what anesthetics the patient will be receiving. The perfusionist is also responsible for inducing hypothermia when needed, and the monitoring technologist must be aware of that as well.

EQUIPMENT

A variety of different machines can be found in the operating room. The NIOM team must know not only their function but also the effect they can have on monitoring. Many machines will produce high-amplitude artifacts that must be recognized.

Electrocautery

The electrocautery (Figure 1.1), also known simply as cautery, is used in almost every operation. The cautery is used to electrically cut skin and to burn bleeding blood vessels closed. It causes a very large artifact that cannot be averaged through (Figure 1.2). The monitoring technologist will need to "pause" the NIOM machine during active cautery.

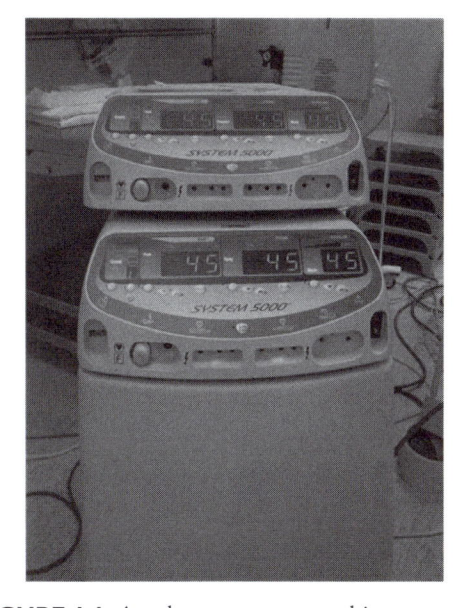

FIGURE 1.1 An electrocautery machine.

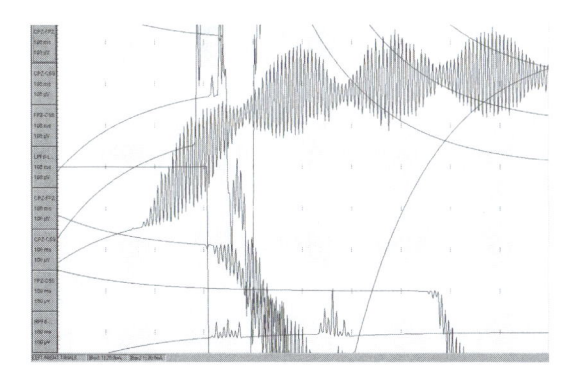

FIGURE 1.2 Example of artifact caused by electrocautery. This was seen when tibial somatosensory evoked potentials were being averaged.

Cardiopulmonary Bypass Machine

The CPB machine is used for aortic surgery (Figure 1.3). In these surgeries, electroencephalography (EEG), somatosensory evoked potentials (SEPs) or motor evoked potentials (MEPs) may be monitored. The perfusionist operates the CPB machine and can administer a variety of anesthetics through it. As noted above, the monitoring technologist must be aware of the drugs being administered through the CPB machine, as they may affect NIOM. The CPB machine can also be used for inducing hypothermia, and when this is being done, the monitoring technologist should make a note, as that will affect the monitoring as well. At times the CPB machine can produce significant artifact that makes interpretation of NIOM difficult. This is particularly true in cases where EEG activity is being recorded at 2 µV/mm to determine electrocerebral inactivity; at such a high sensitivity, artifacts are difficult eliminate.

Microscope and Monitor

The microscope is much used in neurosurgery (Figure 1.4). The monitoring technologist must position his or her equipment and cables in such a way as not to interfere with

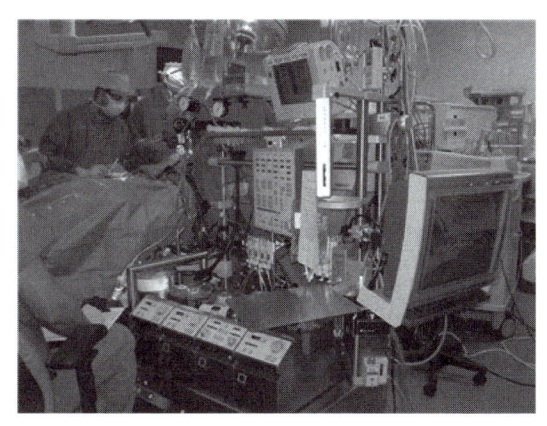

FIGURE 1.3 A cardiopulmonary bypass machine. This machine can also be used to administer anesthetic agents and other drugs as well as for inducing hypothermia.

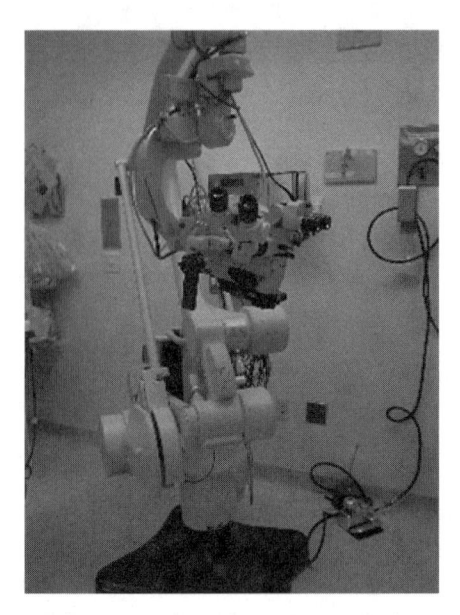

FIGURE 1.4 An operating surgical microscope. During surgery, this microscope will be draped with sterile sheets.

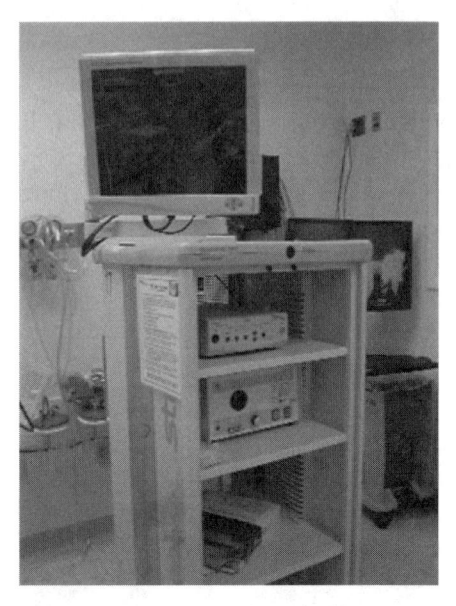

FIGURE 1.5 A monitor that displays images of the surgical microscope.

the microscope moving in and out of the field. There is rarely an artifact problem related to the microscope. The microscope will be sterile and draped prior to the start of the case and should not be touched once draped. Often the microscope is connected to a monitor that displays what the surgeon is seeing through the microscope (Figure 1.5). This is helpful, as all operating personnel can then see what is happening in the surgical field.

Ultrasound

Various types of ultrasound are commonly used in the operating room in a variety of surgeries (Figure 1.6). The ultrasound probes are usually operated by the surgeon, but they can be used by the anesthesiologist as well.

Intraoperative Ultrasound

A standard ultrasound machine is used to precisely locate tumors or other lesions in the surgical field. The ultrasound probe is covered in a sterile sheath and held by the surgeon. This type of ultrasound is used sporadically during the surgery.

Transesophageal Echocardiography

During aortic surgery, a procedure called transesophageal echocardiography (TEE) may be performed by the anesthesiologist. During this procedure, the anesthesiologist often has his or her fingers in the patient's mouth, manipulating the TEE probe. TEE usually does not produce artifact that affects NIOM. However, if MEP monitoring is being performed, it is important to be sure the anesthesiologist does not have his or her fingers in the

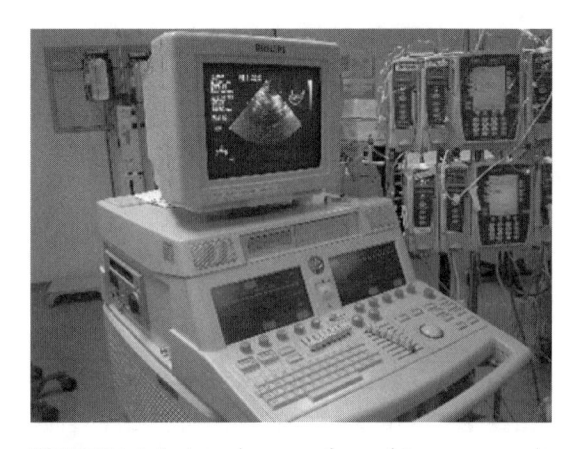

FIGURE 1.6 An ultrasound machine commonly used in the operating room.

patient's mouth, since a transcranial electrical stimulus will cause the patient to bite down. A surprise MEP stimulation could therefore cause injury to the anesthesiologist. It is best to alert both the surgeon and anesthesiologist when a MEP stimulus is about to be delivered.

Laser

A carbon dioxide (CO_2) laser is sometimes used during surgeries in which a tumor, such as a lipoma, must be broken down. This is often done in tethered cord surgery. Special CO_2 goggles must be worn by operating room personnel to protect their eyes against damage. This laser does not often produce an artifact that affects NIOM.

Cavitron Ultrasonic Surgical Aspirator

The cavitron ultrasonic surgical aspirator (CUSA) is another device that uses sound waves to break down tissue, usually tumors. It is used in many different types of surgical procedures. At times it can produce an artifact that makes it difficult to average evoked potentials (EPs).

Anesthesia Equipment

The anesthesia work station includes monitoring equipment, gas delivery devices, a documentation station, storage area, work platform, and a variety of other anesthetic tools (Figure 1.7). This equipment generally does not produce artifact in NIOM. However, the monitoring technologist should learn to identify anesthetics delivered, inspired and expired gases, blood pressures, and temperature, all of which are displayed on the anesthesia equipment.

X-ray

A standard x-ray machine is found most often in orthopedic and neurosurgery to locate bone structures so as to determine surgical

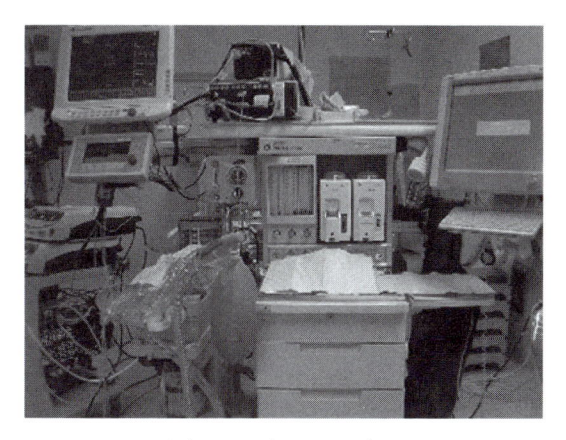

FIGURE 1.7 The anesthesia work station.

starting points. The x-ray machine does not produce an artifact that interferes with NIOM.

Fluoroscopy

Fluoroscopy, a type of x-ray system, is used in the operating room; its images can be visualized immediately without having to be processed. It is composed of at least two parts and, if needed, can be used with an injector for visualizing blood vessels. When fluoroscopy is being used, the monitoring technologist should make sure that he or she is appropriately covered with lead protective garments.

C-Arm

A C-arm is that part of a fluoroscopy device that is brought in close proximity to the patient and through which the x-rays pass (Figure 1.8). It can be used for diagnostic and interventional purposes. Although a C-arm can be wall-mounted, in the operating room it is often mobile so that it can be positioned appropriately. The C-arm can be angulated in any direction so as to provide the best possible imaging study. Mobile C-arm units provide image recording by either spot-film or digital image acquisition.

Monitor

Various image recording devices may be incorporated, including a film changer, cine

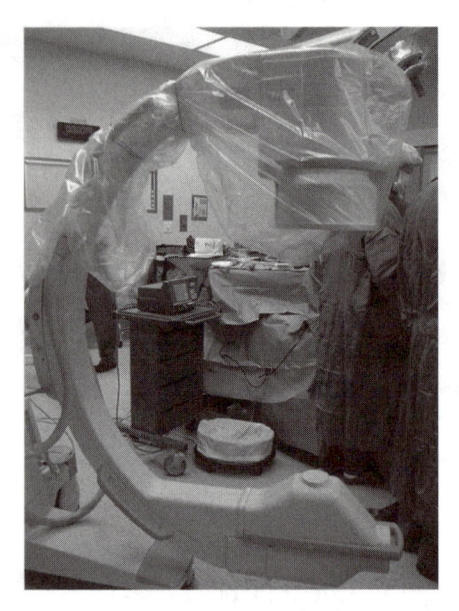

FIGURE 1.8 The C-arm. Notice that it is draped with sterile sheets.

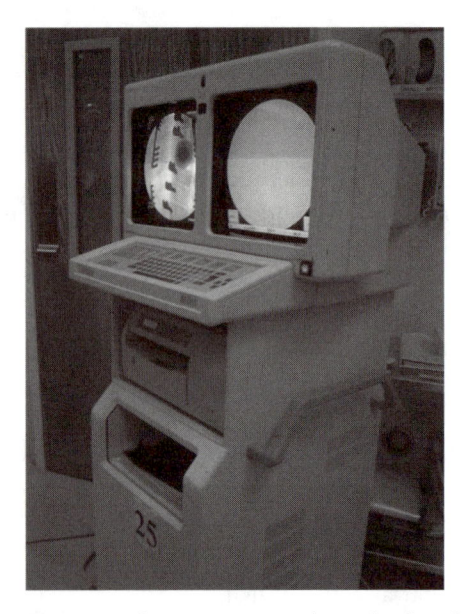

FIGURE 1.9 The monitor used to display fluoroscopy images during surgery.

camera, or digital image acquisition for digital subtraction. Most often a monitor is used to display the digital image (Figure 1.9).

Injector

The injector is the part of the fluoroscopy system through which a dye can be injected to visualize blood vessels. It is used often in endovascular surgeries. Fluoroscopy seldom causes significant artifact that would prevent adequate NIOM.

Cell Saver

The cell saver is used to process the patient's blood and return the red blood cells to the patient (hence the name). At times, especially when grounding is faulty, the cell saver can produce significant artifact that impairs averaging EPs.

Image-guided Surgery Systems

Image-guided surgery systems are sophisticated systems that help surgeons identify and locate structures deep to the surface. They work in a manner similar to global position-ing systems. A magnetic resonance imaging (MRI) study is preloaded in the computer and sensors are attached to the patient. An infrared camera detects the position of the patient's head. Surgical instruments can also have sensors that make them appear on the MRI, making localization easier. An example of this is the BrainLAB, used in neurosurgical procedures (Figure 1.10). Image-guided surgery systems seldom produce artifact that would hamper NIOM.

Surgical Table

Surgical tables are of many different types. They are usually electrically powered and plug into an AC outlet. In addition to moving up and down, they can turn in various directions to help optimize patient positioning. Because they plug into the AC outlet, they can also produce artifact, which can make averaging EPs difficult (Figure 1.11). The artifact can be isolated to the bed if unplugging the bed eliminates the artifact. If this happens, a discussion with the anesthesia team about whether the operating table can remain disconnected must take place.

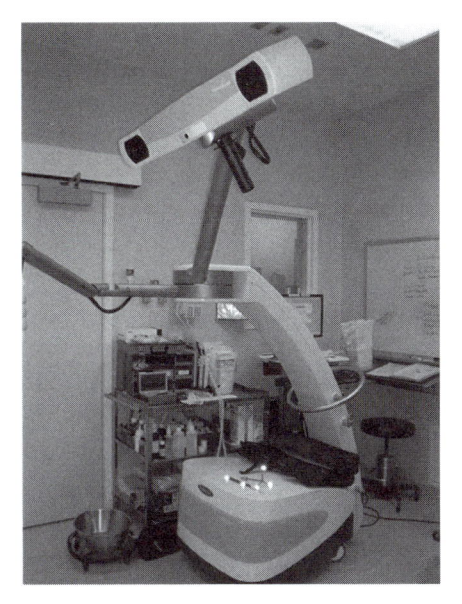

FIGURE 1.10 The BrainLAB, which helps localize structures in the surgical field.

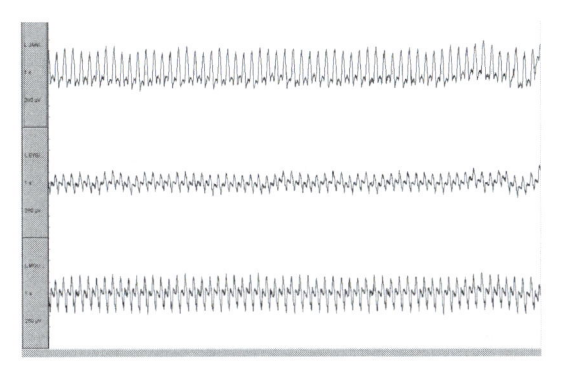

FIGURE 1.11 Example of artifact caused by the operating table. Disconnecting the table eliminated the artifact.

Surgical Drill

Many surgical procedures involving the skull and other bones require the use of a handheld drill by the surgeon. The appearance of such a drill is similar to that of a drill used around the home; however, they are made to surgical specifications and have special drill bits. When a drill is being used, significant artifact is produced, so that EP monitoring is not possible (Figure 1.12). Many times it is best to stop averaging Es

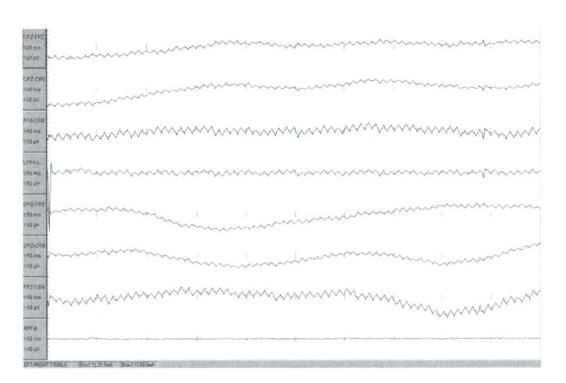

FIGURE 1.12 Example of artifact caused by a surgical drill. This was noted during microvascular decompression surgery for trigeminal neuralgia. After exposure, when the drill was no longer in use, the artifact disappeared.

until after the drilling has been completed. This is commonly seen in retromastoid craniotomies, such as those done for cerebellopontine angle surgeries.

PREPARATION

Preparing for a surgery in which monitoring will be used is among the most important things that the NIOM team does. Thorough planning reduces anxiety during the surgery and ensures that the best possible monitoring is performed.

Preoperative Studies

Preoperative studies are EP or EEG studies performed at least one day prior to surgery. Although it is not always possible to perform preoperative studies, they should be considered if and when possible. The primary reason for performing a preoperative study is verification that the patient has responses that can be monitored during surgery. If any abnormalities exist, these are identified and the surgeon is notified prior to the surgery. This process also allows for a greater degree of confidence in the baseline responses in the operating room.

In certain centers, patients may be screened for preoperative studies based on their medical history. Those with a higher likelihood of abnormal or absent responses may be candidates for preoperative studies. These would include patients with tumors of the central nervous system, patients with peripheral neuropathy, etc.

Contraindications to NIOM

There are very few absolute contraindications to NIOM. The presence of a cardiac pacemaker and cranial and other implants is a contraindication to MEP monitoring. In the past, a history of epilepsy was also considered a contraindication to MEP monitoring. However, recent data suggest that the risk of provoking seizures with MEP is very low (4). There are no contraindications to other types of monitoring.

Supplies

Some of the supplies the monitoring technologist needs can be found in the operating room. Most of them, however, will need to be brought in by the technologist. Usually the technologist will carry a small toolbox, apron, or bucket with supplies needed for any situation. The most important of all is, of course, electrodes. Available electrode types include disposable needles, disposable foam pads, reusable gold cups, corkscrew needles, and a variety of other electrodes found in many supply catalogs. A list of supplies that the technologist should have on hand is presented in Table 1.1. This is not meant to be an exhaustive list but should be a good start for the beginning technologist.

Setup

The type and site of surgery being performed will determine the type of monitoring that is needed. Many centers will have protocols that specify which modalities are to be monitored for each type of case. If a new type of procedure is being performed, the surgeon, anesthesiologist, and neurophysiologist should jointly decide which monitoring modalities are needed. Ideally, this should happen well before the morning of the case.

TABLE 1.1 A List of Supplies that Must be Present in the "Tool Box" of a Monitoring Technologist

Supplies	Applications
A variety of tapes	To attach surface and needle electrodes
Conductive gel	To use for disc electrode conduction
Exfoliant	To prepare the skin prior to application of surface electrodes
Alcohol preps	To disinfect skin before placing needles and also for cleanup afterwards
Skin-marking pen	Head and muscle marking
Collodion	For gluing surface electrodes to head
Acetone	To remove collodion
1-inch gauze	Used with collodion to reinforce the attachment of surface electrodes
Conductive paste	To use for disc electrode conduction
Cotton applicator tips	To apply exfoliant
Syringes	To hold and apply collodion and conductive gel
Tape measure	To measure head and body markings
Air dryer	To dry collodion
Cotton balls	Used with acetone to remove collodion
Blunt-tip applicator	Used with syringe to apply conductive gel into disc electrode hole

Access to the patient should be coordinated with the surgical team, anesthesia team, and the circulating nurse. If there are surface electrodes that need to be applied, it is often easier to apply these in the preoperative holding area or induction room rather than in the operating room. For the patient's comfort, needle electrodes are often placed after the patient has been anesthetized.

It is important to place the electrodes securely, since it will be difficult to access them once the patient is prepped and draped. The wires should be guided along the patient's body, toward the NIOM machine. They should be secured along the operating table and not left to dangle, so that they do not trip the surgeons or get caught in a C-arm or other piece of equipment. The setup is extremely important. It will determine the integrity of the waveforms and the ease with which the technologist can monitor the case.

Anesthetic Considerations

Detailed descriptions of anesthetic applications are given elsewhere in this text. However, it should be mentioned that the monitoring technologist should have frequent, open, and clear communications with the anesthesia team prior to and during the case. A case requiring electromyographic (EMG) monitoring calls for few changes on the part of the anesthesiologist other than restricting the use of neuromuscular blocking agents. Cortical potentials of the SEPs are sensitive to inhalational agents and should be limited to a low and steady concentration if used; subcortical and peripheral SEP responses are less sensitive to these agents. Brainstem auditory evoked potentials (BAEPs) are resistant to most anesthetic agents, so there are few restrictions when monitoring only BAEPs. However, BAEPs are often monitored concurrently with cranial nerve VII (CN VII) EMG during posterior fossa tumor resections. In these cases, neuromuscular blocking agents should be limited. Indeed, many cases involve multiple modalities monitored together.

MEP monitoring is sensitive to inhalational agents. Additionally, neuromuscular blocking agents can obliterate MEP responses. When MEPs are performed, consideration should be given to a TIVA technique, as with propofol and opioids.

EEG monitoring is sensitive to sedative-hypnotic agents such as barbiturates, propofol, etc. These agents can induce a burst-suppression pattern. Low dose of inhalational agent may be preferred when EEG monitoring is being performed. A more complete discussion of anesthetics and their affect on NIOM is presented in a later chapter.

Remote Monitoring

Many times the neurophysiologist who is responsible for interpreting the NIOM is not present in the operating room. In these situations, the neurophysiologist must review the data remotely. It is the monitoring technologist's responsibility to connect the NIOM equipment to a remote monitoring system and ensure its working order. The neurophysiologist must do the same with his or her equipment. It is a good idea for the technologist to have a dedicated telephone line rather than using the operating room phone. The various systems available for remote monitoring are discussed in a later chapter.

SAFETY

Safety is of utmost importance in the operating room. The monitoring technologists must be not only concerned with the safety of the patient but also with his or her own safety and the safety of the other personnel in the operating room. Attention to the issues listed below can help ensure safety for all.

Cords and Cables

It has already been mentioned that electrode wires need to be neatly strung along the side of the bed so that the staff will not trip over them. There are many other cords and cables that the monitoring technologist must deal with. All of these should be run from the bed to the monitoring computer flat along the floor, neatly tied together. Some "no trip" operating room supplies are available to cover these cords for everyone's safety.

Grounding

The patient will have an electrical ground through the electrocautery system. An additional ground will be necessary for NIOM only if the monitoring equipment requires it as a system reference.

Infection Control

The NIOM team should always practice universal precautions for infection control. If needle electrodes are being used, the skin should be prepped with alcohol skin prep. Needle electrodes are for a single use only and should be disposed of in a sharps container. Surface electrodes may be reused and should be cleaned and disinfected using the individual laboratory's protocol.

Burns

Although burns are rare, they do occasionally occur and are most often associated with improper electrocautery grounding. When the electrocautery cannot find proper ground, it seeks another outlet for the current. The next available outlet is usually a monitoring electrode. Needle electrodes cause greater injury than surface electrodes because they are smaller and have a greater concentration of current in a smaller area. To prevent or reduce these types of injuries, the technologist should assist the circulating nurse in placing the electrocautery ground to ensure its proper placement. If a burn occurs, the surgeon and the neurophysiologist should be notified immediately.

Personal Protective Equipment

Personal protective equipment is worn by the monitoring technologist and other personnel in the operating room. If a CO_2 laser is in use, everyone in the operating room should wear proper goggles to protect their eyes. When overhead ultraviolet (UV) lights are in use, a visor or plastic goggles should be worn to protect against UV light. During x-rays, including those taken with the C-arm (fluoroscopy), the technologist should either exit the room or wear lead protection covering at least the reproductive organs and thyroid. Gloves should always be worn when handling a patient, as this is fundamental to universal precautions.

ETIQUETTE AND PROTOCOL

As is true when one goes into any new environment, going into the operating room requires knowledge of etiquettes and protocols that are specific to the operating room. The monitoring technologist should familiarize himself or herself with these etiquettes and protocols so that the surgery can be helped to move along faster.

Patient Access

Access to the patient before a case begins can be somewhat of a competition. The preoperative nurse must check the patient in, get vital signs, place an intravenous line, and perform a variety of other tasks before the patient can go to the operating room. The circulating nurse must meet the patient, check allergies, etc. The anesthesia team must explain anesthetic protocol to the patient, check allergies, answer questions, and perform other tasks before anesthetic procedures are begun. The surgeons need patient access to mark the surgical site, answer last-minute questions, sign consents, etc. The monitoring technologist must meet the patient, explain his or her part of the procedure and why it is important, take a history, and place electrodes. All this must happen in a coordinated manner so that an inordinate amount of time is not spent in this process. The monitoring technologist will likely find it easier to work with other members of the operating room team in a collaborative effort. In other words, it is most effective to introduce oneself to the other team members, explain what needs to be done, and ask when would be a good time to apply electrodes.

Attire

Before entering the operating room restricted area, the NIOM staff must be dressed in the proper hospital-issued scrubs. They are usually supplied in the locker room or by vending machines. If scrubs are not available, disposable paper scrubs or "bunny suits" should be worn over street clothes prior to entering the restricted area. Head covering and shoe covers must be worn into the restricted area. These covers and disposable paper scrubs must be removed when leaving the restricted area. Face masks must be worn when entering the operating room.

Cleanup and Follow-up

The work of the NIOM team does not end with the termination of the surgery. A substantial amount of time is required for disposing of supplies and cleaning others as well as performing follow-up of the service provided.

Disinfecting Equipment and Supplies

Upon completion of the surgery, cables, head boxes, stimulating boxes, and amplifiers should be wiped down with a disinfecting solution and stored neatly on the NIOM machine. Any pencils, tape measures, or other tools that touched the patient or may have been cross-contaminated should be disinfected also. Any reusable electrodes should be scrubbed of any gross contamination and then soaked in a disinfectant. Disposable supplies should be disposed of properly.

Postsurgical Testing

When the patient awakens from surgery, the monitoring technologist should be present for testing of the pathways that were monitored during the case. This includes moving toes, moving hands, feeling touch sensation on the feet and hands, smiling, hearing, or other testing as appropriate. This is especially important if changes were seen during NIOM, as they can be correlated to the neurologic examination. It is important for the technologist to be present for this testing so that, if the patient does not respond as expected, the surgeon can question the technologist (and neurophysiologist) about the NIOM. In addition, if the surgeon finds it necessary to reoperate emergently, the NIOM team may be asked to monitor for the emergent procedure.

DOCUMENTATION

Thorough and complete documentation is of critical importance in NIOM. It serves not only to provide information about what happened during the case but also to protect the NIOM team should postoperative complications occur (5).

Preoperative Documentation

Prior to the date of surgery, if a preoperative EP or EEG study is performed, it must be interpreted and abnormal results communicated to the surgeon. On the day of surgery, the patient's history must be recorded, with particular attention focusing on any contraindications for MEP monitoring. If such a contraindication exists, it must be discussed with the surgeon and noted in the patient's medical record.

Documentation During Surgery

This is the most important documentation performed by the monitoring technologist. The exact modalities being tested and when each test is performed should be noted, along with the measured latencies of the peaks of interest or intensity of current needed to stimulate a particular structure. Many modern NIOM machines allow the technologist to enter notes directly onto the waveforms, making documentation easier. The technologists should also note the anesthetics used, their concentrations, and when they were changed. Physiologic parameters, such as blood pressure and temperature, and important surgical milestones should also be noted. When an alarm based on changes seen in NIOM is sounded, that must be recorded by the technologist. Preferably, the surgeon's response to the alarm should also be noted. Similarly, discussions with the anesthesiologist should be noted as well. These help protect the NIOM team, as the documentation confirms that the NIOM team attempted to alert the responsible parties when problems occurred.

As important as complete and thorough documentation is, noting irrelevant comments in the patient's permanent medical record is not advisable. For example, a discussion between the attending surgeon and the surgical resident about how easy or difficult a particular case is does not need to be noted by the monitoring technologist. Arguments between operating room staff should also not be noted unless they are directly relevant to the NIOM.

Postoperative Documentation

After the surgery is over, the monitoring technologist should make certain that documentation is complete. If certain elements of documentation could not be completed during the case because of concurrent responsibilities, they should be finished at this time. Significant findings noted on the postsurgery examination should also be noted. Per laboratory protocol, data sheets (or waveform sheets/discs) are submitted to the neurophysiologist for report generation and storage. Unlike other types of reports for medical procedures, this NIOM report serves mostly a billing and medicolegal purpose rather than a clinical one. The clinical interpretation is provided in real time and not with the report. As such, the NIOM report should include the reason for NIOM, the modalities performed and how, whether any significant changes were noted and if so, what they were. Documentation that the surgeon was notified of these changes immediately is very important. Finally, the number of hours spent for interpretation should be included. The patient's chart, along with technical (number of hours spent on the case by the monitoring technologist) and professional (number of hours spent interpreting the case by the neurophysiologist) charges are sent to the proper personnel.

CONCLUSIONS

Performing NIOM is not simply performing clinical EP or EEG studies in the operating room. It requires a different knowledge and mind set. The operating room can be an intimidating environment for new NIOM staff. Beginners should learn the etiquettes and policies of their operating rooms. They must know who the other members of the operating team are and their roles. There are many pieces of equipment that may be present in the room, and the technologist must know which one will cause problems with NIOM. Attention to detail in setup, performing the NIOM, and afterwards will help the NIOM team provide a safe and effective service that will help reduce morbidity.

REFERENCES

1. Fortunato NH. *Berry & Kohn's Operating Room Technique*, 9th ed. St. Louis: Mosby, 2000.

2. Turner S, Wicker P, Hind M. Principles of safe practice in the perioperative environment. In: Hind M, Wicker P, eds. *Principles of Perioperative Practice*. Edinburgh: Churchill Livingstone, 2000:17–50.
3. AORN. Recommended practices for perioperative nursing: section 3. In: Fogg D, ed. *Standards, Recommended Practices, and Guidelines*. Denver: AORN, 2004:209–399.
4. MacDonald DB. Safety of intraoperative transcranial electrical stimulation motor evoked potential monitoring. *J Clin Neurophysiol* 2002;19:416–429.
5. Nuwer MR. Regulatory and medical-legal aspects of intraoperative monitoring. *J Clin Neurophysiol* 2002;19:387–395.

2 Basic Neurophysiologic Intraoperative Monitoring Techniques

Robert E. Minahan
Allen S. Mandir

This chapter discusses and introduces the basic techniques of neurophysiologic intraoperative monitoring (NIOM). Techniques for electromyography (EMG), motor nerve conduction studies, somatosensory evoked potentials (SEPs), motor evoked potentials (MEPs), brainstem auditory evoked potentials (BAEPs), and electroencephalography (EEG) are all discussed. A full discussion of all signal acquisition parameters is beyond the scope of this chapter, but Table 2.1 summarizes the data necessary to allow proper configuration of these tests. All recording parameters are selected based on the expected frequency range, size, and latency of target signals while stimulus parameters are provided.

FREE-RUNNING EMG AND MOTOR NERVE CONDUCTION STUDIES

Background

EMG can be monitored in any muscle accessible to a needle, wire, or surface electrode. Mechanical irritation of peripheral nerves or nerve roots results in muscle activity of the corresponding musculature. The consequent EMG recordings provide essentially instantaneous feedback to the surgeon regarding the effects of his or her actions. EMG monitoring is most effective in cases where nerve injury results from repetitive mechanical irritation of a nerve.

Anatomy and Physiology

The most common surgeries in which EMG is monitored are those that place cranial nerves or spinal roots at risk. Therefore it is important that muscles innervated by the elements at risk be assessed. Commonly used spinal root or cranial nerve innervated muscles are listed in Table 2.2. Note that each spinal root innervates many muscles (and this group of muscles is termed the *myotome* for that root); conversely, most muscles are innervated by multiple spinal roots.

In order to understand EMG potentials due to surgical irritation, we need to first consider the motor unit potential (MUP). The MUP is a group of muscle fibers innervated by a single axon. A single axon may innervate as few as three muscle fibers (as in eye muscles) or more than 500 (as in the gastrocnemius). In the typical scenario when surgical irritation of axons is sufficient, axonal depolarization results in the activation of the muscle fibers innervated by those axons. Depolarization of a single axon leads to single MUP, which is recorded as a "spike" on EMG.

For NIOM, EMG is typically presented both visually on a monitor and aurally over a

TABLE 2.1 Recording and Stimulating Parameters

	Filters (Hz)		Typical amplitude (µV)*		Typical latency (ms)*		Stimulation intensity*		Stimulation duration (ms)		Stimulation rate (Hz)	
	Low Freq.	High Freq.	Low	High	Low	High	Low	High	Low	High	Low	High
Free-running EMG	10	2000–5000	20–1000		n/a		n/a		n/a		n/a	
Lumbar pedicle screw testing	10–20	2000–5000	10–150		10–25		0–50 mA		0.2–0.2†		1–4	
Motor evoked potentials (myogenic)	10–40	2000–5000	25–2000		15–75		200 V–1000 V		0.05–1		n/a	
Motor evoked potentials (D-waves)	30	1500	1–30		5–20		100 V–500 V		0.05–1		Manual–1	
SEP-median nerve cortical	30	250–1000	0.5–5		17–23		20 mA–35mA		0.2–0.5		1.3–4.7	
SEP-median nerve subcortical	30	500–1500	0.5–3		11–16		20 mA–35mA		0.2–0.5		1.3–4.7	
SEP-tibial nerve cortical	30	250–1000	0.5–5		35–45		25 mA–50 mA		0.2–1		1.3–4.7	
SEP-tibial nerve subcortical	30	500–1500	0–3		27–35		25 mA–50 mA		0.2–1		1.3–4.7	
EEG	1	50–70	0–100		n/a		n/a		n/a		n/a	
BAER	30–100	1500–3000	0.3–3		1.5–10		75 dB–110 dB		0.1–0.1		5–15	
Neuromuscular junction testing	20	5000	0–10,000		3–7		20 mA–75 mA		0.2–1		2–3	

*Values may fall outside these ranges in atypical, pathologic, or pediatric cases
† Pedicle screw testing at durations other than 0.2 ms change the threshold ranges noted in the text

CHAPTER 2: Basic Neurophysiologic Intraoperative Monitoring Techniques

TABLE 2.2 Muscles Commonly Used in EMG Monitoring*

Cranial nerve–innervated muscles
    III, IV, VI – Extraocular muscles
    V – Masseter, temporalis
    VII –Frontalis, orbicularis oculus, orbicularis oris, mentalis, others
    IX – Stylopharyngeus
    X – Pharyngeal and laryngeal muscles
    XI – Sternocleidomastoid, trapezius
    XII – Tongue

Spinal root myotomes
    C1 – None
    C2 – Sternocleidomastoid
    C3 – Trapezius, sternocleidomastoid
    C4 – Trapezius, levator scapulae
    C5 – Deltoid, biceps
    C6 –Biceps, triceps, brachioradialis, pronator teres, flexor carpi radialis (FCR)
    C7 –Triceps, pronator teres, FCR, forearm extensors
    C8 –Triceps, ulnar forearm muscles, all hand intrinsic muscles (incl. abductor pollicis brevis, first dorsal interosseous, adductor digiti minimi)
    T1 –Hand intrinsic muscles, flexor carpi ulnaris
    T2,T3, T4, T5, T6 – Intercostal muscles, paraspinal muscles
    T6,T7, T8 – Upper rectus abdominis, paraspinal muscles, intercostal muscles
    T8,T9, T10 – Middle rectus abdominis, paraspinal muscles, intercostal muscles
    T10, T11, T12 – Lower rectus abdominis, paraspinal muscles, intercostal muscles
    L1 –Quadratus lumborum, paraspinals, cremaster ± iliopsoas ± internal oblique
    L2 –Iliopsoas, adductor longus, quadriceps, adductor magnus
    L3 –Quadriceps, adductor longus, adductor magnus, iliopsoas
    L4 –Quadriceps, tibialis anterior, adductor longus, adductor magnus, iliopsoas
    L5 –Tibialis anterior, peroneus longus, adductor magnus
    S1 – Gastrocnemius, abductor hallucis
    S2 – Gastrocnemius, abductor hallucis
    S2–S5 – Anal sphincter, urethral sphincter

*This list should not be considered inclusive and additional appropriate muscles for monitoring can be found in any diagnostic EMG text.

speaker. Irritation triggers motor units in a variety of patterns that are influenced by the preexisting condition of the nerve, the degree and mechanism of neural irritation, and the integrity of distal neuromuscular function. An EMG "burst" describes a brief period of polyphasic EMG activity representing the near simultaneous activation of multiple axons (motor units). An EMG "train" describes repetitive firing of one or more motor units lasting from a second to minutes. With intense multiaxonal irritation or voluntary muscle activation, MUPs may fill the recording channel. In this case, MUP overlap and no individual MUPs are distinguishable. When this is seen during diagnostic EMG, it is termed an interference pattern, and in relation to a surgical irritation can be thought of as an extended burst. Typically this activity will cease with removal of the irritating factor, though a train of one or more MUPs may persist, as described in more detail below (Figure 1.1A to D).

Characterization and Interpretation

In order to understand what level of clinical significance a pattern of EMG activity represents, the activity must be characterized beyond a simple burst or train description. The most important feature suggesting significance is a relation to surgical events at the time. In addition, a number of electrical features of EMG activity can suggest greater or lesser degrees of irritation and therefore greater or lesser clinical significance.

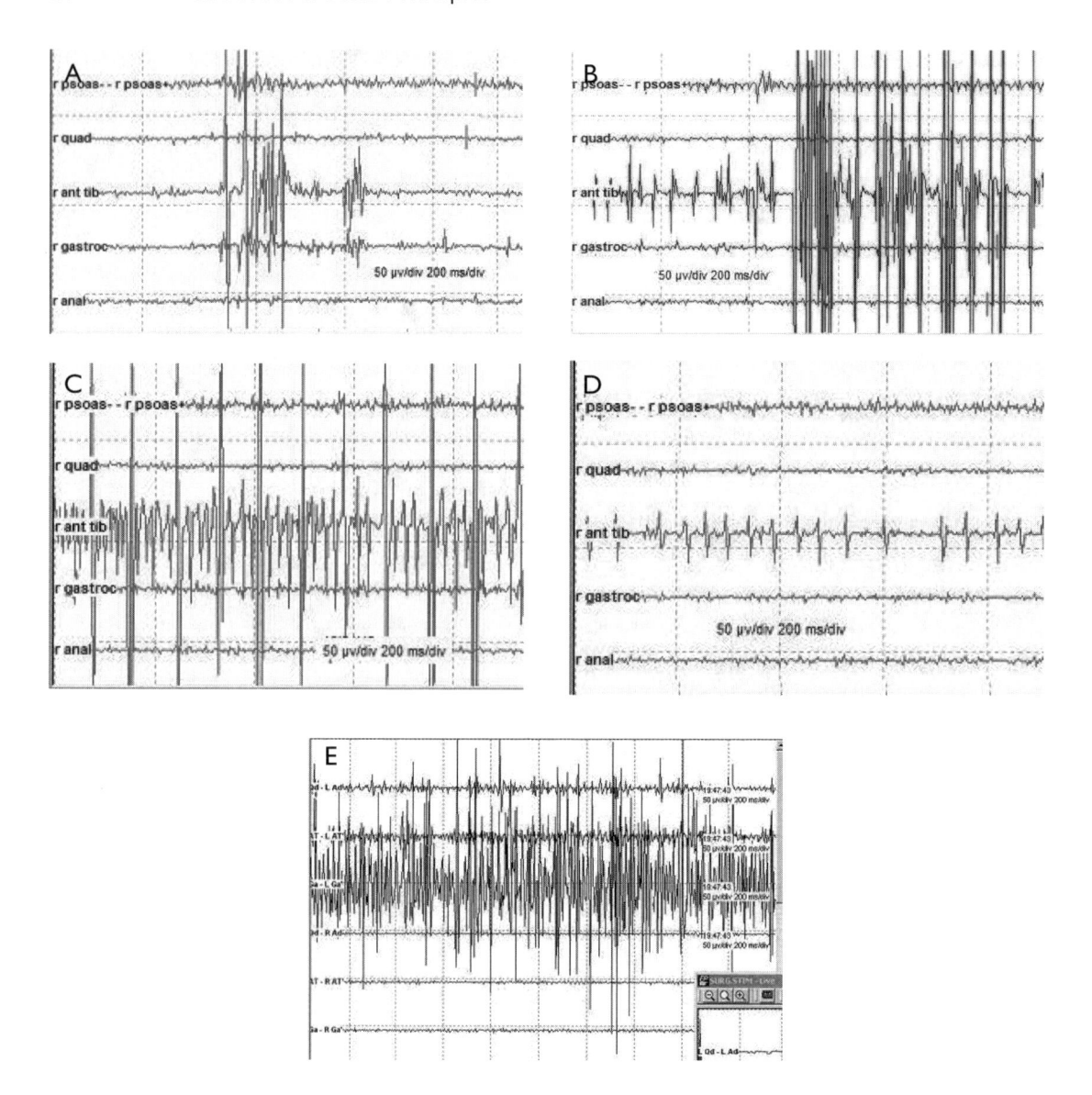

FIGURE 2.1 EMG may be seen in a variety of patterns. A. A minor burst of activity occurring as a lumbar root is manipulated. B. A more intense burst occurring on the background of an ongoing train of activity. C. Intense ongoing trains of activity from multiple motor units (asynchronous activity). D. A residual train of activity as the effect of nerve root irritation wanes. E. An interference pattern in the left gastrocnemius muscle after inadvertent trauma to the corresponding nerve root.

Relation to Surgical Events

The onset of EMG activity with a surgical action suggests a causative role. In addition to mechanical irritation, temperature (cold saline, heat from electrocautery) and osmotic irritation may induce intense EMG activity. Recognition of nonmechanical causes is important, because under usual circumstances these have little or no clinical implication. Mechanical irritation, on the other hand, is associated with a risk of injury to the corresponding nerve either immediately or with repetitive trauma. Mechanical irritation may induce a wide range of EMG patterns, as described in greater detail below; as a rule, however, the degree of irritation will correlate roughly with the intensity of the EMG activity. In addition, EMG activity that persists after the cessation of the irritative maneuver also suggests a relatively intense initial irritation.

EMG activity may occur without apparent modulation related to ongoing surgical activity. The most clinically important but fortunately least common situation in which this might occur is when irritation is due to prior surgical actions that leave the nerve in an irritated state. Examples of such situations include a bone fragment that is in contact with a nerve or a nerve root compressed during tightening of instrumentation. If the causative role is not or cannot be identified immediately, ongoing EMG activity is likely to persist and the source of irritation may remain unidentified. More commonly, EMG activity that is not correlated to surgical events may be attributed to benign causes, such as return of muscle tone and voluntary muscle activity. Muscle tone may return with low levels of neuromuscular blockade and low anesthetic depth. Some muscles are more prone to demonstrate return of tone (e.g., frontalis, anal sphincter), but depending on the patient, this may include other muscles. In the extreme case of low anesthetic depth, voluntary muscle contraction may occur and electrical activity typically precedes gross clinical movement. Finally, EMG activity may be present prior to incision in some patients. Although a number of clinical conditions may lead to continuous muscle activity, in the setting of EMG NIOM, the cause is likely to relate to the reason for surgery (e.g., radiculopathy) and in these patients only increased EMG activity over this baseline is likely to reflect further nerve irritation.

EMG activity may also be correlated to surgical activity when the surgical activity is trivial or remote from the neural elements activated. Once some degree of nerve damage is established (either intraoperatively or preoperatively), minor manipulation of the corresponding nerve or even patient movement may elicit strong EMG activity (see below). For example, in many patients with severe preoperative spinal stenosis, EMG activity may be elicited by trivial surgical actions due at least in part to an increased proclivity of axons to fire. EMG activity in these cases is common and, when associated with surgical actions remote from neural elements, poses a very low risk of further damage to nerves.

Finally, it is possible that reflexive EMG activity may be triggered in myotomes remote from surgical activity through nociceptive input or other mechanisms. Such reflexive mechanisms are not well described in the EMG monitoring literature; however, a clear correlation of EMG activity to surgical activity, even when not in the expected myotomes, should trigger suspicion of a causative role.

Number of MUPs

Each distinct MUP represents a separate depolarizing axon. Thus, greater numbers of axons affected by any irritative source will result in larger numbers of distinct MUPs recorded and a greater intensity of recorded EMG activity.

Firing Rate

The rate at which MUPs fire correlates to the degree of irritation, with higher rates indicating a greater degrees of irritation. Rates of firing for individual units tend to be constant over short periods but may gradually wax (persistent irritation) or wane (irritative source typically removed) over time. Activity may abruptly cease at any time. Most firing patterns are regular for individual MUPs; but when many MUPs are activated, each will have its own onset, offset, and rate. This combination of different rates, initiation, and cessation of MUPs results in what has been described as an "asynchronous" pattern of EMG firing. The extreme case of asynchro-

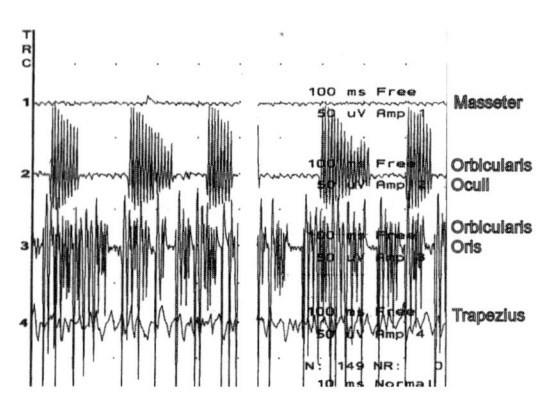

FIGURE 2.2 Repetitive microtrauma to nerves may produce intense EMG activity, as seen in this vestibular neuroma resection. The orbicularis oculi shows myokymia and the orbicularis oris shows asynchronous high-rate trains of activity reflecting significant irritation and likely clinically apparent postoperative neuropathy.

nous firing is the interference pattern, as described above (Figure 2.2).

Shape

The shape of MUPs is largely determined by the distance and orientation of the MUP with respect to the recording electrodes coupled with the number of muscle fibers in the MUP. Some authors have tried to correlate the shape of the MUP with significance (multiphasic being more significant than monophasic), but this distinction is likely to be most useful in distinguishing artifact from MUP. When correctly identified, a monophasic MUP is likely to reflect recording from a distant muscle. The monophasic MUP therefore suggests ongoing axonal depolarization, although the absence of closer units may suggest relatively sparse activity. In addition, the shape and size of any single MUP is usually consistent over time. However, with partial neuromuscular blockade, some variation may be present due to inconsistent activation of component muscle fibers.

Amplitude

High-amplitude EMG activity resulting from the superimposition of multiple MUPs suggests a higher degree of irritation, as discussed above under "Number of MUPs." On the other hand, the amplitude of any single MUP is likely unimportant, as a single MUP represents activation of a single axon. No studies have determined if the axons associated with either large or small MUP are preferentially activated due to mechanical irritation; therefore it may be that small or large units are essentially recruited by chance. In addition, chronic nerve or root denervation may lead to remodeling of motor units, with more muscle fibers innervated by single axons. If this is the case, patients with preexisting chronic radiculopathy are likely to have large motor units. Finally, the recorded amplitude is also a function of how close the motor unit's muscle fibers are to the recording electrode.

Relation of EMG Activity to Degree of Nerve Dysfunction

EMG is the only signal in NIOM in which an absence of activity is the expected state in both normal nerves and with complete loss of function of the monitored neural target. Given this convergence of extremes, one must examine the effect of a given irritative maneuver through the entire spectrum of nerve dysfunction.

Stripping of epineurium, perineurium, and possibly myelin appears to increase the propensity of axons to depolarize in response to irritants. As a result, the undisturbed nerve is less likely to be irritated with minor manipulation than a nerve that has undergone non-axonal damage. Once the axon itself is disrupted, that axon will not produce MUPs with proximal irritation (though the cut end of the distal portion of the axon may retain an ability to depolarize). Thus, as progressive axonal injury occurs, the nerve may once again show lesser degrees of EMG activity with manipulation proximal to the injury. This phenomenon is best illustrated when a nerve is subject to repetitive microtrauma, as with resection of neural tumors. In these cases, first, progressively increasing intensity of EMG activity is often seen. At its maximum, myokymic potentials and very high rates of neurotonic trains may be seen (50 to 100 Hz) (1). When myokymic or high-rate neurotonic patterns are encountered, the gradual subsequent reduction in EMG activity despite continued surgical manipulation may reflect either less irritation or suggest progressive dysfunction of the nerve (Figure 2.2).

Repetitive microtrauma to the nerve nicely demonstrates the spectrum of EMG responses that might be observed with gradual and progressive dysfunction. However, the mechanism of neural injury will determine which if any of the intermediate stages of dysfunction are reached. For example, abrupt transection of a nerve may be associated with a single burst of EMG activity followed by electrical silence thereafter. In fact, sharp transection may not have any EMG correlate. As a result, one must consider the mechanisms of potential injury and the likely timing of associated progression through the range of dysfunction in considering the significance of EMG in relation to the surgical activity at the time (Figure 2.2).

The onset of nerve ischemia may be irritative under appropriate conditions, but under most conditions we consider ischemia to be nonirritative and therefore no EMG may be present. As a result, compressive nerve insults may yield variable EMG correlates if coincident ischemia blocks axonal depolarization. In addition, any source of neuromuscular dysfunction distal to the site of surgical irritation will reduce sensitivity from EMG monitoring and allow false-negative results. These include distal nerve compression or ischemia, distal neuropathy, limb ischemia, excessive neuromuscular junction blockade, or inexcitable myopathy.

Communication with the Surgeon

EMG is considered by many to be the simplest form of NIOM. While this may be the case, the above discussion shows that one must still have a healthy respect for the complexities involved with EMG monitoring. It is the monitoring team's duty to identify the location, pattern, intensity, and duration of this activity and then communicate it to the surgeon when appropriate. At least as important as the type of EMG activity is the relation to surgical activity at the time of occurrence. Thus, the neurophysiologist must maintain awareness of surgical events and give feedback immediately upon occurrence, so that the surgeon understands the relationship of EMG to his or her activities.

Short bursts of activity and low-frequency trains of activity are usually, at worst, low-level irritation with a low risk for persisting injury. The burst is typically a physiologic phenomenon due to the excitation of mechanoreceptors on the axon. The report of brief bursts to the surgeon should suggest manipulation of a nerve but little else. The surgeon may find reports of bursts helpful if he or she is not aware of being in contact with neural structures or if that activity is restricted to simple bursts without more ominous patterns present. Such activity is often described as "minor," so that its typically benign nature is clear.

Activity that persists after the cessation of the offending surgical action suggests some level of ongoing insult or injury (often subclinical) and is more often described as "significant." Persistent trains of one or a few MUP at lower rates are described as moderate activity, and activity with many MUP or particularly high train rates described as intense.

Motor Nerve Conduction Studies ("Triggered EMG")

Electrical Evaluation of Pedicle Holes and Screws

Spinal instrumentation must be anchored to the vertebral column in order to provide support and allow bony fusion. Screws are often placed in the pedicle to provide this anchor; if they are malpositioned, however, they may impinge on exiting nerve roots, causing radiculopathy. Pedicle holes and screws should be electrically tested to assess for perforation of the pedicle wall. If the hole drilled in the pedicle perforates the wall, a low-impedance pathway will be created between stimulation within the hole and nearby exiting nerve roots. When a perforation exists, a relatively low level of electrical stimulation will activate these nerve roots, with resultant activity recorded from their corresponding muscles. Thus the integrity of the pedicle can be assessed based on the minimum level of electrical current needed to activate nearby nerve roots. At lumbosacral root levels using monopolar cathodal stimulation at 0.2-ms duration, thresholds can be interpreted as shown in Table 2.3 (2).

Typically, if pedicle screws stimulate (activate nearby roots) at less than 7 mA, a perforation has occurred, whereas if they stimulate at greater than 10 mA, a perforation is unlikely. For holes, however, if activation is noted at less than 5 mA, a perforation is likely; if they stimulate at greater than 7 mA, perforation is unlikely. In this context, "hole" refers to stimulation of the pedicle hole using a ball-tipped electrode as the cathode. If, instead, the hole is indirectly stimulated via an instrument (e.g., tap), then current shunting may occur if that instrument is in contact with any tissue or fluid and results will be skewed. "Screw" refers to stimulation of the head of the screw shaft after placement. If, instead, the mobile top of a polyaxial screw is stimulated, there may be an inconsistent electrical connection to the shaft and again results may be skewed. In cases where low thresholds are found, the surgeon may choose to remove or redirect the screw at that site. Alternatively, in a situation where redirection is not practical or a screw is particularly important to the success of fusion, the surgeon may leave the screw in place after probing the hole and/or performing fluoroscopy or other radiographic imaging in an attempt to determine if the pedicle wall is likely to be perforated in a clinically significant manner—i.e., there is potential impingement on a nerve root. The presence of free-running EMG activity corresponding to screw placement or probing suggests that a perforation with nerve impingement is present.

Pedicle screws or lateral mass screws at thoracic and cervical levels may also be electrically evaluated, and cutoff threshold values are likely to be similar to those for lumbosacral levels. However, evidence for specific values remains to be fully determined (Figure 2.3).

Motor Nerve Conduction Studies for Purposes Other than Pedicle Screw Evaluation

Motor nerve conduction studies may be used in a variety of settings where motor nerves are accessible to the surgeon and potentially at risk of injury. In these cases, the surgeon will directly stimulate nerves of interest and motor responses recorded in the corresponding muscle. This technique may assess the continuity and function of nerves from the point of stimulation to the muscle and can explore whether neural structures are in or near an area of proposed resection or electrocautery. A common use of these techniques is for vestibular schwannoma resection, where the facial nerve must first be located and then assessed.

Anesthesia

Anesthetic agents have little effect on the recorded muscle responses of EMG or motor nerve conduction studies. Neuromuscular

TABLE 2.3 Threshold Values Indicating the Likelihood of Pedicle Screw Malpositioning

	Perforation probable	Perforation possible	Perforation unlikely
Hole	<5 mA	5–7 mA	>7 mA
Screw	<7 mA	7–10 mA	>10 mA

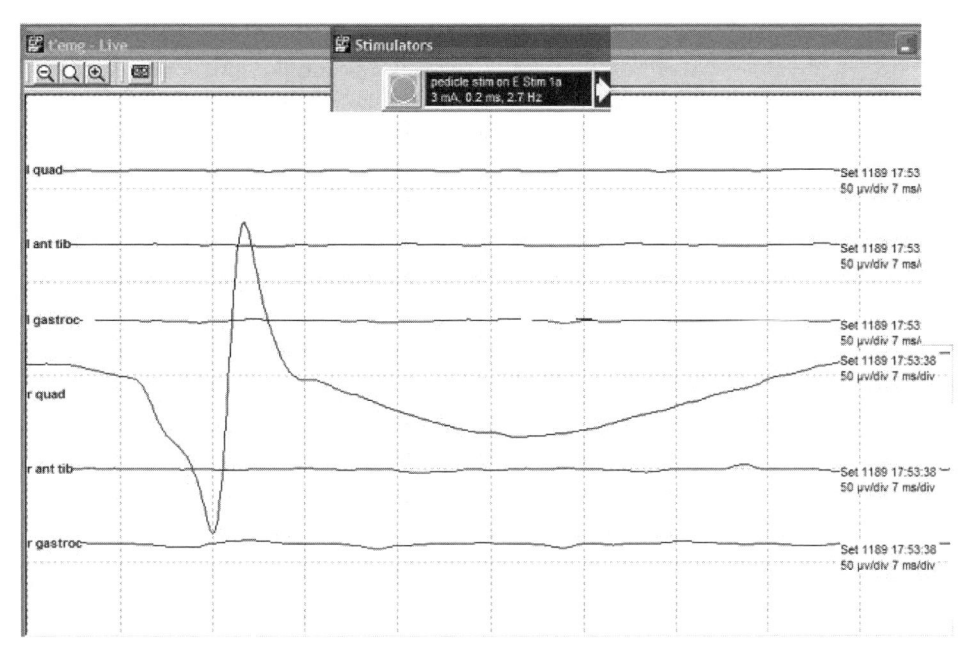

CHAPTER 2: Basic Neurophysiologic Intraoperative Monitoring Techniques

FIGURE 2.3 A CMAP is seen in the right quadriceps muscle after stimulation of the right L3 pedicle screw at 3 mA. This is a low threshold, indicating a low-impedance pathway (pedicle wall perforation) between the screw and exiting nerve roots.

blocking agents, on the other hand, may have a profound effect if sufficient residual neuromuscular function is not present. When partial neuromuscular blockade is used during EMG monitoring or motor nerve conduction studies, we target a level that does not depresses the abductor pollicis brevis compound motor action potential amplitude more than 80% relative to an awake value. This level is reasonably approximated by a train-of-four ratio (ratio of the fourth to first compound motor action potential using repetitive nerve stimulation at 2 Hz) in the gastrocnemius muscle of > 0.3 or the presence of at least two responses in the abductor pollicis brevis exceeding 600 µV in amplitude (unpublished data). If the anesthesiologist is assessing visual responses to train-of-four testing, then four out of four twitches is the only reliable criterion due to the imprecision of that test. However, in most cases, two or three visible twitches will also be adequate, but the confidence in this finding is reduced.

SOMATOSENSORY EVOKED POTENTIALS

Background

SEPs have been the primary spinal cord monitoring modality for decades and have more recently been augmented but not supplanted by motor evoked potentials (MEPs). SEPs remain a ubiquitous form of neuromonitoring because they assess all levels of the neuraxis from the peripheral nerve to the cerebral hemispheres.

SEPs are well suited for NIOM for a number of reasons. First, with modern techniques and equipment, responses have a definable amplitude and latency that can be quantified for comparison throughout a procedure. Second, the signals have reasonable stability, so that injury can be identified with confidence. Third, multiple recording sites can be employed along the course of the assessed somatosensory pathways and the neural generators for each of these sites are known within practical precision. This latter aspect allows localization to peripheral nerve, spinal cord, or brain when a neural insult occurs and thus allows the most appropriate corrective actions to be taken. Finally, an SEP can be elicited from almost any nerve containing sensory fibers, with median, ulnar, and tibial nerves used most frequently.

SEP Generators and Localization

Localization of neural deficits based on patterns of SEP changes relies on an understanding of the neural generators producing the observed waveforms. If the generators are known, it is a simple matter to understand that after stimulation of a single nerve, loss of signals at a point along the course of its propagation to the brain suggests an insult between the most proximal generator with a retained signal and the next most proximal generator with a degraded signal. Table 2.4 shows generators for median and tibial nerve SEPs.

The cervicomedullary signals generated by upper extremity SEPs are among the most complex, because multiple signal components contribute to the response recorded at 13 to 14 ms when using standard recording techniques. In recording with an electrode over the posterior neck, there are negative components contributed by the cervical spinal cord.

TABLE 2.4 Neural Generators for Median and Tibial Nerve SEP Generators

	Median Nerve SEP Generators			Tibial Nerve SEP Generators			
Label	Generator	Common channels used	Alternate labels	Label	Generator	Common channels used	Alternate labels
N9	Brachial plexus	EPi-EPc	Erb's	**Popliteal**	Tibial nerve action potential	Popliteal	
N11	Spinal nerve root	Crv-Fpz		N23	Dorsal horn interneurons	T12-iliac cr.	Lumbar point
N13a	Dorsal horn interneurons	Crv6-Fpz	Cervical, subcortical	**P31**	Medulla	Crv-Fpz, Mast-Fpz	Cervical, sub-cortical
N13b	Dorsal column	Crv2-Fpz	Cervical, subcortical	N34	Primary sensory cortex	Cc-Fpz	N37
P13	Spinomedullary junction	Crv-Fpz, Mast-Fpz	Cervical, subcortical	**P38**	Primary sensory cortex	Ci-Fpz, Cz'-Fpz, Ci-Cc, Cz'-Cc	P39, P40, cortical
P14	Lemniscal paths, cuneate nucleus	Crv-Fpz, Mast-Fpz	Cervical, subcortical	N38	Primary sensory cortex	Cc-Fpz	
N18	Brainstem/thalamic	Ci-noncephalic					
N19	Primary sensory cortex	Cc-Fz, Cc-Ci	N20, cortical				
P22	Primary motor cortex	Cc-Fz, Cc-Ci					

EP = Erb's point; Crv = electrode over spinous process, Crv2 and Crv6 refer to the vertebral level; Cc = C3' or C4', whichever is contralateral; Ci = C3' or C4', whichever is ipsilateral; Bold = more important and more consistently recorded signals.

At roughly the same latency there are positive components recorded from Fpz that are contributed by the medulla. Referencing these electrodes together summates the component signals and produces the observed "subcortical" response. When a surgery is performed at the cervical level, it is best that the entire subcortical signal be generated above the level of surgery so that it will be reliably affected should a cervical-level cord injury occur. For this purpose a mastoid or ear electrode is referenced to FPz to record a signal that is generated at or above the foramen magnum. In this case a cervical-level electrode is omitted so that the associated spinal cord generators do not contribute to the recorded subcortical signal. This prevents a portion of the subcortical signal to persist in the presence of a cervical cord injury and avoids recording novel generators that may arise with an injury (far-field signals due to abrupt termination of axon conduction). As an example, an anterior cervical spine procedure may be associated with a number of different SEP changes reflecting different events (Table 2.5).

Localization must also include information from other monitoring modalities. Figure 2.4 is a demonstration of bilateral loss of tibial nerve SEP signals during lower thoracic decompression and fusion in a patient with spinal stenosis due to Pott's disease. The loss of cortical SEP signals following tibial nerve stimulation occurred in the setting of intact signals at the popliteal fossa, intact SEPs following median nerve stimulation, and intact MEP signals. These findings suggest dysfunction of large fiber somatosensory pathways above the level of the knee and below the cervical cord. This was presumed to result from thoracic posterior column dysfunction at the level of surgery, and the surgeon elected to expeditiously decompress the spine at that level. Signals returned as decompression was achieved.

Interpretation

The most commonly used criteria for identifying a significant degradation of the SEPs are drop in amplitude below 50% of the baseline and/or a latency prolongation of 10% over the baseline value. These criteria are based on clinical experience and standards may vary among NIOM groups. Application of these "standard" criteria may need to be modified in cases where signals are of poor initial quality or where confounding systemic factors exist, such as alteration of anesthetic gases, low level of neuromuscular blockade, dramatic blood loss, or other metabolic derangements.

When a "significant" SEP degradation meets the above criteria, it must, of course, be interpreted within its clinical context. Once again, localization of the dysfunction allows appropriate action and may prevent warnings to the surgeon in cases where anesthetic, positioning, or technical issues are present. In addition, correct localization can help direct the surgeon to the most appropriate course to correct dysfunction due to surgical events. Finally, timing of the SEP changes in respect to surgical events is helpful in identifying a culprit surgical maneuver. This latter statement

TABLE 2.5 Localization of Neural Dysfunction Based on Pattern of SEP Changes*

Locus of neural insult	Associated pattern of SEP degradation
Spinal cord dysfunction	Loss of subcortical and cortical signals, Erb's point intact
Limb malpositioning	Unilateral loss of Erb's point, subcortical and cortical signals
Cerebral ischemia (carotid retraction)	Unilateral cortical loss, intact subcortical signal
Anesthetic effect	Global cortical loss, intact subcortical signals

*This allows identification of a number of different sources of insult during an anterior cervical procedure.

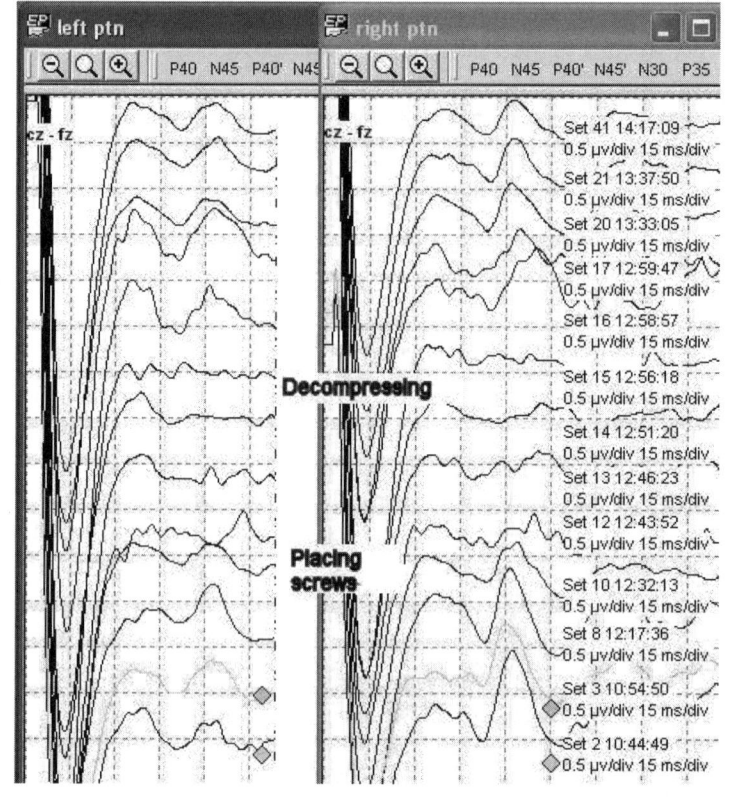

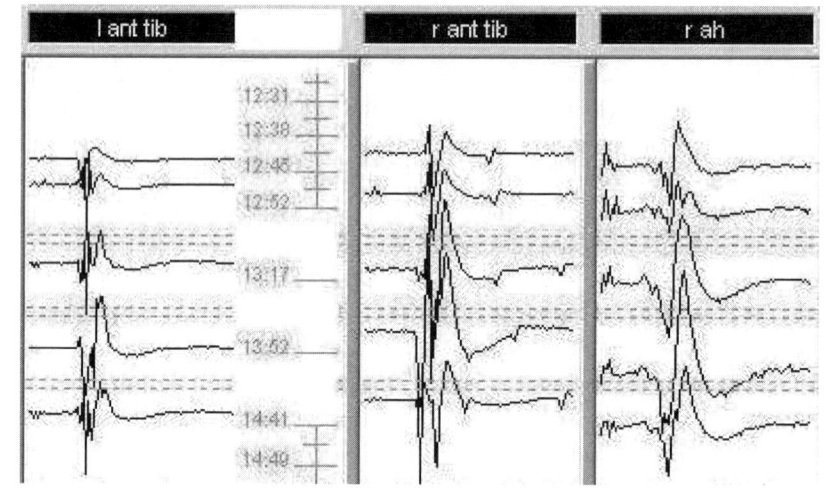

FIGURE 2.4 Tibial SEP signals were lost during a posterior thoracic decompression and fusion in a patient with spinal stenosis due to Pott's disease. The signals were lost early in the procedure (A) and recovered with decompression. The MEP signals (B) were stable at the time, suggesting an isolated posterior column effect.

comes with the caveat that the advent of MEP testing has made clear that SEP changes may be significantly delayed when dysfunction primarily affects the anterior spinal cord.

Indications

Given that SEP assess all levels of the neuraxis, it is not surprising that SEPs are a staple part of most neuromonitoring configurations. Any surgery that places somatosensory pathways at significant risk is likely to benefit from monitoring with SEPs if a corrective action is possible when dysfunction is identified. A review of SEP monitoring at all levels of the neuraxis is beyond the scope of this chapter, but appropriate cases include cervical or thoracic-level spinal surgeries, posterior fossa surgeries, hemispheric and deep brain surgeries, and surgeries that place the peripheral nerve at risk. The SEP has poor sensitivity at the level of the spinal nerve root. SEPs from peripheral nerves are typically mediated by multiple nerve roots and, as such, have poor sensitivity to monoradiculopathies. Despite this, surgeries that place multiple roots at risk simultaneously (e.g., the cauda equina) may still benefit from SEP monitoring.

The most common use of SEPs is for spinal cord monitoring; thus this deserves special note. A 1995 Scoliosis Research Society poll found that there was a 50% decline in major neurologic deficits associated with scoliosis surgery after introduction of NIOM, that SEP identified insults with a sensitivity of 92% and a specificity of 98.9%, and that participation of experienced monitoring teams was associated with half the rate of neurologic deficits compared to results with inexperienced teams (3).

Anesthesia

Anesthetic considerations for SEP monitoring are discussed in greater detail in another chapter. As a general principle, volatile anesthetics suppress cortical SEP signals in a dose-dependent manner. On a "per MAC" basis, this effect is similar for nitrous oxide and potent inhalation agents; however, the rapid onset and offset of nitrous oxide's effects when its concentration is altered make its suppressive effect potentially more difficult to distinguish from neural insults. Propofol also may suppress SEP signals, but with less potency than the volatile agents.

Rigid cutoff values for anesthetic levels are not necessary for the management of SEPs, although guideline targets may be helpful to the anesthesia team. Levels must be sufficiently low that robust and stable signals are obtained at a postequilibration baseline. From that point forward it is the stability of the anesthetic regimen that is most important.

TRANSCRANIAL ELECTRICAL MOTOR EVOKED POTENTIALS

Background

Traditional NIOM of the spinal cord has relied upon SEPs despite the fact that motor dysfunction is the most feared form of spinal cord injury. SEPs allow monitoring of signals that traverse the dorsal columns of the spinal cord, whereas motor function is only indirectly assessed, relying on coexisting dysfunction in sensory pathways to predict motor injury. Unfortunately, motor pathways may be injured while sparing sensory pathways for at least two reasons. First, there is anatomic separation between motor and dorsal column sensory pathways, with motor structures residing in the anterior cord. Second, the vascular supply to the anterior spinal cord is distinct from that to the posterior columns. The anterior spinal cord may be selectively vulnerable to ischemia due to a less robust vascular anastomotic network that does not compensate as well as the posterior vasculature in the face of hypoperfusion. In addition and possibly more importantly, motor gray matter (neurons) in the spinal cord is far more sensitive to ischemia than the dorsal column sensory white matter (axons) and thus is selectively vulnerable for this reason as well.

The lack of direct anterior cord monitoring with SEP is problematic, and cases of isolated injury with preserved SEP spinal cord monitoring have occurred. In addition, it is now clear that MEP signal changes may precede SEP signal changes, allowing earlier identification of spinal cord dysfunction and thus better correlation to surgical events with more timely intervention. At the same time, SEPs remain useful in identifying sensory dysfunction and in providing a second, independent test of cord function. In addition, posterior columns may also be injured while anterior cord pathways are spared (see Figure 2.4). Thus, MEPs are almost always performed in conjunction with SEP monitoring, and these test modalities function as complementary tests.

MEP Technique

Recording

Transcranial stimulation nonspecifically activates motor fibers subserving many or all levels of the spinal cord, and choosing appropriate muscles for recording is important to localize motor tract deficits. Ideally, recording is performed from at least two muscles on each side below the surgical level and one muscle above it to serve as a control signal. Common muscles used for this purpose are abductor pollicis brevis, tibialis anterior, and abductor hallucis. Other muscles may be added as needed for redundancy and greater localization precision (see Table 2.2 for commonly used muscles).

Alternatively, averaged "D-wave" responses may be obtained from the spinal cord white matter tracts using an electrode placed in the epidural or subdural space. This technique allows high-quality signals without significant degradation from anesthetic agents or neuromuscular blockade. D waves are not discussed in detail in this chapter but excellent references are available (4,5).

Stimulation

Transcranial activation of subcortical motor tracts is elicited most efficiently with anodal stimulation. A number of electrode configurations may be used for transcranial stimulation, but all utilize anodal stimulation with the anode placed over or adjacent to the targeted portion of the motor strip. Although an optimized configuration is yet to be agreed upon, usually one electrode is placed on C1 (expanded International 10–20 System) and the other on C2, with the anode being on the side of the targeted brain and the other electrode used as cathode. In any given patient the optimal location of these electrodes is variable and more lateral placement at C3 or C4 for one or both of the electrodes may be attempted.

MEPs are best elicited using a train of stimuli, which serves to overcome anesthetic inhibition of the synapse at the anterior horn cell of the spinal cord. Trains of four to nine stimuli are delivered with an interstimulus interval of 2 to 4 ms.

Signal Optimization

Myogenic MEP signals are frequently variable in their amplitude and morphology, making interpretation of changes challenging compared to other NIOM methods. If MEP signals are poor, there are three general types of causes to consider: signal acquisition methods, anesthetic/systemic variables, and patient pathophysiology.

Signal acquisition methods relate to factors controlled by the monitoring team and the monitoring system must be confirmed as working correctly with electrode positions and stimulation parameters optimized. Anesthetic and systemic variables are those factors managed by the anesthesiology team, such as anesthetic agents, blood pressure, temperature, oxygenation, neuromuscular blockade, and myriad others. Finally, patient-related factors may relate to physiologic or pathophysiologic sources of poor MEP signals. Preexisting dysfunction of motor pathways such as stroke, myelopathy, or neuropathy may limit the initial quality of signals, while deterioration of MEP signals may reflect surgical injury to motor pathways or benign causes such as alteration of stimulation efficiency resulting from scalp edema or cerebrospinal fluid (CSF) drainage (Figure 2.5).

Degradation of signals is often multifactorial, and adjustments or allowances must be made for factors within any or all of these general categories. A full discussion of all possibilities within these categories is beyond the scope of this chapter, but at minimum, each category should be considered in detail when MEP signals are suboptimal or deteriorating.

MEP Interpretation

There are no universally accepted criteria for identification of significant myogenic MEP signal changes. While this may be a source of frustration for those looking for easy "rules" by which to interpret MEPs, it should come as no surprise. Initially, obtained MEP signals in one patient may be robust and stable, may be widely variable in their amplitude and morphology in another, and may be absent in another despite an optimized regimen. For a given patient, initial signal quality may fall anywhere along the continuum from robust to absent. If excellent monitoring techniques are assumed to be used, the variability among different patients stems from varying anatomy, degrees of preexisting motor pathway dysfunction, and sensitivity to anesthetic agents used.

More importantly, one should not expect to apply the same interpretative criteria to signals that are robust initially as to those that are initially barely present. A number of criteria have been proposed, including a specific percentage of signal loss, presence vs. absence of signals, an increase in stimulation threshold necessary to obtain signals, and complexity/polyphasia of the recorded response. Any criterion must be applied in a manner that makes sense based on initial signal quality and variability as well within the context of changes in systemic variables that may occur.

For robust signals, the authors use complete loss of a signal or abrupt significant decrease in amplitude of 80% or more in the absence of an explanation other than surgical injury. Gradual changes in signals more commonly reflect systemic factors or an "anesthetic fade" phenomenon, so gradual changes might be given less credence unless the onset

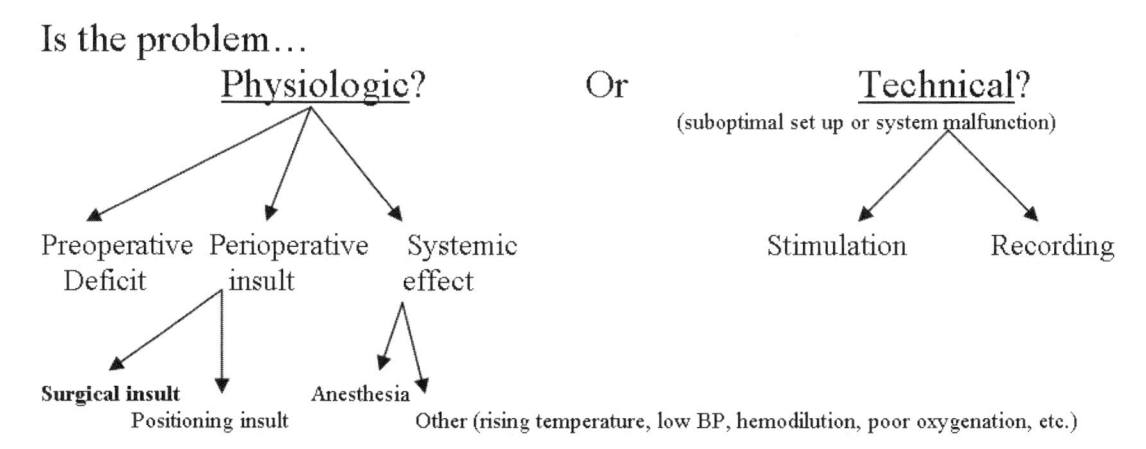

FIGURE 2.5 Poor-quality MEP signals may be due to suboptimal signal acquisition methods, unfavorable anesthetic or systemic variables, and/or the patient's physiology or pathophysiology.

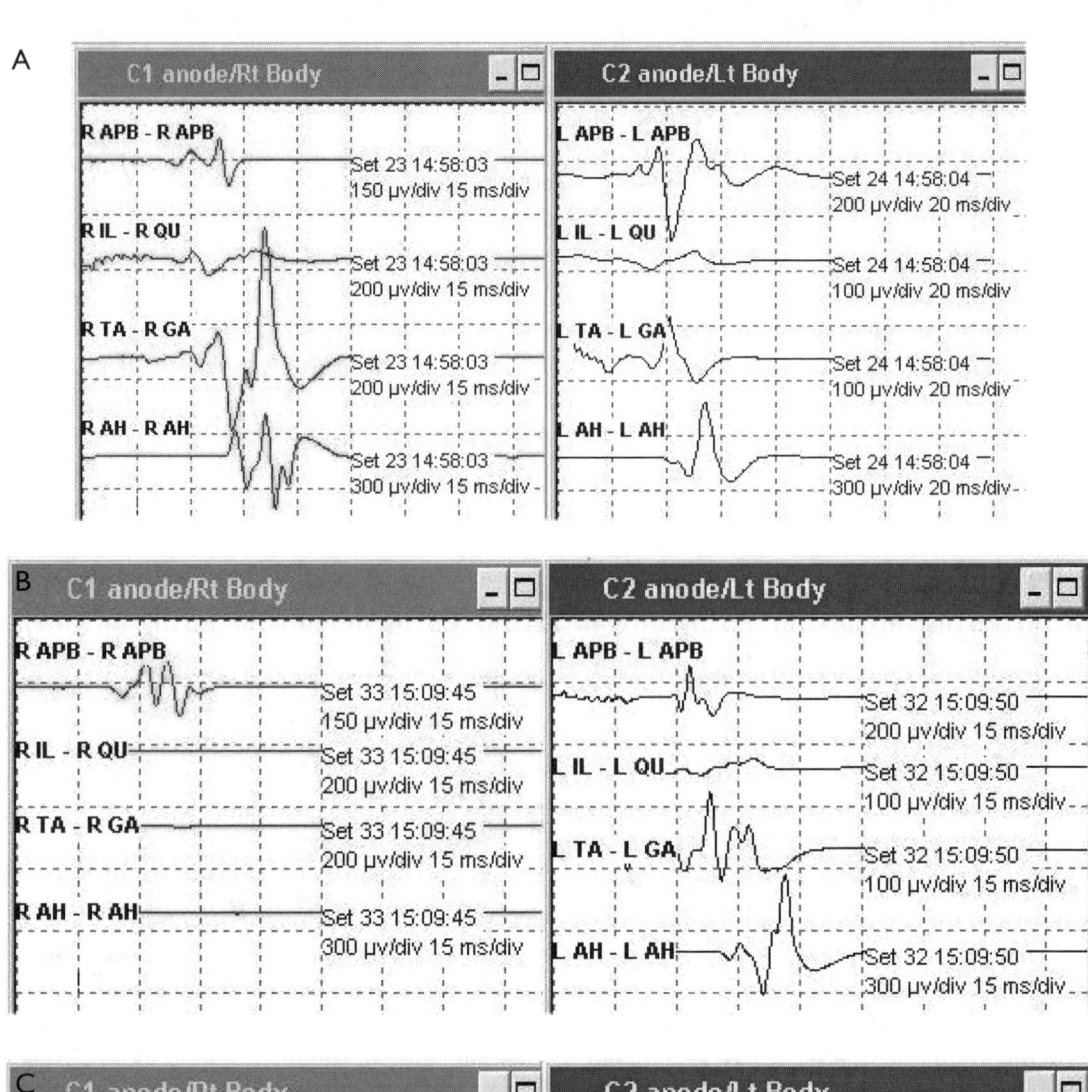

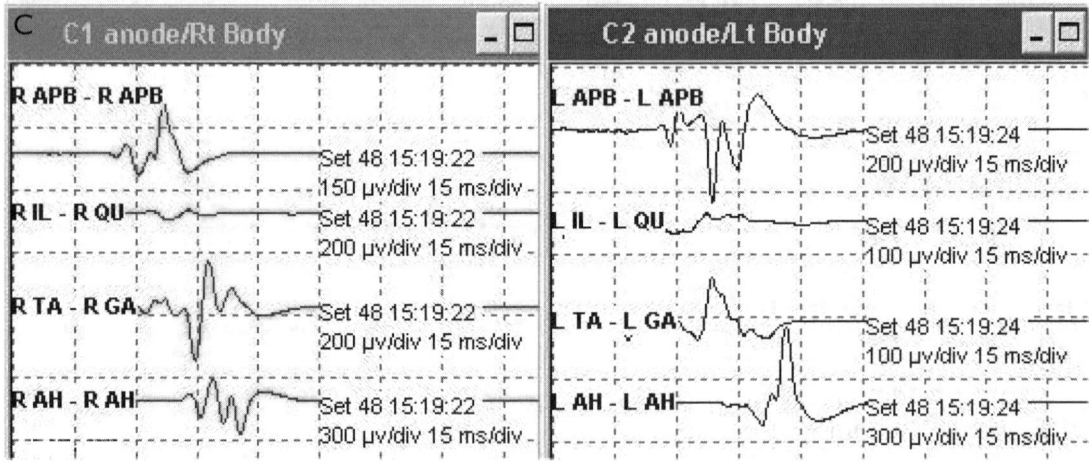

FIGURE 2.6 Right-body MEP signals are lost during scoliosis correction. MEP signals are robust immediately preceding spinal correction (A). Lower extremity right-body MEP signals are lost soon after correction was initiated, while the left-hand and left-body signals are preserved (B). Signals immediately started to improve after corrective forces were relaxed and were comparable to baseline minutes later (C). APB = abductor pollicis brevis, IL = iliopsoas, QU = quadriceps, TA = tibialis anterior, GA = gastrocnemius, AH = abductor hallucis.

of the change can be related to a surgical event that may result in gradual dysfunction (6). For poor initial signals, the criterion used is usually limited to the presence or absence of the signal. This criterion risks false-negative findings but represents a balance with what would otherwise be an untenable false-positive rate (Figure 2.6A to C).

MEP Complications and Contraindications

The most common complication of MEP testing is tongue laceration due to contraction of the masseter muscle triggered by transcranial stimulation. This can be minimized by routine use of a soft bite block. Another near universal aspect of MEP monitoring is patient movement due to muscle contraction after transcranial stimulation. This is an expected part of MEP, although it could lead to complications if movement occurs unexpectedly during a delicate portion of a surgery. As a result, the surgeon is typically warned prior to stimulation, and testing is delayed if there is an objection from the surgeon. These and the following less common complications have been reviewed by McDonald (7), who reported one case of mandibular fracture, presumably due to masseter contraction. Seizures have rarely been seen intraoperatively in the setting of MEP testing, with the review by McDonald finding 5 instances in 15,000 cases. Cardiac arrhythmia was reported in one case, but there was no clear relation to the MEP stimulation. Interference with cardiac pacemaker programming is a theoretical concern, but no reports of interference have been made and the magnetic fields produced by MEP stimulation are likely to be small relative to routinely used electrocautery. The authors' practice in the setting of a pacemaker is to proceed with MEP testing but to discuss this low risk with the anesthesia team, so that they are prepared should any cardiac anomaly arise.

Contraindications to MEP testing include the presence of indwelling deep brain stimulation electrodes and cochlear implants. In addition, the presence of plegia in the target limbs obviates the need to attempt MEP testing and makes successful acquisition unlikely. Finally, we avoid MEP testing in patients with recent craniotomy or skull fracture for two reasons. First, we do not want to cause damage by shifting unstable skull elements due to scalp muscle contraction, and second, we do not want to place electrodes into skull defects. There are few data on patients under 2 years of age, and similar skull stability concerns should be considered.

MEP Indications

MEP monitoring adds sensitivity and confidence to more traditional SEP monitoring protocols. MEPs are used in those cases with a reasonable probability of motor injury that spares dorsal columns sensory pathways and/or in high-risk procedures where a second independent test of spinal cord function is desired. For spinal cord monitoring, some will argue that MEPs should be used in every case where the spinal cord is at risk, while others are still more selective. Although this debate cannot be resolved here, there is good evidence for addition of MEP monitoring in intramedullary spinal cord tumor cases, most cervicothoracic spinal deformity cases, thoracic aortic aneurysm surgeries, and complicated cervical-level cases. In addition, MEP monitoring may also be useful at other levels of the nervous system, as for selected intracranial tumors or cerebral aneurysms. Finally, the use of MEP for lumbar-level procedures is usually not recommended on a routine basis due to a low likelihood of disassociated sensory and motor injury and imperfect sensitivity of MEPs to individual root injury.

Anesthesia

The stimulus for transcranial electrical MEPs activates subcortical white matter, which effectively bypasses the cortical effects

TABLE 2.6 Anesthetic Agents Inhibit MEPs with Varying Levels Of Potency

Degree of MEP inhibition	Anesthetic agent
High	Potent volatile agents, N_2O
Moderate	Propofol, benzodiazepines
Little or none	Etomidate and derivatives, ketamine, narcotics

of anesthetic agents. Unfortunately, anesthetics are also potent inhibitors of the synapses at the anterior horn cell in the spinal cord, and this is the primary locus of the undesirable inhibition of MEPs. In a simple sense, one can stratify these agents according to the extent of their effect on the anterior horn cell, as in Table 2.6.

Ideal anesthetic regimens for MEP monitoring are a matter of significant debate. However, grouping into potent, moderate, and little inhibition is widely accepted. As one shifts from more a potent inhibition to less potent group (at similar depths of anesthesia), MEPs will tend to improve (if originally present) or be more likely to appear (if originally absent). At some centers, those anesthetic regimens with low levels of inhibition may be less familiar to the anesthesia team and therefore more difficult to manage compared to standard anesthetic regimens. In general, the acquisition of robust and therefore reliable MEPs will be dramatically aided when anesthesiologists experienced in MEP anesthesia are available. Finally, lower inhibition regimens may also be slightly more expensive, but cost differences are minor.

Ideally, anesthetic regimens can be adjusted and tailored to the individual patient based on MEP quality during the early portions of the procedure. However, given limited available time, this may not be feasible in all cases; in most cases, a gradual, stepwise shift will not allow adequate acquisition and evaluation of signals before critical portions of the procedure begin.

Neuromuscular blockade will also impact MEP signals. In general, neuromuscular blockade has a more predictable and linear effect on MEPs, whereas volatile anesthetics have an unpredictable nonlinear effect. Typically, at reasonable levels of partial neuromuscular blockade, MEPs will be obtainable if the anesthetic agents are appropriate. However, if only low-amplitude MEP signals can be obtained, it may be necessary to forgo the use of partial neuromuscular blockade.

ELECTROENCEPHALOGRAPHY (EEG)

Background

EEG is a measure of cortical activity in real time. As it is applied in NIOM, EEG often is useful to detect widespread, gross changes in cortical function and does not require the high spatial resolution typically found in diagnostic EEG studies. Since it is not an evoked potential, EEG cannot make use of averaging techniques to increase its signal-to-noise ratio. However, the recorded EEG is typically much larger (tens of microvolts) compared to evoked responses like SEPs.

Generators

EEG recordings comprise postsynaptic potentials from cerebrocortical neurons. Surprisingly, cortical action potentials, though larger in amplitude than postsynaptic potentials, do not contribute to the EEG waveform due in part to physiologic filtering through tissue and bone as well as the longer duration of postsynaptic potentials. Furthermore, not all cortical neurons are represented in recorded EEGs from the scalp; it is the large pyramidal cells in cortex layer V that are primarily represented in scalp EEGs. This is due to the relatively large postsynaptic potentials produced in layer V of the cortex and the vertical dipoles created, which are more likely to be recorded at the scalp. Finally, patterns and distribution of synchronous firing also favors these large pyramidal cells to be represented in surface EEGs.

Classification of Frequency

Frequencies of EEG waveforms are classically divided into ranges as follows: delta < 4 Hz; theta 4 to 7 Hz; alpha 8 to 12 Hz, and beta 13 to 30 Hz. In normal individuals without the presence of anesthesia, states of wakefulness correlate to frequency, with the higher ranges expressed in states of wakefulness. During NIOM, however, when anesthetics are present, the depth of anesthesia will influence the EEG frequency. As a general rule, as anesthesia is induced, the EEG goes through a stage of activation (beta activity) early on, which then gives way to slowing. As the depth of anesthesia increases, slowing potentiates, which leads to burst suppression and eventually to electrocerebral inactivity.

Recording Montages

The choice of EEG montage may need to be tailored according to the surgery at hand. Reasons for modifying the montage may result from physical limitations in electrode placement or the need to focus on a region of interest. For intracranial surgeries, the location of the sterile field may necessitate adjustment of a standard electrode placement. To increase focus on an area of interest, additional scalp or subdural electrodes may be placed, including the use of cortical electrode strips. For uses in extracranial surgeries, as in carotid endarterectomies (CEAs), EEG may be employed to monitor cortex directly at risk for ischemia. In other procedures where only more general assessment of cerebral function is required (e.g., in MEP anesthetic assessment), a simpler montage may be used. In addition, EEG monitoring is often performed along with other modalities, including SEP, where electrodes are placed that may also be used as part of the EEG montage.

For CEA surgeries, the authors employ a modified eight-channel montage that takes advantage of C3' and C4' electrodes placed for SSEP recordings, with good sensitivity for quickly detecting gross changes (Figure 2.7). The eight channels represent anterior and posterior derivations with lateral and medial representations (Fp1 to P3; P3 to O1; Fp1 to C3'; C3' to O1; Fp2 to P4; P4 to O2; Fp2 to C4'; C4' to O2). A more complex montage may be used, but with the trade-off that real-time monitoring may be more difficult to follow without clear benefits of sensitivity.

For MEP monitoring, only a simpler, more general setup is required, with montages utilizing existing derivations of existing SEP scalp electrodes to assess for burst suppression (Figure 2.8).

Patterns

As in other NIOM modalities, EEG changes are assessed compared to the patient's baseline and particular attention is paid to

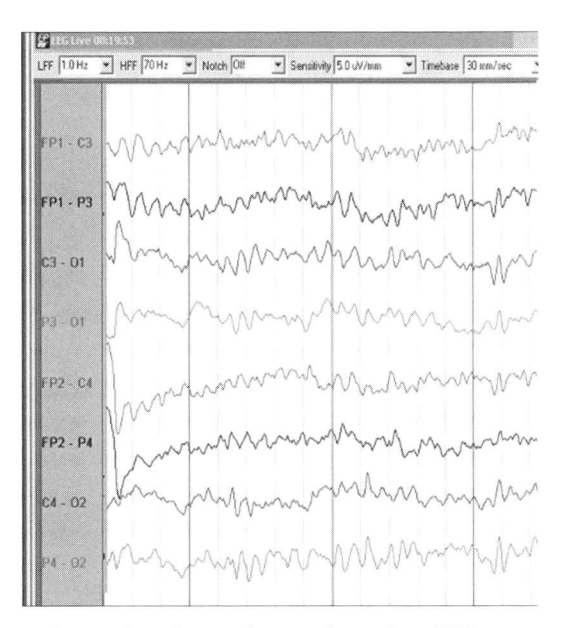

FIGURE 2.7 A sample snapshot of an EEG montage used in carotid endarterectomy procedures employing eight channels to include frontal and posterior channels on medial and lateral aspects.

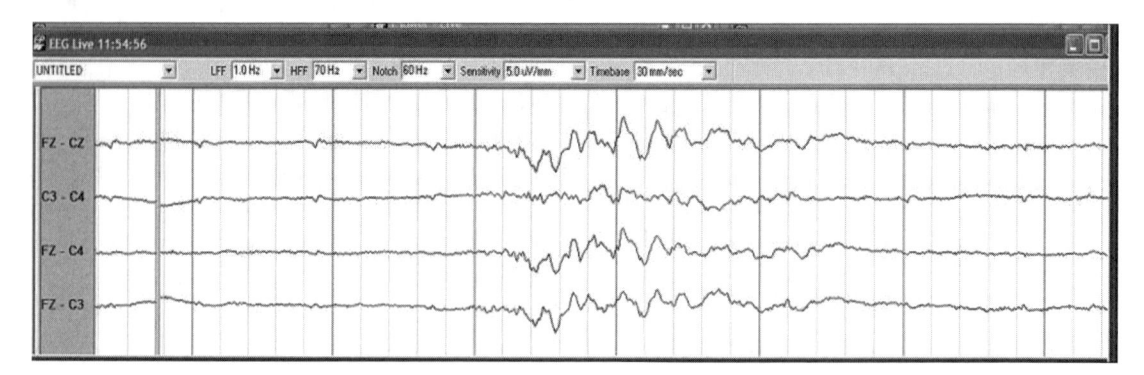

FIGURE 2.8 In MEP cases, a simplified EEG montage may be employed for purposes for monitoring for presence and levels of burst suppression. This sample demonstrates a burst suppression pattern.

new asymmetries that develop during the operative procedure. Both amplitude and frequency composition may change from an intraoperative insult. As cortex is depressed, say from ischemia, lower frequencies may be observed (delta or theta), while higher frequencies (alpha or beta) are reduced or lost. Conversely, the amplitude of the EEG may initially increase as the underlying cortex becomes more synchronous under these adverse conditions. As ischemia progressively worsens, amplitudes will depress, as in conditions of suppression or cerebral silence. The sequential pattern change from normal EEG to slowing to suppression to silence reflects predictable underlying levels of cerebral hypoperfusion (8).

During CEA procedures, increased slowing ipsilateral to the surgical side may be seen following carotid cross-clamping, typically with a frontal predominance. However, bilateral changes may also result from unilateral occlusion and it is helpful to ensure a stable anesthetic regimen around the time of cross-clamping to help distinguish surgical- from anesthetic-induced changes. In order to ensure reasonable sensitivity for detecting changes in EEG, levels of anesthesia should ideally not induce a level that overly suppresses EEG waveforms. Particular attention may be paid to timing of delivering boluses of anesthetic agents (e.g., around time of anticipated carotid clamping during CEA procedures) to prevent undue EEG suppression.

The burst suppression pattern is characteristic of anesthetic boluses or of excessive anesthetic depth. (Figure 2.8). Burst suppression seen during MEP procedures can alert the anesthetist to excessive anesthetic and explain degraded MEPs due to inhibition at the anterior horn cell. For intracranial procedures, a state of burst suppression or silence may be chosen as a means of cerebral protection. In these cases, EEG monitoring may be helpful in titrating the depth of this suppression.

Artifact

As with other NIOM modalities, achieving acceptable signal-to-noise ratios may be a challenge within the operating room. Common sources of NIOM external electrical noise include those devices, leads, and cables located near the head of the patient. Especially during periods of electrocautery, EEG monitoring is precluded. In addition, mechanical artifacts from surgeon movement of EEG leads, adjacent wires, or the patient while working near or on the skull may also contribute to EEG artifacts.

Processing Methods

Continuous EEG patterns are sufficient for the experienced examiner to follow during

NIOM to detect changes and patterns of interest. However, several methods of EEG processing exist that may assist in interpreting the EEG for changes. These methods should not replace monitoring raw, real-time EEG in order to avoid misinterpretation of artifact that may mask changes or result in false-positive results. A common method of processing is to transform the raw EEG signal into frequency spectra to separate out the EEG frequency ranges graphically. Fourier analysis is applied to the raw EEG traces and the power of the signal at a frequency is plotted and updated over time. Other processing methods have been introduced that are meant to process EEG and analyze for the depth of anesthesia, the details of which are beyond the scope of this chapter.

Applications

EEG may be used in NIOM for procedures where the cortex is directly at risk or, as discussed earlier, as a means to indirectly assess anesthetic effects. Procedures such as the resection of an arteriovenous malformation (AVM), aneurysm repair, and carotid endarterectery (CEA) are examples where vascular supply to the cortex is at risk for compromise. Often EEG is combined with other modalities such as SEPs in these procedures.

When burst suppression is induced, as for cerebral protection, EEG can identify the presence of that state and its depth. The depth of burst suppression can be roughly estimated by the length of interburst suppressive period, with a typical target range of 10 to 15 seconds.

Direct cortical EEG recording (electrocorticography) may be used to direct resection of epileptogenic tissue in epilepsy surgery or as part of eloquent cortex mapping techniques used to guide resection of dysfunctional brain.

Changes of Significance

Once a reliable EEG baseline is obtained and an anesthetic regimen stabilized, changes in amplitude and frequency composition will give clues to surgically induced changes affecting the cerebral cortex. As with all NIOM modalities, the timing and nature of the change as well as correlative evidence assist with interpretation of a clinically significant event. When looking for evidence of significant cerebral hypoperfusion, as during carotid endarterectomy, typical criteria indicating the need for carotid shunting are 50% loss of overall amplitude, 50% loss of alpha and beta activity, or a doubling of low-frequency activity (9).

BRAINSTEM AUDITORY EVOKED RESPONSES

Background

BAEPs reflect peripheral and brainstem generators within the pathway following vestibulocochlear nerve (CN VIII) activation. The first five waves of the response are resistant to anesthesia and therefore well suited to NIOM. Furthermore, the multiple generators represented allow relative localization of insults during brainstem and CN VIII pathway procedures. In addition to classic BAEP recordings, direct recording of a CN VIII nerve action potential may be performed and allows robust and rapidly acquired auditory-induced signals.

Auditory Pathways

Although exact generators may be in dispute, the auditory pathways involved in classic BAEP recordings include the distal CN VIII (wave I of the BAEP) to the cochlear nucleus (wave II; with perhaps contribution in part from cochlear nerve), superior olivary nucleus (wave III), lateral lemniscus (wave IV), and inferior colliculus (wave V). For NIOM, waveforms I to V may be reliably followed, representing a pathway from cochlear nerve to midbrain. Later waveforms generated in BAEP recordings presumably arise from thalamus and cortical radiations to auditory cortex, but these are typically absent or unreliable, especially under conditions of anesthesia. The later components may be useful as a marker of depth of anesthesia, but these uses are still investigational.

Stimulation and Recording Techniques

BAEPs are elicited by delivering a click stimulus to the ear being monitored. To avoid contribution from the contralateral ear, masking white noise is introduced to the contralateral ear at approximately 60 dBnHL. Many hundreds of averaged trials are required to record reliable potentials; thus long acquisition times must be balanced against the loss of waveform resolution that occurs as the stimulation rate is unduly increased. A rate of approximately 11 Hz provides a reasonable balance. As with all signal-averaging techniques, stimulation rates should avoid divisors of 60 so as to avoid incorporation of 60-Hz noise within the average. BAEP morphology is dependent upon the polarity of the square-wave pulse delivered. A rarefaction (pulling pulse on the eardrum) or condensation (pushing pulse) may be chosen with typically an enhanced wave I from the former.

Two channels are used to record BAEPs (1: ipsilateral ear – Cz; 2: contralateral ear –Cz), and others may be added as desired (e.g., ipsilateral ear–contralateral ear). Wave I is a negative potential recorded at the ipsilateral ear, while the later waves are positive potentials widely distributed across the scalp and recorded at the vertex for ease of electrode application and to minimize EMG interference. The channel from the contralateral ear is reflective of the ipsilateral channel, but without the presence of wave I and typically with better separation of waves IV and V. This information may be helpful in elucidating the different waveforms, especially for an ear with deficits that exhibits dispersed and delayed peaks.

If CN VIII is at risk and exposed during surgery, as may be the case with cerebellopontine angle tumor procedures, a specialized recording electrode may be placed directly on the nerve. This allows an averaged CN VIII nerve action potential to be directly recorded using the same click stimuli as described above. However, far fewer stimuli are required in recording a stable averaged response (10).

Interpretation

As with other NIOM modalities, BAEPs are compared throughout the procedure to baseline recordings performed during early stages of the procedure. It may also be helpful to have preoperative BAEP studies to help with identification of waveforms and to provide reasonable expectation as whether signals will be present intraoperatively. A pretest expectation of signals may be particularly helpful when an intraoperative absence of all waveforms is identified at baseline. As may be reasoned, BAEPs are similarly affected by the inability to deliver an effective sound stimulus to the cochlea and by dysfunction of the cochlea. Thus the absence of wave I and subsequent waveforms is equally explained by either poor transduction of the sound pulse through the ear or dysfunction of the cochlea. The former may arise from a myriad of technical issues, including too low or absent a stimulus intensity from the sound generator, dislodgement of the tubal insert, or fluid/wax within the ear dampening the sound pulse. Thus a prior expectation of signal presence may prompt additional steps to identify and correct technical issues, while an expectation of an absence of signals can avoid extraordinary troubleshooting measures.

Similarly, if all waveforms including wave I are degraded intraoperatively, technical issues must be distinguished from pathophysiologic conditions. Given the potential nonphysiologic causes, a full evaluation of stimulus and recording systems is performed. However, when abrupt loss of wave I occurs and is correlated to surgical events, it often reflects loss of cochlear function; the most common cause is compromise of the internal auditory artery. When this loss of all waveforms is due to surgical action, the risk of deafness is high.

Persistence of wave I with loss of all later components suggests dysfunction at the level of the cochlear nerve. This pattern may reflect total nerve transection, transient conduction block, or desynchronization of the conducted auditory activity. Thus prognosis is more variable in this case and will depend on the underlying cause.

Waves subsequent to wave I are generated in the brainstem, with waves III and V being the most reproducible. Changes in latencies and amplitudes of these components help to localize dysfunction of corresponding brainstem structures. Tracking the interpeak latencies of waves I to III and III to V assists in discerning anatomic areas of dysfunction. A signal delay within the cochlear nerve, for instance, may present with prolongation of waves I to III, while isolated prolongation of the III to V interpeak latency may be seen with brainstem retraction.

In general, a loss of wave V amplitude greater than 50% or a 0.5-ms prolongation of its latency is considered a significant change in BAEP. However, refinement of these arbitrary levels is likely needed and may be have to be tailored to the type of surgery (11). As with other modalities of NIOM, the timing of observed changes is important in interpreting changes in relation to both surgical events and other monitored signals. For example, if changes in BAEP accompany changes in SEP, a brainstem insult is likely.

Indications

Operations that involve the cerebellopontine angle are the most common ones requiring BAEP monitoring as part of a multimodality monitoring regimen. Brainstem tumor and vascular procedures, microvascular decompression, vestibular neurectomy, and other posterior fossa procedures may benefit from BAEP NIOM. Changes in BAEPs may be seen from irreversible actions (e.g., cochlear nerve transection) or from reversible causes (such as brainstem retraction), so that timely information to the surgical team may be of assistance to spare function. Indeed, the duration of deteriorated waveforms is suggested to have a predictive correlation to clinical outcome (12). The use of direct recordings of cranial nerve VIII allows more rapid feedback and may allow for additional information when artifact would interfere with BAEP identification or when BAEPs are poorly formed but hearing is preserved.

Anesthesia and Other Factors Affecting BAEP

Commonly used anesthetics including volatile agents have little or no effect on BAEP, making these waveforms relatively unique in their resilience to fluctuating anesthetics. However, BAEPs are susceptible to influences of auditory noise sources in the operating room that may not affect other NIOM modalities. Sound and electrical sources that affect the BAEPs include the presence of drilling, ultrasonic aspirators, electrocautery, intraoperative microscopes, and EMG artifact. The first three on this list are the most common offenders of interference and BAEP acquisition may need to be paused during their use. Frequently BAEPs are performed during acoustic nerve surgeries, where facial nerve EMG is also monitored and thus neuromuscular blockade is low or absent. The placement of recording electrodes at the vertex and either ear helps to minimize EMG interference, as little muscle mass exists under these electrodes. Body temperature will influence BAEP latency. In particular, with aggressive cooling conditions (e.g., < 27°C), the BAEP will be obliterated.

CONCLUSIONS

Many different neurophysiologic testing modalities can be used for NIOM. Often more than one modality will be needed during a surgical procedure. It behooves the neurophysiologist to understand the surgical procedures and know which neural structures will be at risk. Based on this assessment, a combination of various modalities should be chosen for NIOM. A clear understanding of the various neurophysiologic tests in the diagnostic laboratory helps the neurophysiologist interpret them when they are used in the operating room.

REFERENCES

1. Prass RL, Luders H. Acoustic (loudspeaker) facial electromyographic monitoring: Part 1. Evoked electromyographic activity during acoustic neuroma resection. *Neurosurgery* 1986;19:392–400.
2. Calancie B, Madsen P, Lebwohl N. Stimulus-evoked EMG monitoring during transpedicular lumbosacral spine instrumentation. Initial clinical results. *Spine* 1994;19:2780–2786.
3. Nuwer MR, Dawson EG, Carlson LG, et al. Somatosensory evoked potential spinal cord monitoring reduces neurologic deficits after scoliosis surgery: results of a large multicenter survey. *Electroencephalogr Clin Neurophysiol* 1995;96:6–11.
4. Kothbauer K, Deletis V, Epstein FJ. Intraoperative spinal cord monitoring for intramedullary surgery: an essential adjunct. *Pediatric Neurosurgery* 1997;26:247–254.
5. Sala F, Niimi Y, Berenstein A, Deletis V. Neuroprotective role of neurophysiological monitoring during endovascular procedures in the spinal cord. *Ann N Y Acad Sci* 2001;939: 126–136.
6. Lyon R, Feiner J, Lieberman JA. Progressive suppression of motor evoked potentials during general anesthesia: the phenomenon of "anesthetic fade". *J Neurosurg Anesthesiol* 2005; 17:13–19.
7. MacDonald DB. Safety of intraoperative transcranial electrical stimulation motor evoked potential monitoring. *J Clin Neurophysiol* 2002;19:416–429.
8. Sundt TMJ, Sharbrough FW, Piepgras DG, et al. Correlation of cerebral blood flow and electroencephalographic changes during carotid endarterectomy: with results of surgery and hemodynamics of cerebral ischemia. *Mayo Clin Proc* 1981;56:533–543.
9. Nuwer MR. Intraoperative electroencephalography. *J Clin Neurophysiol* 1993;10:437–444.
10. Møller AR, Jannetta PJ. Monitoring auditory functions during cranial nerve microvascular decompression operations by direct recording from the eighth nerve. *J Neurosurg* 1983;59: 493–499.
11. James ML, Husain AM. Brainstem auditory evoked potential monitoring: when is change in wave V significant? *Neurology* 2005 22;65: 1551–1555.
12. Nakamura M, Roser F, Dormiani M, et al. Intraoperative auditory brainstem responses in patients with cerebellopontine angle meningiomas involving the inner auditory canal: analysis of the predictive value of the responses. *J Neurosurg* 2005;102:637–642.

3 Remote Monitoring

Ronald G. Emerson

Optimal supervision of neurophysiologic intraoperative monitoring (NIOM) and the ability to respond in a timely manner to problems and emergencies require that the clinical neurophysiologist have real-time access to NIOM data. When the neurophysiologist is not present physically in the operating room (OR), a remote data connection can provide suitable access. Indeed, many vendors of NIOM equipment also supply remote monitoring software. In hospitals with modern network infrastructures, remote monitoring within the facility can be as simple as installing these programs. Monitoring from more distant sites or from sites with suboptimal or more complex data connections can be more complicated. Nonetheless, in most cases a suitable solution is available.

BACKGROUND

Although it is not the intent here is not to offer a tutorial on the computer networking or the Internet, a few necessary basics are covered. Today's Internet is a direct descendent of an initiative from the Cold War era to develop a robust communication network that would survive wartime damage. In contrast to traditional telephony, where communication is continuous between two points, data transmitted across the Internet are broken into discrete packets that can follow different routes between sender and receiver. Internet data packets are even permitted to arrive out of order, to be resequenced at the destination. The influence of the Internet is so pervasive that protocols evolved to serve it govern almost all computer networks regardless of whether they actually connect to the Internet.

Networked computers are identified by their IP (Internet Protocol) address. Much like a street address, an IP address indicates the location of the computer on the network. IP addresses are usually assigned by special servers that are part of the network infrastructure; the network infrastructure also implements a set of rules for routing data packets between computers based on their IP addresses.

Just as the NIOM team needs to be able to detect and resolve technical problems that compromise monitoring, it is helpful for the team to be able to recognize and fix simple problems with remote monitoring. To determine the IP address of a Windows-based NIOM system, simply click Start > Programs > Accessories > Command Prompt and type "ipconfig" (Figure 3.1A). The IP address of the NIOM machine may remain constant, or it may change from day to day; within an institution, changes usually affect only the

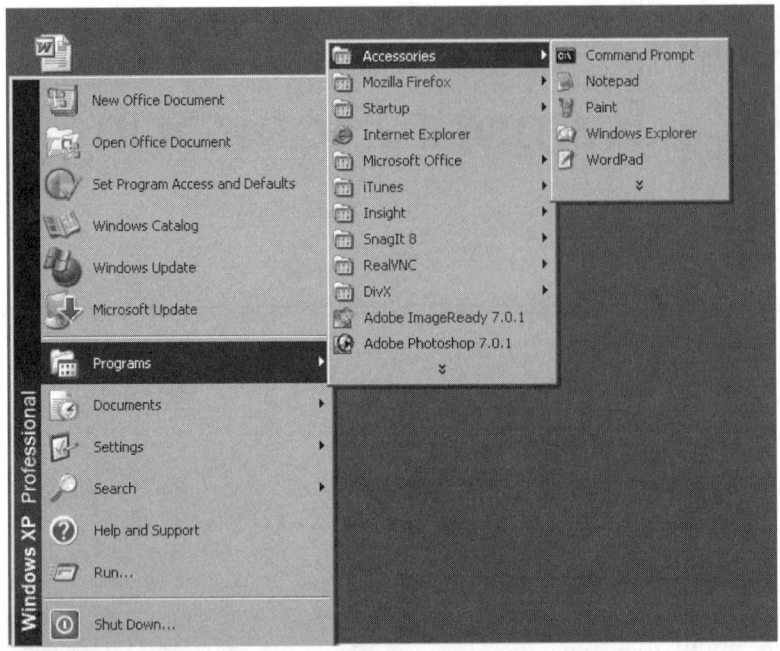

FIGURE 3.1 To determine the IP address of a Windows computer, (A) first open a Command Prompt Window by clicking Start à Programs –> Accessories –> Command Prompt. (B) in the Command Prompt Window, type "ipconfig." The system will respond with information that includes the IP address of your machine and also the IP address of your default gateway.

rightmost digits (e.g., 21 in Figure 3.1B). An IP address of 0.0.0.0 or, by convention, 169.254.x.x[1] is invalid and usually indicate that your computer was unable to obtain a proper address. An easy way to verify connection to the network and that the network is working is to send a test message (or "ping") to some other machine on the network. If the message is received, the target machine will respond with the time it took for the test message to be received. If the message is not received, the ping will fail.

---

[1] In this notation, x is an integer from 0 to 255.

FIGURE 3.2 To ping a machine, open a Command Prompt Window (see Figure 3.1), and type "ping," followed by the IP address of the target system. In this example, the target is 10.2.2.16. The ping is successful, with times between 1 and 2 milliseconds.

The "default gateway," the device that typically connects the computers on a floor or building with a larger network or to the Internet, is often a good choice for pinging. "Ipconfig" also displays a machine's address (Figure 3.1B). In Figure 3.2, the command "ping 10.2.2.16" sends a series of four test messages to the default gateway; in each case the gateway machine responds promptly. In contrast, in Figure 3.3, the connection has been lost and the ping fails.

On Window machines, the network connection can be partially tested by clicking on the network icon in the system tray, usually at the lower right of the screen (Figure 3.4). A bad network connection may return a message indicating "limited connection" or "network cable unplugged." A defective network cable can be physically plugged in but functionally disconnected; loss of resilience with use of the plastic tab on the network connector is a common cause of an unreliable or

FIGURE 3.3 Example of a failed ping, returning the message "request timed out."

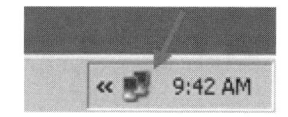

FIGURE 3.4 Network icon in the System Tray, usually at the lower-right-hand corner of a Windows computer.

intermittent connection on portable equipment (Figure 3.5).

Local networks are generally designed to permit data to flow freely between all connected devices. At points where a local network joins a larger network or the Internet, routers and firewalls may selectively limit the flow of data. Some types of data may be permitted to reach only specific destinations, while others may be excluded entirely. Generally, institutional firewalls have a "deny all" policy for inbound traffic, with exceptions provided for special data types. The firewall illustrated in Figure 3.6 block all inbound traffic but web and mail data; designated servers are the only permitted destinations.

Filtering by data type is easily accomplished because, in addition to the data "payload" and the IP addresses of sending and receiving computers, data packets also specify source and destination "port numbers," which effectively specify the type of data car-

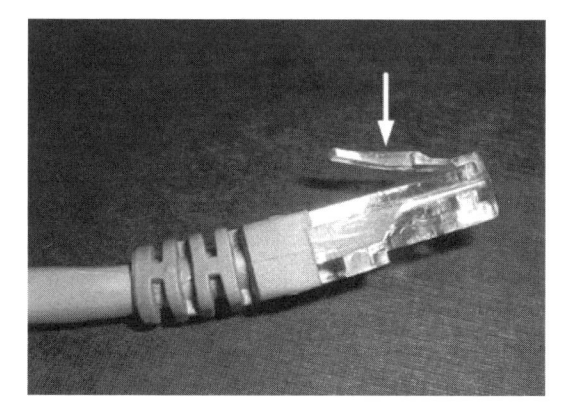

FIGURE 3.5 Ethernet cable connector. The arrow points to a plastic tab that commonly loses resilience with age, causing an unreliable electrical connection.

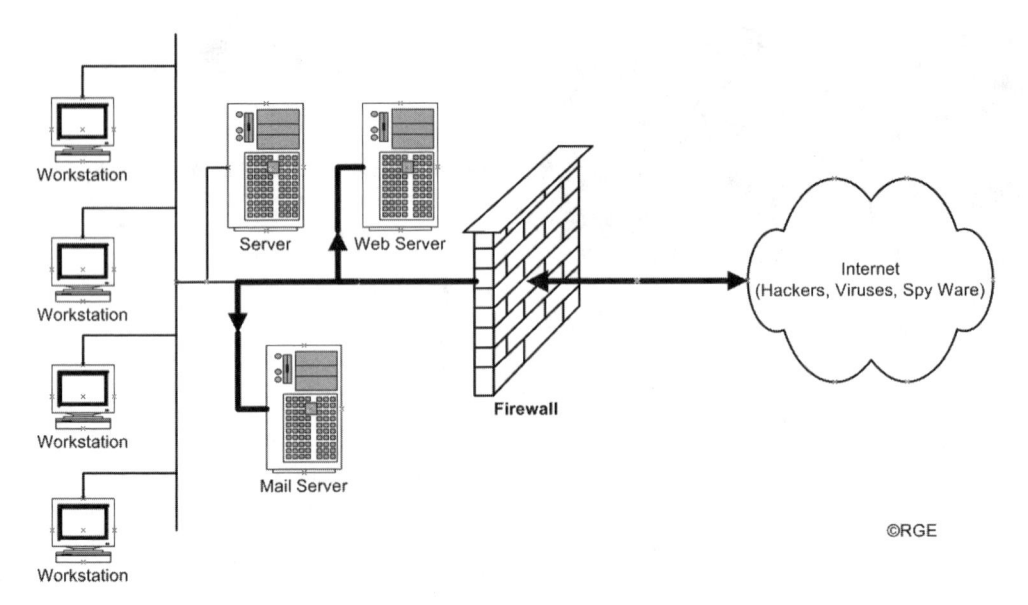

FIGURE 3.6 Institutional firewall blocks all inbound traffic except for packets bound for the mail and web server. Packets that are inbound but are responding to messages sent by inside computers are also permitted.

ried in the payload (Figure 3.7). In Figure 3.6, the firewall is configured to permit inbound traffic only to the web server on Port 80 and the mail server on Port 25.

By convention, IP numbers in the 192.168.x.x and 10.x.x.x ranges are nonroutable on the Internet and reserved for use on private networks. Commonly, institutions make use of nonroutable IP numbers internally; the network address translation (NAT) protocol is used by the firewall to enable internal machines to communicate with external hosts. This arrangement makes internal machines invisible to the Internet unless communication is initiated by the internal system or special firewall provisions are made to "map" specific internal machines to additional, routable IP addresses.

FIGURE 3.7 Typical data packet consisting of a "data payload" plus the source and destination IP addresses and ports.

REMOTE CONNECTION TECHNIQUES

Various options exist for remote data connections. The best choice will depend on the type and quality of the remote Internet connection and the services and policies of the hospital.

Virtual Private Networks

One approach entails the use of a virtual private network (VPN). A VPN is effectively a secure tunnel through the Internet connecting the hospital's internal network and a remote site. A VPN makes the computer (or an entire remote site) appear as if it were within the hospital, behind its firewall (Figure 3.8). If the hospital uses private (192.168.x.x or 10.x.x.x) IP addresses, these can be directly accessible on a VPN. Technically, virtual private networking is accomplished by wrapping the internal network packets (including both internal IP addresses and the data payload) inside another packet whose IP addresses specify the ends of the tunnel (Figure 3.9). In this arrangement, the remote computer has

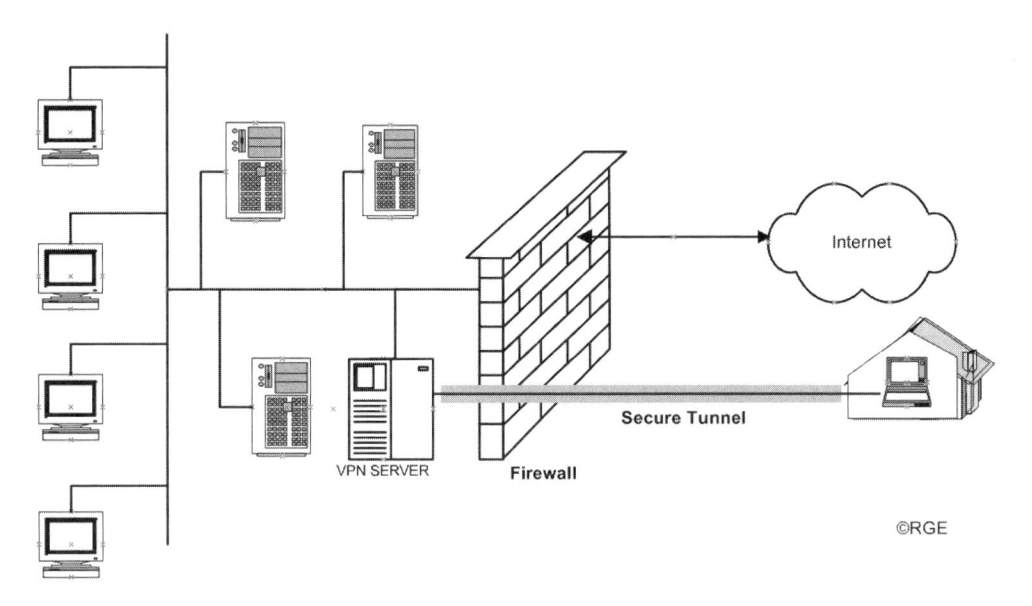

FIGURE 3.8 A VPN creates a secure tunnel through the Internet, allowing an external computer to function as if it were behind the institutional firewall.

two IP addresses: a normal Internet IP address and an IP address that is actually part of the hospital network. Generally, the internal network packets are encrypted before they are wrapped inside the VPN packets and are decrypted as they emerge from the tunnel.

Security concerns may cause some institutions to not offer or restrict remote VPN connections. Since a VPN logically moves the remote computer to within the institutional firewall, it also exposes the internal network to viruses and other potentially dangerous software that may be present on remote machines. Although desktop computers within an institution may be actively managed, kept up to date with antivirus software and security patches, and restricted to running properly vetted software, a similar level of control of home computers is likely to be more difficult.

VPN tunnels can be intolerant of suboptimal network connection. Communication glitches, common on the Internet, may interrupt VPN traffic, requiring the user to reestablish connection. VPN may not work in some settings (e.g., on some hotel guest networks).

Remote Application Servers

An alternative approach to remote access is to run the applications to be accessed remotely on special remote application servers. When remote users connect, their computers become the virtual keyboards and monitors of a remote server on which the application actually runs. Only the image to be displayed plus keyboard and mouse clicks are transmitted between the server and the

Internet Source IP and Port	Internet Dest IP and Port	Encrypted data payload		
		Internal Source IP and Port	Internal Destination IP and Port	Data Payload

FIGURE 3.9 VPN data packet. An internal data packet is encrypted and becomes the data payload carried by the VPN "wrapper."

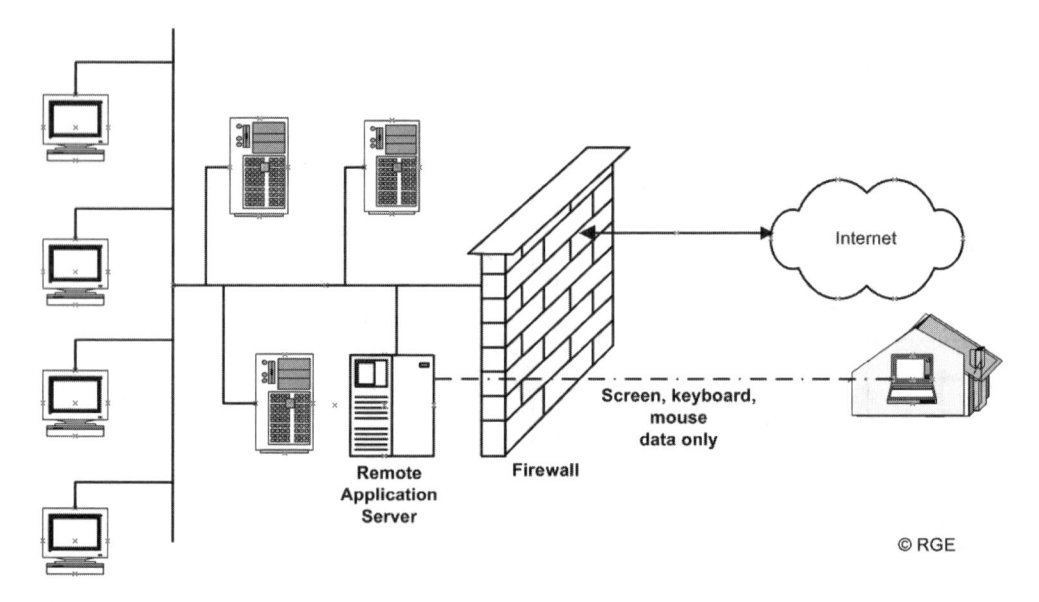

FIGURE 3.10 Only virtual screen images plus keyboard and mouse clicks travel beyond the institutional firewall in this remote application server implementation. Although it appears to the user that applications are running on the remote computer, they are really running on the remote application server.

remote user (Figure 3.10). If desired, remote users can be permitted to view documents but prohibited from transferring files.

In contrast to VPN, which can expose internal networks to viruses and other security threats posed by unmanaged remote computers, the remote application server solution can fully shield the internal network. Additionally, remote application systems can require less bandwidth and can offer better performance under suboptimal Internet conditions. Conditions that would cause a VPN to disconnect may cause remote application systems to simply stutter or become momentarily unresponsive. On the other hand, given sufficient bandwidth and stable Internet connectivity, some software may perform better over a VPN. Although remote desktop systems require special client software to be present on the remote system, this client software often requires minimal or no user configuration.

Microsoft's Windows Servers 2000 and 2003 support remote application services. Citrix Systems offers a well-known remote application solution based on Microsoft's Windows Terminal Services but may provide better security and performance (1,2). Citrix also provides a web-based interface that also checks for the client software on the remote machine; if it is not there, the user is directed through a very simple one-time installation process.

REMOTE NIOM REVIEW SOLUTIONS

In addition to establishing a remote connection with the NIOM machine, a technique must exist to transmit the data being collected for remote NIOM review. Several techniques are available for such review.

Vendor-Specific Remote Display Software

Vendors of NIOM systems commonly provide companion programs for remote display of NIOM data in real time over a network connection. These programs typically emulate the display and review functions of the NIOM machine. They permit the remote user to view ongoing recordings in real time as well as to review prior data from earlier in a case. Since the actual physiologic waveform data are sent to the remote site, the user is typically able to manipulate the remote display (e.g., to change gains and filters independently of the technologist in the OR).

In-Hospital Use of Vendor-Specific Remote Display Software

Vendor-specific remote software generally functions seamlessly on internal hospital networks. There are, however, a few important technical points of which the user should be aware. If the NIOM or remote machines have "personal firewalls," it will probably be necessary to open the port used by the remote software. Personal firewalls are enabled by default in Windows XP service pack 2.

To use the remote software, the user typically needs to know the IP address or name of the NIOM machine. Depending upon institutional policy and whether the NIOM machines is used in more than one location within the hospital, the NIOM machine will be assigned either a fixed IP address or will receive a "dynamic" address that may change from day to day. In the latter case, the technician in the OR will need to make the remote user aware of the machine's IP address.

The remote software may also permit the user to specify the NIOM machine by name. A machine may be identified by an official "fully qualified" name (e.g., NIOM2.neuro.columbia.edu), by a simple shorter name (NIOM2), or by both. Depending upon how the NIOM machine is configured and the network naming protocols in use, the remote user may have better success using the IP number than the name.

Remote Use of Vendor-Specific Remote Display Software

Special provisions are likely to be necessary for using vendor-specific remote software from beyond the hospital firewall. Typically, the firewall will prevent software running on an outside computer from initiating communication with the NIOM machine in the OR. A VPN is commonly used to access to a hospital's internal network from outside its firewall.

Vendor-specific remote client running over a VPN can be the ideal remote monitoring solution, providing the remote monitoring station with full functionality—the same as would be available from within the hospital. The requirements are (a) support of the VPN by the hospital, (b) installation of both VPN "client" and vendor-specific remote software on the remote computer, and (c) a stable, high-quality Internet connection to the remote site.

Use of a remote application server can be a reasonable alternative if it is compatible with the vendor-specific remote application. Because one remote system will effectively be running on top of another, remote monitoring may seem somewhat sluggishly responsive to key and mouse clicks. Nonetheless, a remote application server implementation has the advantages of (a) only a single license for the vendor—supplied remote software may be necessary, (b) less software—and no NIOM specific software—needs to be installed on the remote computer so that virtually any Internet-connected computer can be a remote monitoring station, and (c) it may function more reliably than a VPN if the Internet connection is slow or otherwise suboptimal.

Screen Capture Remote Control Software

Generic screen-capture software is an alternative to a vendor-specific remote program. Typically, the "server" version of the software is installed on the NIOM machines and the "client" version on the remote machine. Rather than transmitting waveform data to the remote site, screen-capture software simply transmits an image of the NIOM machine's screen. An obvious limitation to this is that the remote station can see only what is happening in the OR in real time; the user cannot replay past events or change settings independently. The corresponding advantage is that the remote station displays exactly what is happening in the OR without requiring the user to choose settings or make adjustments. Assuming that the remote user has simultaneous voice or "instant messaging" communication with the technician in the OR, it is simple to say "show me."

A wide selection of screen-capture remote control software is commercially available. One of the more ubiquitous is virtual network computing (VNC). Several variants of VNC are available free under the General Public License.[2] VNC is platform-independent, meaning that you can, for example, run a Windows version on the NIOM machine in the OR and monitor remotely using an Apple or Linux machine. Although the basic version of VNC does not support encryption, remote communication can be secured by simply running VNC (or other screen-capture remote control software) through a secure VPN tunnel.

Rather than using a VPN, the screen-capture client software may be installed on a remote application server. Again, performance here may be sluggish because two layers of remote software are in use. Yet if a VPN connection is not available or suitable and if vendor-specific software is either not available or not compatible with the remote application server, this arrangement may be acceptable.

pcAnywhere and other similar commercial products support secure, encrypted remote connection. Proper configuration of this software is critical, since it is possible to configure it in a nonsecure manner. Also, it is likely that specific ports will need to be opened in the hospital's firewall. Users should therefore consult with appropriate authorities at their institutions.

An important caution when using screen-capture software for remote monitoring is to avoid inadvertently granting control permission to the remote site. By design, VNC and similar software packages allow the remote user to control the host system—i.e., a user at home could control the NIOM machine in the OR. If that is not intended, this option should be disabled.

Reverse-Connection Remote Software

A popular variant of the screen-capture remote control software makes it easy to connect from a remote computer to a target computer behind a hospital firewall. Programs such as GoToMyPC circumvent firewall restrictions by reversing the direction of communication initiation (3). As discussed above, most firewalls are generally configured to permit only very specific inbound connections and block all others. However, they are more permissive with outbound connections, and almost all institutional firewalls permit outbound web traffic (port 80 for unencrypted and 443 for encrypted). Once an outbound conversation has been initiated, associated inbound traffic is permitted (otherwise one could not browse the web).

In the reverse-connection scenario, special software on the target computer (e.g., the NIOM machine in the OR), in addition to performing screen capture and remote server functions, also establishes and maintains a continuous connection with an outside third-party server by sending it periodic "keep alive" packets (Figure 3.11). When a remote user wants to contact the target computer, it instead contacts the third-party server; the remote user is then able to communicate with the target machine by effectively joining a conversation already in progress, initiated from within the firewall!

Reverse-connection remote systems can offer elaborate security, including remote user authentication, end-to-end data encryption so

---

[2] Supported by the Free Software Foundation (www.fsf.org), the General Public License grants users access to run, to study how a program works, and to modify it and distribute it; it and also provides that these right will be preserved in derivative works.

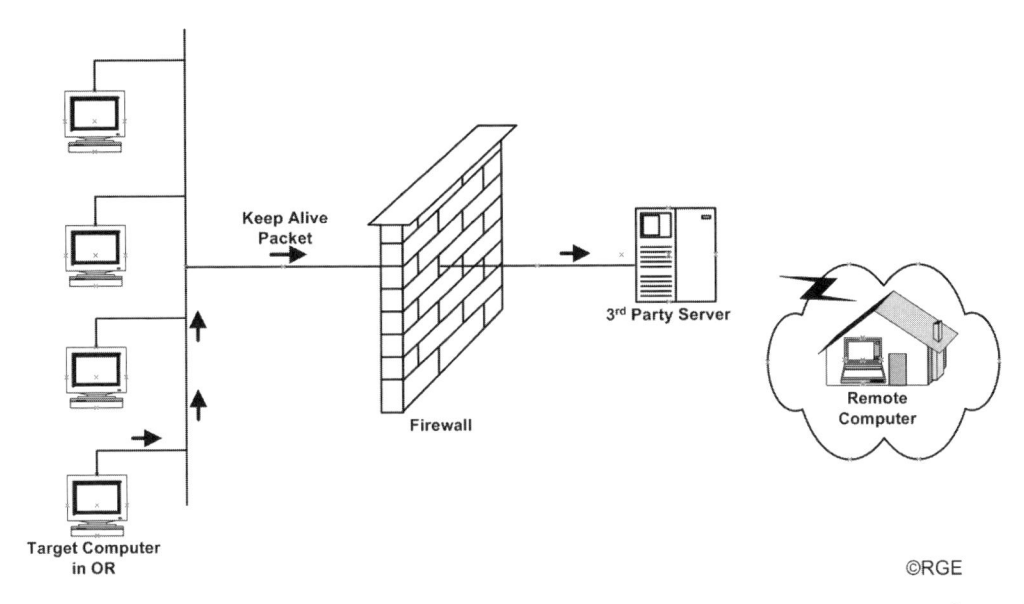

FIGURE 3.11 Reverse-connection remote system software on the target computer (e.g., the NIOM machine) sends "keep alive" packets to a third-party server, which waits for the remote system to connect.

that the third party cannot decipher the data being transferred between the target and remote machines, and provisions to prevent target systems from becoming unknowing hosts to reverse-connection remote software. Nonetheless, this technology does provide a mechanism for potentially violating the intent of institutional firewall and security policies; in any case, it transfers responsibility for the security of data protected by the Health Insurance Portability and Accountability Act (HIPAA) to a third party. Accordingly, some institutions may block access to these third-party servers. For these reasons, it is suggested that users consult with their institutions prior installing this type of software for remote NIOM monitoring.

Image Capture/Web Server

A "solution of last resort," one that will work in almost any environment, is to install software on the NIOM machine that periodically takes a picture of the screen display (or a portion of it) and automatically sends it to a web server. The web server can be located behind the institutional firewall or, if external access to an internal web server is not easily arranged, on the Internet using an independent Internet service provider. Inexpensive programs, such as Snagit, can be set to automatically capture screen images at preset intervals (e.g., twice a minute) and output them, for example, using the file-transfer protocol (FTP). A very simple script causes the image displayed by the browser to be refreshed at corresponding intervals. Configuration of the remote server as both a web server to display the images and an FTP server to receive them, while beyond the scope of this chapter, is simple and is well within the capabilities of many computer novices.

A disadvantages of this technique is that screen images are captured periodically (e.g., once of several times a minute, not continuously). Further, unless secure, encrypted protocols are used for both the web connection and transfer of the images from the NIOM machine to the web server (FTP is not secure), it is critical that no patient identifiers (e.g., the patient's name, unit number, etc.) be inadvertently captured in the image.

An advantage of this technique is that it will work well with just about any remote computer with an Internet connection. No special software needs to be present on the remote system; a web browser is all that is necessary. Web connections are, by design, not continuous; when you browse the web, each mouse click typically initiates an independent conversation with the server that ceases once the page is transmitted. Accordingly, this type of connection is suitable when Internet connectivity is slow or unreliable, and it works well with handheld wireless devices.

CONCLUSIONS

In today's NIOM environment, remote review of data by the neurophysiologist is common. The NIOM team must be knowledgeable not only about monitoring techniques but also about Internet connectivity to ensure that data are adequately transmitted from the acquisition system to the remote review system. There are several different ways in which connection to the host computer can be established, both from within the hospital and from the outside. There are many different methods that allow data from the acquisition system to be reviewed at a remote site. Each has advantages and disadvantages and each NIOM team must pick a system that works well for them.

REFERENCES

1. Montoro M. Microsoft RDP man in the middle vulnerability. Available at: http://www.securiteam.com/windowsntfocus/5EP010KG0G.html. Accessed November 20, 2006.
2. Frequently Asked Questions—Citrix ICA and man-in-the-middle attacks. Available at: http://support.citrix.com/article/CTX101737. Accessed November 20, 2006.
3. Citrix GoToMyPC security white paper. Available at: https://www.gotomypc.com/downloads/pdf/m/GoToMyPC_Security_White_Paper.pdf. Accessed November 20, 2006.

4 Anesthetic Considerations

Michael L. James

The practice of anesthesia has historically relied on the induction of a reversible state of amnesia, analgesia, and motionlessness. With the improvement of medical technology, advancement of knowledge, and practice of evidence-based medicine, modern anesthesiology comprises a great deal more. It has become the role of the anesthesiologist during surgical, obstetrical, and diagnostic procedures to provide anesthesia, optimize procedural conditions, maintain homeostasis, and, should it be necessary, manage cardiopulmonary resuscitation. Additionally, anesthesiology has found itself branching out into chronic and acute pain treatment as well as the intensive care unit. Obviously there has been an expansion of expectations for the practice of anesthesia over the last few decades; however, ultimately, anesthesiology is the practice of manipulating a patient's neurologic system and physiology to effect some beneficial end.

PRINCIPLES OF ANESTHESIA

There are four basic types of "anesthesia": general anesthesia, regional anesthesia, local anesthesia, and sedation. For the purposes of neurophysiologic intraoperative monitoring (NIOM), general anesthesia (the creation of reversible coma) is nearly always required and consists of four basic stages: premedication, induction, maintenance, and emergence. Prior to entering the operating suite, "premedications" may be administered to prepare the patient for the perioperative period. Usually this takes the form of mild sedation for anxiolysis, analgesics for preprocedural pain, antihypertensives, antiemetics for patients with a high likelihood of postoperative nausea and vomiting, antisialagogues to facilitate intubation, etc. In the operating room the historic principles of anesthesia are still the foundation of practice, and analgesia (i.e., painlessness), amnesia (i.e., memory loss), motionlessness, and hemodynamic stability can be obtained and maintained by a variety of means. Commonly, general anesthesia is induced through the administration of a large bolus dose of an intravenous sedative-hypnotic (e.g., propofol). A dose of intravenous opioid (e.g., fentanyl) and a paralytic agent (e.g., vecuronium) may be given at this time as well to facilitate endotracheal intubation. After induction, anesthesia maintenance usually consists of some amount of inhaled volatile anesthetic agent (e.g., isoflurane) in a mix of oxygen and either air or nitrous oxide and some dose of intravenous opioid. The amount of volatile agent is quantified in terms of mean alveolar concentration (MAC). MAC is expressed as a percentage of inhaled gas and is defined as the alveolar partial pressure of a gas at which 50% of patients will not move with a 1-cm abdominal surgical incision. However, in practice the necessary amount of volatile agent is determined by effect. It is during anesthesia maintenance that NIOM occurs (as does the surgical procedure). After the procedure is finished, the expectation is that the anesthetic coma will be completely reversible, and the patient must emerge from anesthesia without experiencing lasting effects from the agents. Emergence is usually accomplished by reversing any residual neuromuscular blockade and allowing the patient to eliminate volatile agent via breathing. Volatile anesthetic agents are minimally metabolized and largely removed from the body in the same manner they were introduced: ventilation.

In terms of NIOM, special considerations for general anesthesia are discussed later; however, it is important for neurophysiologists and technologists to have a clear expectation of the step-by-step nature whereby anesthetic and surgical procedures are undertaken, and it is important to remember that the operating room is generally a highly active environment with people, monitors, equipment, and electrical cords all moving about at once. Any change in the NIOM may be due to many factors, not the least of which is the surgical procedure, and every attempt should be made to regain fading or lost waveforms, as permanent loss may indicate postoperative impairment (1). Therefore the entire process becomes most efficient when each individual in the room understands all the steps, including those of every other individual, required to prepare for, perform, and enable emergence from a procedure in an environment of open communication and respect for each other's responsibilities.

NONPHARMACOLOGIC FACTORS: ANESTHETIC CONSIDERATIONS

Physiologic function of the human body plays a major role in neuronal functioning; it is arguably the most important factor, and a great deal of human physiology is influenced by actions of the anesthesiologist. The manner in which these physiologic functions are manipulated often directly determines measurable neurophysiologic function. Further, it is reasonable to assume that physiologic function determines, in large part, the survivability of nerves and their supporting structures.

Temperature

It is well established that temperature plays a significant role in nerve function, especially in the axon. Changes of a fraction of a degree can drastically alter latencies and amplitudes of neuronal potentials with cortical structures being more affected than peripheral nerves (2). Relative hypothermia produces changes that invariably present as slowed latencies from slower nerve conduction. In addition there are predictable, characteristic effects of profound hypothermia that, at least initially, begin with slowing to a delta frequency (3). The opposite is true with relative hyperthermia for both evoked potentials (EPs) and electroencephalograms (EEGs). It is important to note that regional temperature changes are invariably difficult to predict, for a variety of reasons. General anesthesia causes an overall cooling effect in the body core due to peripheral vasodilatation, which is usually opposed by active surface warming and warmed intravenous fluids. Additionally, cold and/or warm irrigants are nearly always applied to the surgical field. As a result, the extremities, brain, and spinal cord are being heated or cooled depending on where they lie in relation to warmed air blankets, intravenous fluid lines, the surgical field, etc. Therefore, unless it is individually measured, the actual temperature of a given region is impossible to know, but the potential effects should be kept in mind during the course of monitoring. It is very common for patients to experience a decrease in core body temperature for the first 15 minutes after anesthetic induction. With active warming during the administration of most anesthetic agents—unless the surgical procedure requires an alternative strategy—the patient's temperature will then be kept greater than 36°C by the anesthesiologist.

Blood Flow

Logic dictates that ischemic nerves do not function normally; therefore measurable neural potentials would become abnormal. In fact it has been demonstrated that somatosensory evoked potentials (SEPs) can be lost when cerebral blood flow falls below 15 mL/min/100 g (2). This can be assumed to be true for the spinal cord and peripheral nerves as well. Unfortunately, it is difficult to actually measure blood flow to any given structure, so systemic blood pressure is often used as a surrogate. Furthermore, systemic blood flow does not necessarily dictate regional blood flow, especially in the brain, which makes it even more difficult to predict. Monitors are becoming available that purport to quantify regional blood flow (e.g., cerebral oximetry, microdialysis), but a discussion of these is beyond the scope of this chapter. Essentially then, there are two main considerations for the neurophysiologist: systemic hypotension and decreased regional blood flow. When profound, systemic hypotension results in globally reduced blood flow, which translates into tissue ischemia of varying degrees based largely on autoregulation. For example, during spinal surgery, controlled deliberate hypotension is often requested of the anesthesiologist so as to assist in controlling blood loss; however, surgical traction and hypotension can aggravate each other with deleterious effects to the patient, and NIOM can assist in determining the acceptable limit of systemic hypotension (4). There are many examples of causes of decreased regional blood flow, and almost all are due to some interruption in blood supply either due to compression from surgical instruments (intentionally or unintentionally), patient positioning, tourniquets, vasospasm, vascular ligation, etc. Anecdotally, some have reported discovering incidental ulnar nerve ischemia secondary to compression during routine monitoring for spinal fusion. When the compression was released, the nerve potentials returned to normal.

Ventilation

Optimal neural functioning depends on maintenance of a homeostatic extracellular environment. Hypo- or hypercapnea can alter cellular metabolism by changing the acid-base status of the individual. In general individuals tolerate relatively profound acid-base derangements, especially upward trends in pH. Unless the pH of a patient drops below 7.2, neuronal mechanisms are maintained. Additionally, there is a suggestion that extremes in hypocarbia (< 20 mmHg partial pressure) can alter SEP monitoring (5). Alternatively, profound hypoxia is poorly tolerated, especially in the surgical setting of ongoing blood loss and potential hypotension.

Hematology

Like hypoxia, profound anemia can contribute to neural dysfunction. Normally, anemia is well tolerated to levels of hemoglobin less than 7 g/dL. However, in the surgical setting of possible large volume blood loss, hypotension, and hypoxia, it is generally accepted that hemoglobin levels should be kept above 8 g/dL and may require optimizing at 10 g/dL. At approximately 10 g/dL of hemoglobin, oxygen delivery appears to be maximized and transfusion above this threshold does not appear to improve augmentation. There are animal data that support this supposition in SEP monitoring (6).

Intracranial Pressure

Increase in intracranial pressure is a relatively well documented cause of shifts in cortical responses of EPs and prolongation of motor evoked potentials (MEPs), presumably due to compression of cortical structures. There is a pressure-related increase in latency and decrease in amplitude of cortical SEPs and as intracranial pressure becomes pathologic, uncal herniation occurs with subsequent loss of subcortical SEP responses and brainstem auditory evoked potentials (BAEPs) (7). Alleviation of this pressure can return EPs to normal.

Other Factors

Neuronal function depends on maintenance of a homeostatic intra- and extracellular environment determined by potassium, calcium, and sodium concentrations. It is logical to assume that alteration in these concentrations would result in dysfunction and possible changes in measurable neuronal potentials. The concentration of these ions is largely in the control of the anesthesiologist, and maintenance within ranges of normal values is necessary. In addition, profound hyper- or hypoglycemia should be avoided, as either extreme can result in cellular dysfunction; although there is no evidence that they result in intraoperative changes in NIOM, there are data to suggest that both can lead to poor outcomes (8).

EFFECTS OF SPECIFIC ANESTHETIC AGENTS

In general the anesthesiologist and neurophysiologist are constantly at odds in that nearly all anesthetic agents, given in high enough doses, cause depression of NIOM potentials. However, with open communication and mutual understanding of each other's activities, NIOM can be successful with nearly any anesthetic technique. The crucial concept is that any change in either anesthetic or NIOM must be communicated to the team, so that every person in the operating room is acting under appropriate assumptions.

Inhalation Agents

Despite being the oldest form of anesthesia, the exact mechanism of action of inhalation agents remains unclear. Inhalation anesthetics consist of two basic gases available in the United States: halogenated agents (halothane, isoflurane, sevoflurane, desflurane) and nitrous oxide. Doses of gas are given as percentage of inhaled mixture, and effective doses are expressed as some amount of MAC. As discussed before, one MAC of an agent is sufficient to prevent 50% of patients from moving to the stimulation of surgical incision (Tables 4.1 and 4.2).

TABLE 4.1 Effects of Inhaled Agents on Evoked Potentials

	BAEP		SEP		MEP	
Agents	Latency	Amplitude	Latency	Amplitude	Latency	Amplitude
Desflurane	Inc	0	Inc	Dec	Inc	Dec
Enflurane	Inc	0	Inc	Inc	Inc	Dec
Halothane	Inc	0	Inc	Dec	Inc	Dec
Isoflurane	Inc	0	Inc	Dec	Inc	Dec
Sevoflurane	Inc	0	Inc	Dec	Inc	Dec
Nitrous oxide	0	Dec	0	Dec	Inc	Dec

Inc = increased; Dec = decreased; 0 = no change.

TABLE 4.2 Effects of Anesthetics Agents on Electroencephalogram

INCREASED FREQUENCY	SUPPRESSED
Barbiturate (low dose)	Barbiturates (high dose)
Benzodiazepine	Propofol (high dose)
Etomidate	Benzodiazepine (high dose)
Propofol	
Ketamine	
Halogenated agents (< 1 MAC)	

INCREASED AMPLITUDE	ELECTROCEREBRAL SILENCE
Barbiturate (moderate dose)	Barbiturates
Etomidate	Propofol
Opioid	Etomidate
Halogenated agents (1–2 MAC)	Halogenated agents (> 2 MAC except halothane)

Inc = increased; Dec = decreased; 0 = no change.

Halogenated Agents

The halogenated agents consist of the historic agent halothane, which is still used in most countries outside the United States, and the modern agents consisting of isoflurane, sevoflurane, and desflurane. Each has its own MAC, onset and offset times, and metabolism based on the inherent properties of the gas. Their use results in a dose-related decrease in amplitude and slowing of latency of SEPs, with the least effect seen in peripheral and subcortical responses (2). BAEPs are minimally affected by halogenated anesthetics at usual doses but can be ablated at high doses.

MEPs are enormously affected by the use of halogenated agents and can be entirely ablated even with doses of 0.5 MAC. It appears that this effect occurs proximal to the anterior horn cell due to evidence that waves recorded distal to the anterior horn cell and proximal to the neuromuscular junction remain recordable even at high doses of anesthetic (9). MEP monitoring may also occur through spinal or epidural stimulation with minimal effect on recorded responses; however, cord stimulation results in stimulation of the sensory and motor pathways, and halogenated gases preferentially block the motor responses (10). Therefore it is important to remember that NIOM utilizing spinal cord stimulation may not reliably monitor motor function in the presence of halogenated gases. For this and reasons mentioned above—namely, easy ablation when MEP monitoring is essential—halogenated gases should usually not be part of the anesthetic regimen when using this modality.

The EEG is affected but usually without hindrance to monitoring. All halogenated anesthetics produce a frontal shift of the rhythm predominance when used at induction doses (two to three times MAC doses). The gases then produce a dose-dependent reduction in frequency and amplitude. It is important to note that both isoflurane and desflurane can produce burst suppression and electrocerebral silence at clinical doses. For practical purposes, however, all halogenated agents can be used for maintenance anesthesia when NIOM requires EEG monitoring.

Nitrous Oxide

Nitrous oxide is similar to halogenated anesthetic agents and causes a dose-related decrease in amplitude and prolongation of latency of cortical SEPs and ablation of MEPs. This effect seems somewhat limited in subcortical and peripheral potentials of the SEPs. At equipotent doses to halogenated agents, nitrous oxide may, in fact, cause greater EP depression (2). Additionally, nitrous oxide has somewhat indeterminate effects on the EEG that is highly dependent on other agents and doses being used simultaneously. The effects on the EEG are not wholly predictable, but generally, there is frontally dominant high-frequency activity and posterior slowing. Despite this, a frequent anesthetic technique used during NIOM is a "nitrous-narcotic" technique. The modern version of this technique consists of a high-dose remifentanil infusion (0.2 to 0.5 µg/kg/min) with 60% to 70% inhaled fraction of nitrous oxide. A high, but constant, amount of nitrous oxide is delivered with varying amounts of remifentanil based on surgical stimulation. As long as the percentage of inhaled nitrous oxide is held constant, this practice generally allows recordable responses for most NIOM except transcranial MEPs, although even then 50% to 60% nitrous oxide may be used. The benefit of using nitrous oxide is that brain concentrations vary rapidly with inhaled concentrations, so that if NIOM is problematic and needs maximizing intraoperatively, discontinuance of nitrous oxide will quickly result in the its elimination from the brain and body.

Intravenous Agents

Intravenous anesthetic agents are generally used to induce anesthesia and afterwards to supplement inhalation maintenance anesthesia. Most modern anesthetic techniques consist of a variety of agents, intravenous and inhaled; nearly always an intravenous opioid is administered to augment other agents for either tracheal intubation at induction or intense surgical stimulation exceeding a stable maintenance anesthesia. If halogenated agents are contraindicated or NIOM becomes problematic with their use, a complete anesthetic can consist of intravenous drugs, or total intravenous anesthesia (TIVA). TIVA exists in many forms. The most common regimen is based on continuous propofol infusion and supplementation with intravenous opioid. However, all manner of TIVAs have been described, including the use of ketamine, barbiturate, midazolam, dexmedetomidine, etc., with drug selection depending on utilizing specific attributes of an agent to effect a specific outcome (Tables 4.2 and 4.3).

TABLE 4.3 Effects of Intravenous Agents on Evoked Potentials

	BAEP		SEP		MEP	
Agents	Latency	Amplitude	Latency	Amplitude	Latency	Amplitude
Barbiturate						
Low dose	0	0	0	0	Inc	Dec
High dose	Inc	Dec	Inc	Dec	Inc	Dec
Benzodiazepine	0	0	Inc	Dec	Inc	Dec
Opioid	0	0	Inc	Dec	0	0
Etomidate	0	0	Inc	Inc	0	0
Propofol	Inc	0	Inc	Dec	Inc	Dec
Ketamine	Inc	0	Inc	Inc	0	0

Inc = increased; Dec = decreased; 0 = no change.

Barbiturates

Some of the oldest intravenous anesthetics include barbiturates (e.g., thiopental, pentobarbital, phenobarbital, methohexital). These drugs exist in alkaline salt solution and exert their mechanism of action at the GABA$_A$ receptor. Of these, thiopental remains in common use, in certain surgical cases, as an induction agent and as a means of achieving neuroprotection through "burst suppression." Additionally, methohexital is frequently used to facilitate electroconvulsive therapy (ECT). However, much like halogenated agents, barbiturates will produce EEG slowing and, at higher doses, burst suppression and electrocerebral silence. There appears to be little class effect of barbiturates on SEPs, with each agent producing somewhat different results. Thiopental produces transient decreases in amplitude and increases in latency with bolus dosing for induction, but phenobarbital produces little effect until doses causing cardiovascular collapse are reached (11). As with inhaled agents, SEP cortical potentials seemed to be most affected, with relative sparing of subcortical and peripheral responses. In contrast, whether with low-dose continuous infusion or single-bolus dosing, MEP responses can be entirely abolished with the use of barbiturates. Any anesthetic given for a surgical procedure requiring MEP monitoring should exclude the use of barbiturates in any form unless their use (i.e., neuroprotection) supersedes the benefit from MEP monitoring.

Benzodiazepines

Midazolam is a common intravenous benzodiazepine used in preoperative areas prior to transfer to the operating suite. Benzodiazepines also have their site of action at the GABA receptor and have the desirable effects of amnesia, sedation, and anxiolysis. In general, single one-time doses of midazolam given prior to induction have little effect on NIOM during critical portions of the procedure. However, induction doses of midazolam (0.2 mg/kg) or continuous infusions of the drug can slow SEP latencies and decrease amplitudes (12). Furthermore, as with most other anesthetics, even small doses of benzodiazepines (1 to 2 mg) can lead to a marked reduction in MEP responses. However, owing to relatively rapid metabolism of single adminstration, if small doses of midazolam are given preoperatively, their effects on NIOM are usually minimal. Of note, benzodiazepines are anticonvulsants and will all produce slowing of the EEG into the theta range; however, at small doses they create beta-rhythm predominance in frontal leads, which is also seen with chronic oral administration.

Propofol

Propofol remains one of the most common agents used for the induction of anesthesia and is the most common agent used for maintenance anesthesia during TIVA. It is packaged in a lipid-soluble solution and its site of action is also at the GABA receptor. Owing to rapid redistribution after dosing, propofol is easily titratable to the desired effect, which makes it very useful for TIVA techniques. Induction doses of propofol (2 to 5 mg/kg) cause amplitude depression of EEG, SEP, and MEP responses, as does high-dose continuous infusion (80 to 100 µg/kg/min). However, there is generally rapid recovery after termination if long infusion times (>8 hours) are avoided (13). In recording SEPs or MEPs from the epidural space, there seems to be limited effect of the drug on the EPs; this seems to hold true for recordings from the scalp or peripheral muscle as well (14). Propofol is also notable as an agent that can produce burst suppression and electrocerebral silence on the EEG. Despite profound EEG suppression at high dose, propofol retains its relatively quick termination, allowing for an awake, alert, and neurologically testable patient at the end of a surgical procedure.

Opioids

Intravenous opioids represent a critical mainstay in the practice of modern "balanced" anesthesia to control perioperative pain. Nearly all general anesthetics will have some form and dose of intravenous opioid as a central component. Intravenous opioids in current use during the perioperative period include morphine, hydromorphone, fentanyl, alfentanil, sufentanil, and remifentanil; they are administered for various indications and at a wide variation in dosing regimens. All intravenous opioids have almost no effect on NIOM even at very high doses, making them of essential importance during anesthesia for procedures requiring NIOM. Even when given in the epidural or intrathecal space, they have minimal effect on EPs (2). It has been noted that generous application of opioids can result in improved MEP monitoring owing to the reduction of spontaneous muscle contraction and lowering of the MAC for other anesthetic agents. With regards to the EEG, opioids produce a mild slowing into the delta range without effect on amplitude. Opioids will not produce burst suppression or an isoelectric EEG even at the highest doses. Of particular importance, the development of remifentanil has revolutionized opioid use in TIVA. Remifentanil is an ultra-short-acting opioid with a half-life on the order of 5 minutes regardless of dose. This allows for very rapid titration of analgesia with little or no effect on emergence times, thus permitting high-dose opioid TIVA to minimize the dose of an associated sedative-hypnotic.

Ketamine

Ketamine is one of the older anesthetic agents and has undergone a recent resurgence of use owing to the finding that it helps to alleviate postoperative pain and chronic pain states. Ketamine influences a variety of receptors and has the unique characteristic among anesthetic agents of enhancing EP responses, especially in the cortex and spinal cord (15). Whether given as single bolus at induction or as continuous infusion, ketamine can increase EP amplitude in SEP, MEP, and BAEP recording, making it an attractive agent for use during NIOM. Additionally, the use of ketamine can produce larger amplitudes, with mild slowing into the theta range on the EEG, and there is anecdotal evidence that ketamine may be proconvulsant. The downside to ketamine use (and the reason ketamine fell out of favor prior to the last 5 years) is the occurrence of emergence delirium and dissociative hallucinations. Additionally, increase in intracranial pressure from enhanced cerebral blood flow due to ketamine makes it of limited use in neurosurgical patients with intracranial hypertension as well as in some other patient populations. Ketamine has been found particularly useful as a low-dose infusion (10 to 20 µg/kg/min) to supplement a propofol/opioid TIVA technique in procedures that require anesthetic-sensitive NIOM (e.g., MEP). The addition of low-dose ketamine to a propofol-based TIVA allows for a substantial reduction in propofol infusion doses and enhancement of EP responses while minimizing the undesirable side effects of ketamine. For procedures requiring NIOM techniques that are highly sensitive to the effects of anesthetics (e.g., transcranial MEP), the use of ketamine in the anesthetic armamentarium should be considered.

Etomidate

Etomidate represents another contradiction to the general rule that anesthetic agents cause EP depression. Induction doses and continuous intravenous infusion enhance both MEP and SEP recordings (16). Etomidate has been used in the past as a component of TIVA during procedures that require anesthetic-sensitive NIOM (e.g., transcranial MEPs). Etomidate is also somewhat contradictory in its EEG effects; at low doses it may be somewhat proconvulsant, and it is occasionally used for ECT or epilepsy surgery; although at higher doses it may produce burst suppression. However, among its many unpleasant side effects, concerns have been raised regarding etomidate-induced adrenal suppression, which can occur with even single-bolus induction doses (0.2 to 0.5 mg/kg). Increased mortality has been seen with prolonged infusion of etomidate, mainly in the intensive care setting (17). Nevertheless, etomidate remains valuable in cases where NIOM responses are difficult to obtain and otherwise may not be recordable.

Dexmedetomidine

Dexmedetomidine is a relatively new agent used in human anesthesia. This selective alpha-2 agonist has seen widespread use in veterinary medicine and has found its way into intensive care units and operating rooms because of its desirable effects of sedation, analgesia, and sympatholysis without respiratory depression. Though increasing ancedotal reports are emerging, there are limited data on the effects of dexmedetomidine on NIOM; however, animal data suggest that there is little effect (18). It may be used as a low-dose infusion (0.2 to 0.5 µg/kg/hr) to augment any anesthetic technique, and it allows for the use of considerably less volatile or intravenous anesthesia or opioid. Its definitive role in anesthetic techniques for highly sensitive NIOM remains to be determined.

Paralytics

Neuromuscular blockers exert their effect by blocking acetylcholine at the nicotinic receptor in the neuromuscular junction. They have no effect on monitoring modalities that are not derived from muscle activity (e.g., EEG, BAEPs, and SEPs). They will completely negate MEP monitoring if intense neuromuscular blockade is utilized. However, employing partial blockade will allow substantial reduction in patient movement with testing, improved surgical retraction, and favorable MEP monitoring. There are many ways to monitor the amount of neuromuscular blockade; the most common is the "train of four" (TOF) technique. It consists of measuring muscle responses, or compound muscle action potentials, after four 2-Hz peripheral nerve stimuli. MEP monitoring is acceptable when neuromuscular blockade is maintained at a TOF of two responses. In using MEP monitoring, it is important for the neurophysiologist and surgeon to know whether the patient is paralyzed. If the patient is not paralyzed, MEP stimulation must be done at times when patient movement is acceptable. If the patient is paralyzed, there are likely to be brief periods when MEP responses are not recordable owing to intense paralysis; it is then imperative to communicate when a neuromuscular blocking agent is redosed. However, either practice, paralysis or not, is acceptable; the main principle is, again, effective and open communication with all parties in the surgical suite.

ANESTHETIC TECHNIQUES

A variety of anesthetic techniques are acceptable for use during NIOM; the type of anesthetic should be tailored to the type of NIOM and the requirements of the surgical procedure. There are, however, a few general principles. First, the least amount of anesthetic agent necessary should be utilized as long as there is little possibility of awareness or discomfort on the part of the patient. The liberal use of opioids can allow for a significant decrement in MAC. Second, the more stable an anesthetic dose can remain for the duration of the case, the less likely that the anesthetic agent might be contributing to intraoperative changes in NIOM waveforms. Supplementation of baseline anesthetic drugs with opioids or less NIOM-offending agents can be made at times of more intense surgical stimulation. Overall, there are essentially four classes of NIOM based on how easily the monitoring technique is ablated by anesthetic agents. As the relative sensitivity of NIOM to anesthesia increases, the anesthetic technique should be adjusted to maximize the least offending agents. Each group and its anesthetic implications are discussed below.

Relative Insensitivity

NIOM that is relatively insensitive to anesthetic agents in general includes BAEPs and SEPs recorded from the epidural space. With these monitoring methods, nearly all anesthetic practices can be used with the understanding that the general objective is to maintain a constant level of anesthesia supplemented with intermittent opioid dosing to control increased surgical stimulus. Of course the least amount of anesthetic necessary to ensure amnesia and analgesia should be used. Generally all patients have baseline EPs, so that once in the operating room, deviation from that baseline can be assessed. If needed, anesthetic level or technique can then be adjusted to refine NIOM recordings.

Sensitivity to Paralytics

Forms of NIOM that are sensitive to neuromuscular blockade include all monitoring that requires elicitation of muscle action potentials (i.e., electromyography, MEP, spinal reflex testing, etc.). For these cases, if very fine control of the amount of neuromuscular blockade can be maintained through vigilant monitoring and drug dosing, neuromuscular blocking agents can be employed. Otherwise they should be entirely avoided once the patient has been intubated. In fact, there are some practices that utilize intraoperative neuromuscular blockade reversal when critical monitoring periods approach. In general, with the exception of MEP recording, which is exquisitely sensitive to anesthetic technique, other forms of anesthetic agents are acceptable. For cases that rely on an unparalyzed patient, relatively "deep" anesthesia (e.g., high doses of anesthetic agents) can be used to offset lack of patient paralysis, allowing optimal surgical conditions of immobility and relaxation while maintaining the integrity of NIOM. However, the general principle of stable, though relatively high, anesthetic dose should be maintained.

Sensitivity to Anesthetics without Sensitivity to Paralysis

NIOM that is not negated by neuromuscular blockade but is sensitive to anesthetic agents includes SEP monitoring. Care must be taken to minimize offending anesthetic agents and optimize non-anesthetic variables (i.e., temperature). Generally, volatile or intravenous anesthesia is acceptable if relatively low doses are maintained (0.5 MAC for anesthetic gases or less than 80 µg/kg/min of propofol). The use of neuromuscular blockade in this situation allows for a modest decrement in anesthetic dose, as patient movement and relaxation then become improbable. However, care must be taken that anesthetic dose is not so low as to permit patient recall or discomfort.

Relative Sensitivity

The need for MEP monitoring can initiate some of the more challenging anesthetic issues. Designing an anesthetic technique to optimize MEP monitoring adds to an already complex surgical procedure. A TIVA technique that limits the amount of sedative-hypnotic agent (i.e., propofol, barbiturate) is usually required. Limiting the dose of sedative-hypnotic to allow for optimal response recording of NIOM requires the use of a second agent, usually opioid, to supplement and augment the anesthetic properties. For instance, using a propofol-based anesthetic requires the addition of opioid, ketamine, or dexmedetomidine infusion to allow a much smaller dose of propofol to be administered. Additionally, if neuromuscular blockade is used, it must be tightly controlled so that profound paralysis does not preclude MEP responses from the muscles. It is not uncommon for the patient to be unparalyzed during critical monitoring portions of the procedure. Therefore the anesthesiologist is often faced with an unparalyzed patient, whose monitoring requires relatively low doses of an anesthetic, and whose airway and accessibility is often remote. One current practice is to utilize high-dose remifentanil infusion to supplement a low-dose propofol-ketamine based anesthetic. This allows very low dose propofol (20 to 30 µg/kg/min), which has minimal effects on MEP responses, to be offset by low-dose ketamine (10 to 20 µg/kg/min), which enhances MEP responses, and an amount of remifentanil that keeps the patient motionless and relaxed.

CONCLUSIONS

In developing an anesthetic plan, the type of NIOM is often as important a consideration as the type of surgical procedure. The crucial factor for a successful procedure is open and candid communication between the operating room staff, neurophysiologist, anesthesiologist, and surgeon. The majority of problems with intraoperative monitoring arise when operating room communication does not allow for each individual to have a clear understanding of the actions of each of the other members. When everyone involved in the procedure is knowledgeable about reasonable expectations and aware of the current situation, the patient benefits from an operating team that is poised and fluid in its execution. With that understanding, it is imperative for the neurophysiologist to understand the limitations produced by an anesthetic and for the anesthesiologist to understand the effects of certain medications on monitoring. Without that fundamental knowledge, there can be little coordinated activity between the two parties, resulting in ineffective monitoring. However, with the knowledge of the basic effect of a given anesthetic agent on monitoring modalities, nearly any anesthetic technique can be administered safely and effectively with all types of monitoring.

REFERENCES

1. James ML, Husain AM. Brainstem auditory evoked potential monitoring: when is change in wave V significant? *Neurology* 2005;65: 1551–1555.
2. Sloan TB. Evoked potentials In: Albin MS, ed. *A Textbook of Neuroanesthesia with Neurosurgical and Neuroscience Perspectives*. New York: McGraw-Hill, 1997:221–276.
3. Stekker MM, Escherich A, Patterson T, et al. Effects of acute hypoxemia/ischemia on EEG and evoked responses at normothermia and hypothermia in humans. *Med Sci Monit* 2002;8:CR223–CR228.
4. Dolan EJ, Transfeldt EE, Tator CH, et al. The effect of spinal distraction on regional spinal cord blood flow in cats. *J Neurosurg* 1980;53: 756–764.
5. Grundy BL, Heros RC, Tung AS, et al. Intraoperative hypoxia detected by evoked potential monitoring. *Anesth Analg* 1981;60: 437–439.
6. Nagoa S, Roccaforte P, Moody RA. The effects of isovolemic hemodilution and reinfusion of packed erythrocytes on somatosensory and visual evoked potentials. *J Surg Res* 1978; 25:530–537.
7. Mackey JR, Hall JW III. Sensory evoked responses in head injury. *Central Nerv Syst Trauma* 1985;2:187–206.
8. McGirt MJ, Woodworth GF, Brooke BS, et al. Hyperglycemia independently increases the risk of perioperative stroke, myocardial infarction, and death after carotid endarterectomy. *Neurosurgery* 2006;58:1066–1073.
9. Gugino LD, Aglio LS, Segal NE, et al. Use of transcranial magnetic stimulation for monitoring spinal cord motor paths. *Semin Spine Surg* 1997;9:315–336.
10. Deletis V. Intraoperative monitoring of the functional integrity of the motor pathways. *Adv Neurol* 1993;63:201–214.
11. Drummond JC, Todd MM, U HS. The effects of high dose sodium thiopental on brainstem auditory and median nerve somatosensory evoked responses in humans. *Anesthesiology* 1985;63:249–254.
12. Sloan TB, Fugina ML, Toleikis JR. Effects of midazolam on median nerve somatosensory evoked potentials. *Br J Anaesth* 1990;64: 590–593.
13. Kalkman CJ, Drummond JC, Ribberrink AA. Effects of propofol, etomidate, midazolam,

and fentanyl on motor evoked responsesto transcranial electrical or magnetic stimulation in humans. *Anesthesiology* 1992;76:502–509.
14. Angel BA, LeBeau F. A comparison of the effects of propofol with other anesthetic agents on the centripetal transmission of sensory information. *Gen Pharmacol* 1992;23: 945–063.
15. Schubert A, Licina MG, Lineberry PJ. The effect of ketamine on human somatosensory evoked potentials after high frequency repetitive electrical stimulation. *Electroencephalogr Clin Neurophysiol* 1998;108:175–181.
16. Kochs E, Treede RD, Schulte AM, Esch J. Increase in somatosensory evoked potentials during induction of anaesthesia with etomidate. *Anaesthetist* 1986;35:359–364.
17. Ledingham IM, Watt I. Influence of sedation on mortality in critically ill multiple trauma patients. *Lancet* 1983;1:1270.
18. Li BH, Lohmann JS, Schuler HG, Cronin AJ. Preservation of the cortical somatosensory-evoked potential during dexmedetomidine infusion in rates. *Anesth Analg* 2003;96: 1150–1160.

5 Billing, Ethical, and Legal Issues*

Marc R. Nuwer

Professional administrative policies and procedures assure patient safety, efficient organization, and clear communication. Well-defined policies discourage self-interested motives and clarify limits. Public policies on health care include laws and regulations about billing, coding, reimbursement, staffing, devices, and liability, among others topics.

This chapter describes some public policy issues that apply to neurophysiologic intraoperative monitoring (NIOM). Issues pertaining to billing apply specifically to the United States. Other ethical and legal issues are general principles and applicable to NIOM wherever monitoring is conducted. Of course, in some legal jurisdictions, other locally specific laws and regulations may apply too.

CODING AND BILLING

These coding and billing rules apply to the United States. This coding system specifies the particular work conducted on a particular patient. In the U.S. medical reimbursement system, these codes allow for reimbursement proportional to the time, effort, equipment, supplies, and risk involved in a procedure. Each specific procedure has its own code number, assigned in the American Medical Association's Current Procedural Coding (CPT).

CPT specifies more than 7,500 medical, surgical, and diagnostic procedures. Cost accounting for each CPT code is determined by the typical work, equipment, supplies, etc., involved in carrying out that procedure. These costs are systematically summarized in the Resource Based Relative Value System (RBRVS), which is used to set the Relative Value Units (RVU) for each CPT. Most U.S. healthcare insurance carriers use RVUs for payment. Other organizations use physician work RVUs to judge the annual work productivity of group physicians.

CPT codes used for most NIOM are presented in Table 5.1. The vast majority of cases use the hourly NIOM code CPT 95920. Other specialty codes are used for certain electroencephalograms (EEG) and functional mapping procedures. The codes also allow for a systematic set of additional policies. The most relevant ones are those that specify the degree of supervision required for each type of procedure.

---
* This chapter is based in part on Nuwer MR. Regulatory and medical-legal aspects of intraoperative monitoring. *J Clin Neurophysiol* 2002;19:387–395.

TABLE 5.1 Intraoperative Neurophysiology CPT Codes

95920	Intraoperative neurophysiology testing, per hour
95829	Electrocorticogram at surgery
95955	Electroencephalogram during nonintracranial surgery (e.g., carotid surgery)
95961	Functional cortical and subcortical mapping by stimulation and/or recording of electrodes on brain surface, or of depth electrodes, to provoke seizures or identify vital brain structures
	Initial hour of physician attendance
95962	Each additional hour of physician attendance

Code 95920 (Intraoperative Neurophysiology Testing)

This code is billed once for each hour of routine NIOM. Time begins when the physician is called to the operating room and ends when he or she leaves. However, the time taken to interpret the baseline testing for each primary base procedure is excluded, since those are billed separately. Time is rounded to the nearest hour. For remote on-line monitoring, the code is used for each hour monitored.

Supervision rules require direct supervision, which may be done remotely online. Direct supervision ordinarily requires the clinical neurophysiologist to be present nearby in the building, readily available to come into the surgery suite on short notice when a problem or need arises. Remote on-line monitoring allows for the equivalent done at a distance, with available interaction by phone or instant messaging. In either case, the clinical neurophysiologist still must be available to respond on short notice if problems occur.

Code 95920 is used along with base codes that specify what modalities were monitored or tested. The base (primary) procedures codes are billed once per procedure. The allowable base procedure codes for code 95920 are listed in Table 5.2. Only these base codes are allowed. At least one must be used for any procedure when code 95920 is used. More than one code may be used when more than one modality is monitored. For example, monitoring resection of an acoustic neuroma may include upper extremity somatosensory evoked potentials, facial nerve electromyography (EMG), and brainstem auditory evoked potentials. Those base codes are 95925, 95868, and 92585, and they are coded with one unit of service each. Code 95920 is billed one unit of service for each monitoring hour

TABLE 5.2 Primary Procedures Allowed as Base Codes for Code 95920

92585	Auditory evoked potential
95822	EEG recording in coma or sleep
95860	Needle EMG
	One extremity
95861	Two extremities
95867	Cranial nerve muscles, unilateral
95868	Cranial nerve muscles, bilateral
95970	Limited
95900	Nerve conduction study, each nerve
	Motor
95904	Sensory
95925	Somatosensory evoked potential
	In upper limbs
95926	In lower limbs
95927	In trunk or head
95928	Central motor evoked potential
	In upper limbs
95929	In lower limbs
95930	Visual evoked potential
95933	Blink reflex
95934	H reflex
	Gastrocnemius/soleus muscle
95936	Muscle other than gastrocnemius/soleus muscle
95937	Neuromuscular junction testing (repetitive nerve stimulation)

after excluding the time taken to interpret the baseline portions of each monitoring modality.

Other procedures can be performed on the same day. For example, laryngeal EMG is coded as CPT 95865. Although it is not a base code for 95920, it can also be coded in addition to other codes if laryngeal EMG was monitored.

Code 95829 (Electrocorticography)

Code 95829 is used for electrocorticography (ECoG). The intraoperative evaluation and medical decisions during an ECoG go well beyond simple monitoring. Code 95920 is used generally to screen for any changes compared to baseline where changes lead to raising an alarm. By contrast, in ECoG, the physician identifies regions to be removed and to be left intact during cortical resections. The difference between monitoring (95920) and deciding what to remove (ECoG) justifies a separate procedure code. Because this procedure requires medical decision making of a high degree, this code and service require the personal supervision of the physician in the operating room.

Code 95955 (Nonintracranial EEG)

For historical reasons, intraoperative EEG during nonintracranial surgery has its own code, 95955. This can be used for EEG during carotid endarterectomy or cardiothoracic surgery. Traditionally this was a "general supervision" service. In that traditional supervision system, an advanced or specialized technologist conducted the EEG monitoring without immediate physician supervision.

When a physician provides a greater degree of supervision throughout the procedure, code 95920 can be used, together with the base procedure code 95822 for intraoperative EEG monitoring. The difference between 95955 and 95920 is the degree of supervision.

Codes 95961 and 95962 (Cortical and Subcortical Localization)

Codes 95961 and 95962 are used when localizing cortical or hemispheric function. This can be localizing motor or language cortex or when placing deep brain stimulator (DBS) electrodes. Code 95961 is used for the first hour. Code 95962 is used for each additional hour. These same codes are used for testing cortical functions in monitoring epilepsy patients with subdural grids. In the operating room, these codes are used in identifying language regions with direct cortical stimulation in an awake patient during a craniotomy.

Codes 95970 to 95979 (Neurostimulator Programming and Analysis)

Neurostimulator programming and analysis use the same codes, 95970 to 95979, inside and outside the operating room. The several neurostimulator codes are listed in Table 5.3. The codes come in simple and complex types. A *simple* neurostimulator pulse generator/transmitter has three or fewer adjustable parameters. A *complex* neurostimulator pulse generator/transmitter is one capable of affecting more than three of the above. Modern DBS systems involve the complex codes. Code 95970 is used when one is just checking the integrity of an implanted neurostimulator without programming it. For DBS brain programming, code 95978 should be used for the first hour and 95979 for each additional 30 minutes. For vagus nerve stimulator programming, code 95974 should be used for the first hour and 95975 for each additional 30 minutes.

In some surgical DBS placements, codes 95961 to 95962 are used to identify the correct locations for the electrodes. Then, the 95870 code is used to assure that the DBS stimulating device is working properly.

TABLE 5.3 Neurostimulator CPT Codes

95970	Implanted neurostimulator analysis
95971	Simple neurostimulator programming
95974	Complex cranial nerve neurostimulator programming
	First hour
95975	Each additional 30 minutes
95978	Complex brain stimulator programming
	First hour
95979	Each additional 30 minutes

STAFFING

Most states and hospitals require a licensed physician to supervise each technologist. Such public policies limit the practice of nonphysician healthcare providers.

Interpreter Staffing

A technologist cannot provide NIOM without any supervision. Many lack the suitable skills, knowledge, ability, training, and experience to provide interpretations and respond to the more challenging moments of monitoring. Many technologists have insufficient medical knowledge to advise the surgeon on the medical meaning of signal changes. Based on such limitations, most hospitals and states require physician supervision.

Surgeons generally cannot supervise the technologist for NIOM. Most surgeons lack suitable skills, knowledge, abilities, training, and experience in clinical neurophysiology to assure high-quality monitoring services, which can lead to mistaken interpretations. They lack an understanding of the technical procedures involved, normal variations and peak identification procedures, artifacts and other technical problems, and the meaning of changes when they occur. The National Correct Coding Initiative (NCCI) precludes billing for both the surgery and the NIOM by the same physician.

A monitoring physician must be available to intervene as needed when problems arise in any case. The monitoring physician also must be able to pay close attention to the individual cases when monitoring simultaneous procedures. For those reasons a limit of three simultaneous cases per monitoring physician is recommended (1).

A nonphysician healthcare provider sometimes does supervise intraoperative monitoring technologists. Any provider must have advanced skills, knowledge, ability, and training, as well as extensive experience to assure quality services and patients' safety. Measuring that can be difficult. The judgment must be made by reasonably independent observers and based upon objective guidelines and standards. There is in place a professional process for assessing physicians' credentials for hospital privileging. These processes can serve as a model or outline of processes to assess nonphysician providers.

Each hospital's medical staff office must assure that each professional meets appropriate standards to practice in that facility. Privileging determines whether an individual practitioner at a given institution should be allowed to practice and for what procedures. The institution checks for medical board and DEA certification, professional disciplinary actions, licensure, training, experience, proof of insurance, malpractice claims, and criminal convictions. Individual proctoring checks that actual practice performance currently meets local community standards. Credentialing evaluates an individual's specific fields of practice and particular techniques for which he or she should be allowed to practice at the institution in question. This examination must be conducted even more thoroughly for any nonphysician than for a physician because there is no state licensure agency also overseeing such practitioners.

Technologist Staffing

Not all technologists are suitable for NIOM. Registration by the American Board of Electroencephalographic and Evoked Potentials

Technologists (ABRET) as an R. EEG T. (registered EEG technologist), R. EP T. (registered evoked potential technologist), and Certificate in Neurophysiologic Intraoperative Monitoring (CNIM) provides one type of check on an individual's NIOM knowledge. More is needed.

Hospitals' neurodiagnostics departments should evaluate each technologist for the his or her skills, knowledge, abilities, training, and experience relevant to NIOM. The lab medical director should establish suitable policies and procedures. Each technologist should be privileged to perform just the NIOM procedures for which he or she is suitably trained. A technologist well skilled in one type of procedure is not necessarily qualified to conduct all types of procedures. Privileging should be subject to annual review and renewal. For example, NIOM without immediate supervision might be restricted to technologists with 3 to 5 years of experience with that technique outside the operating room. An extended period of proctoring would involve a period of immediate supervision followed by a period with less supervision until the individual becomes fully qualified.

Some procedures require a physician to be in the room. These include ECoG, functional cortical localization, and other testing for deliberate decisions about what to resect or spare. A technologist can conduct more routine monitoring without supervisory backup in the room. A physician is commonly available on-line (2). Typically, monitoring technologists are given specific policies and procedures outlining their responsibilities for specific kinds of monitoring services. These policies and procedures can script the specific instances in which the technologist is expected to report adverse changes to the surgical team or to physician or supervisory backup.

MEDICAL-LEGAL ISSUES

Lawsuits can occur after any surgical procedure, even if the monitoring community's practice standards were met. Monitoring does not necessarily eliminate adverse neurologic events; it just reduces their incidence (3).

Yet errors do occur in medical or surgical care. The Institute of Medicine reported that between 48,000 and 98,000 Americans die each year after incidents associated with medical errors (4). Such errors include prescribing or dispensing the wrong medication. Many other problems occur too.

Intraoperative monitoring is a situation where one can encounter communications errors. The NIOM team needs to keep the surgeon aware of the state of nervous system monitoring. In turn, the surgeon needs to know the role of monitoring and realize the possibility of neurologic injury despite monitoring.

Monitoring should be conducted by well-trained staff. Recording quality must be maintained. When quality is poor or results become irreproducible, the surgeon should be told that the monitoring cannot be trusted.

Documentation includes labeling the pages with the patient's name and the time the tracings were collected. A flow sheet should be maintained during the case, summarizing the status of the peaks and any comments to the surgeons.

CONCLUSIONS

Monitoring teams should adhere to proper professional quality and standards. Services should function with appropriate policies on supervision, staffing, privileging, credentialing, and certifying clinical neurophysiologists and monitoring technologists. These should assure each individual's skills, knowledge, abilities, and training relevant to monitoring. Good record documentation and clear communications are also important.

The goals remain to serve the patients first, do no harm, and protect the trust that the public places in us as professional caregivers. NIOM can protect patients, enhance good outcomes, and encourage more thorough surgical procedures.

REFERENCES

1. Nuwer MR. Intraoperative monitoring of the spinal cord. *Clin Neurophysiol*, 2008;119(2): 247–248.
2. Nuwer JM, Nuwer MR. Neurophysiologic surgical monitoring staffing patterns in the USA. *Electroencephalogr Clin Neurophysiol* 1997;103(6):616–620.
3. Nuwer MR, Dawson EG, Carlson LG, et al. Somatosensory evoked potential spinal cord monitoring reduces neurologic deficits after scoliosis surgery: results of a large multicenter survey. *Electroencephalogr Clin Neurophysiol* 1995;96(1):6–11.
4. Kohn LT, Corrigan JM, Donaldson MS, eds. *To Err Is Human: Building a Safer Health System*. Washington, DC: National Academy Press, 1999.

6 A Buyer's Guide to Monitoring Equipment

Greg Niznik

The title of this chapter is a bit of a misnomer, as any modern commercially available NIOM machine will, in fact, fulfill its stated purpose, which is to monitor the nervous system during surgery. Therefore this chapter provides a review of the minimum requirements of NIOM equipment as outlined in the 2006 ACNS guidelines (1). These guidelines and their importance as they relate to NIOM machines are discussed. By having a better understanding of the workings of the NIOM machine, the reader will be better able to make an informed decision in selecting a NIOM machine for his or her practice and be better able to utilize it to its full capability.

A SHORT HISTORY OF A BURGEONING TECHNOLOGY

In the early days of NIOM, most equipment was designed and built by the investigator, either from the ground up or from individual stand-alone components. For example, the author's first clinical evoked potential (EP) system consisted of a one-channel signal averager, battery-powered amplifiers, a constant-voltage stimulator, an analog oscilloscope to display the data, and a pen plotter to provide hard copy of the data. The system was so susceptible to extraneous noise that all testing was done with the subject seated in a Faraday cage, basically a room completely lined with copper wire mesh that was grounded to both the electrical circuit ground and the signal averager. The Faraday cage/room was borrowed from the neurophysiology laboratory, where intra-and extracellular recordings of neural preparations were made. It was only big enough to hold a recliner and a rack for the amplifiers. The amplifiers were so unstable that they had to be reset and have the DC offset zeroed before each trial. The stimulators, signal averager, oscilloscope, and plotter were rack-mounted just outside the Faraday cage.

In the early 1980s, the first multichannel evoked potential (EP) machines became available. These were portable (at least they had wheels) and had integrated, fairly stable amplifier and stimulator systems. More importantly, they were true digital machines that could display and store banks of data. These machines were, for the most part, large and cumbersome towers or consoles weighing several hundreds of pounds. They were a far cry from today's laptop-based systems but they represented a giant leap forward in technology. Having a four- or eight-channel machine with at least two electrical, an auditory, and visual stimulators made the development of NIOM techniques possible. Having stable amplifiers and good filters made the recording of microvolt signals in the electrically hostile environment of the operating room feasible. These machines also had paradigms for signal rejection, which ensured that electrocautery or movement artifact did not destroy the averaged response acquired over the preceding several minutes. Many had available programming languages that facilitated some very basic automation.

These early machines performed only EP testing. If cortical brain function had to be monitored along with EPs, a separate electroencephalography (EEG) machine had to be brought into the operating room. Therefore the space requirement in the operating room for NIOM was not insignificant.

As personal computers became more powerful and as the technology for shrinking digital components improved, more powerful and compact NIOM equipment came on the market. With these, NIOM techniques improved in leaps and bounds. Towers became carts and the number of channels increased, so that eight channels was now the norm. Four electrical stimulators meant that the upper and lower spinal cord could be monitored simultaneously. Amplifiers became even more reliable and stable, reducing the downtime that was previously suffered by saturated amplifiers. True interleaving became available, where data could be collected from several stimulators simultaneously, greatly improving the safety and efficacy offered by NIOM. Prior to this, stimulators were chained, which meant that a set of averages for one stimulator was completed before the next stimulator was activated. Now, with interleaving, each stimulator collected its data simultaneously, so that a complete set of averages was performed for all modalities at once. NIOM machines now were able to perform not only EP testing but also EEG, electromyography (EMG) and nerve conduction studies (NCS) all in one machine. This greatly reduced the amount of space that the NIOM team took up in the operating room. Digital filtering and smoothing made it possible to improve the fidelity and readability of NIOM waveforms.

Today truly portable laptop-based machines are available; 16- and even 32-channel machines are becoming the norm. Automation of data collection, ability to monitor numerous modalities simultaneously, and extremely stable amplifiers coupled with noise-reduction paradigms have taken NIOM technology and techniques to a whole new level. These advances reduce the time that the technologist spends troubleshooting, allowing him or her to concentrate on monitoring the function of the nervous system. Creative ways of displaying and trending data makes identifying significant changes easier and allow earlier intervention. The advent of on-line, real-time supervision of the technologist's work by the neurologist or neurophysiologist has greatly increased the efficacy of NIOM, making surgery safer for the patient.

NIOM is still in its infancy. The technology and techniques used have certainly grown by leaps and bounds over the last 30 years. As technology continues to improve, it is exciting to speculate where the field will be over the next several decades. One thing is certain: improvements in technology and technique will make surgery on and around the nervous system more efficacious and safer.

BASICS OF THE NIOM MACHINE

An NIOM machine consists of three basic parts: some type of stimulator to activate a portion of the nervous system, an amplification system, and a central computer system to digitize, analyze, display, and store the resulting waveform. Each of these parts is discussed separately.

NIOM Stimulators

NIOM stimulators are used to activate that portion of the nervous system which is at risk during surgery. In clinical EP, these are electrical stimulators that activate the somatosensory system, auditory stimulators that activate the auditory system, and visual stimulators that activate the visual system. Monitoring visual EPs is unreliable in the operating room. They are not used routinely; therefore intraoperative visual EPs are not dealt with in this chapter.

Electrical Stimulators

The NIOM machine has electrical stimulators to activate neural structures during somatosensory EPs (SEP), transcranial electrical motor EPs (tceMEP), evoked EMG, and NCS. Typically square-wave pulses of varying intensity, duration, and frequency are delivered. The NIOM machine's central computer controls these functions. In general an NIOM machine will have multiple stimulators available. A minimum of four stimulators is needed to provide simultaneous upper and lower extremity SEPs. Additional electrical stimulators are often available to handle special functions, such as low-power stimulators for direct nerve activation in situ and high-voltage stimulators for tceMEPs.

Stimulus Intensity

An NIOM machine must be versatile in its ability to deliver an electrical stimulus to activate nerves. It must be powerful enough to activate deep neural structures through transcutaneous stimulation, as when the nerves in the arms and legs are being stimulated for SEPs. It must also be able to deliver the fine stimuli needed when neural tissue is being teased away from a tumor mass. It must be able to deliver the stimulus with fidelity and have fine control over the intensity delivered. This control should be in at least 10% increments of the stimulus delivered. For example, for low-current stimuli of less than 1 mA, control over the stimulus intensity in 0.1mA increments is necessary. For stimuli in the tens of mAs, 1 mA increments suffice.

Stimulus Duration

The NIOM electrical stimulator must be able to vary its stimulus duration to meet the needs of each specific surgery. Stimulus duration should be variable from 0.5 to 500 μs. Energy delivered to a nerve is the product of the stimulus intensity and pulse width. This product is known as power (P), which is represented as the area under the stimulus curve (Figure 6.1A). The same power can be delivered to a nerve by using a high intensity and short pulse width or by using a lower intensity and longer pulse width (Figure 6.1B). The maximum power that the NIOM machine can deliver must be limited so that burns do not occur.

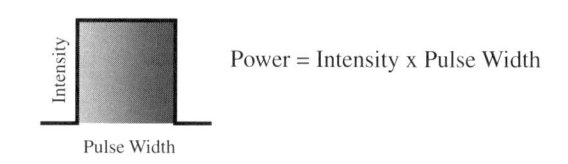

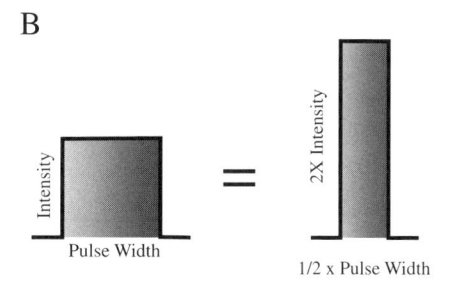

FIGURE 6.1 A. The power of an electrical stimulus is the product of the intensity and pulse width. Power is represented by the area under the square-wave pulse. B. The same stimulus power can be delivered by varying the pulse width and stimulus intensity. These two stimuli have the same power; the first has a long pulse width and low intensity, the second has a short pulse width and high intensity.

Stimulus duration has a direct effect on the presence and magnitude of the stimulus artifact. Using a short stimulus duration, especially when stimulating and recording over short segments, can help minimize the presence of stimulus artifact. As shown in Figure 6.2, the electrical properties of skin can be modeled using electrical components. Subcutaneous tissue acts as a capacitor, which charges and discharges with every electrical pulse. The greater the pulse width of the delivered electrical pulse, the longer the charge and discharge of the capacitor. This then leads to a larger capacitive stimulus artifact in the waveform. By keeping the pulse width of the stimulator relatively short, the capacitive effect of the skin is minimized, thus minimizing the capacitive artifact that may impinge on the recorded signal. Some equipment manufacturers provide stimulators that, instead of delivering a square wave, deliver a biphasic pulse in which the amplitudes of the positive and negative portions of the stimulus can be varied by the technologist. The biphasic pulse minimizes the buildup of charge across the skin, therefore minimizing the presence of a capacitive stimulus artifact.

Constant Voltage vs. Constant Current

The NIOM machine should be able to deliver both constant-current and constant-voltage stimuli. Generation of an action potential in a neuron is initiated by depolarization of the relative charge across it membrane. By passing a negative current across the outer surface of the neuronal membrane, the inside of the neuron becomes relatively more electrically positive until threshold is reached and the all-or-none cascade of events known as the action potential leads to propagation of an electrical signal along the neuron. In order to ensure that activation of a nerve is consistent for each stimulus delivered during repetitive stimulation, the current delivered at each pulse should be held constant. Therefore, in general, constant-current stimulation is the preferred method of electrical stimulation during NIOM. As explained in Ohm's law, V = IR, voltage and current are related by the resistance within the stimulation circuit. For purposes of NIOM, this resistance is primarily skin resistance. Constant-current stimulation varies the stimulus voltage in order to ensure that the required and requested current is delivered at each pulse regardless of changes in skin resistance.

Two exceptions are detailed in the literature where constant voltage is the preferred method of stimulation during NIOM procedures. These are during stimulation of cranial nerves during tumor resection and in tceMEP. Some authors have suggested that constant-voltage stimulation is preferred over constant-current stimulation when nerves in a wet field are stimulated, as it overcomes the problem of current shunting through fluid (2). When a nerve immersed in fluid is being stimulated, current flows through the path of least resistance, primarily through the fluid, and there is

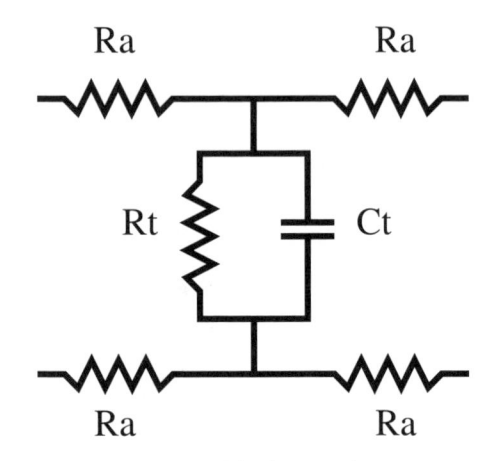

FIGURE 6.2 A simplified equivalence circuit of current flow across a membrane can be used to model how a stimulus current flows across the skin and subcutaneous tissue. The circuit consists of resistance to axial flow of current (Ra); that is, current flow along the surface of the skin and subcutaneous tissue. Current flowing through skin and subcutaneous tissue is represented by a resistor and capacitor in parallel (Rt, Ct).

no way of determining how much current actually reaches the nerve. Furthermore, current shunting varies depending on how wet or dry the field is and how much is shunted through the adjacent fluid. It has been suggested that using constant-voltage stimuli should ensure adequate current delivery across a nerve regardless of whether the field is dry or wet. This theoretically would ensure that adequate depolarization would occur during all phases of surgery and under all stimulating conditions.

Transcranial Electrical Motor EP

Until a few years ago, tceMEP stimulators were experimental and not approved by the FDA for use in routine clinical settings. Use of stand-alone stimulators or using a machine's integrated constant-voltage stimulator to stimulate the motor cortex transcranially was considered an off-label use of this equipment. In late 2002, Digitimer Ltd. received the first FDA approval for their D185 stimulator for use as a transcranial electric stimulator. Since then other manufacturers have acquired FDA approval for their transcranial electrical stimulators. These subsequent approvals are based on the stimulus output specifications of the Digitimer D185. The D185 is a constant-voltage stimulator with a maximum output voltage of 1,000 V. Its maximum current output is 1.5 A. It has a fixed pulse width of 50 μs and a fast rise time of 0.1 A/μs. TceMEP methods employ trains of stimuli to activate the motor cortex. The D185 delivers up to nine pulses per train at an interstimulus interval of 1.0 to 9.9 ms in 0.1 ms increments.

Prior to using either a stand-alone tceMEP stimulator or a tceMEP stimulator integrated into a NIOM machine, one must determine whether the stimulator is FDA-approved for transcranial stimulation. If it is not, its use as a tceMEP stimulator is considered off-label. The use of a medical device for an off-label application may involve a series of regulatory procedures specific to individual institutions. At the very least, it may involve making the surgeon aware that the tceMEP stimulator is not approved for transcranial stimulation. The surgeon deeming it necessary for the surgery prescribes its use and accepts responsibility for its safe and prudent operation. However, the institution may hold that off-label use of a stimulator requires Institutional Review Board (IRB) approval under a research protocol, that the patient be informed of the potential risks and benefits of this investigational procedure, and that the patient's consent be obtained before this equipment is used. The bottom line is that one must check with the given institution as to what the requirements are for off-label use of medical equipment.

Auditory Stimulation

Sound and the Decibel Scale

Before embarking on a discussion of the specific properties needed in NIOM auditory stimulators, a clear explanation of the way sound is measured must be presented. The decibel, the often misunderstood unit of measurement of sound, pressure, power, and voltage is discussed first. This discussion of the decibel is also relevant to discussions of other aspects of the NIOM machine; for example, in describing how efficiently analog filters eliminate unwanted noise.

The decibel (dB) is 1/10 bel, a basic unit of sound, named after Alexander Graham Bell. The decibel describes the relative strength of a sound. In other words, it describes how loud a sound is relative to another sound. Therefore if a sound has an intensity of 80 dB, its intensity is 80 dB above some reference value (i.e., the subject's threshold of hearing, the threshold of hearing of a normal population, or background noise). It is always a comparison.

What is perceived as sound is the result of a wave of air pressure that displaces the eardrum and is subsequently transduced into an electrical signal. Therefore sound intensity is in reality a measurement of air pressure on the eardrum. In terms of sound intensity, a decibel, then, is a measure of relative sound pressure. A 1-dB change in sound intensity approximates a just perceivable change in sound level by the human ear under ideal conditions. The ear perceives sound in a nonlinear fashion; in fact, it perceives sounds logarithmically. Therefore the decibel is a logarithmic measure.

If the power of two sounds, such as those coming out of a loudspeaker, is measured, the decibel difference in their power is described by the following equation:

$$dB = 10 \log_{10} (P2 / P1)$$

where P = power.

In this equation, doubling the power of a loudspeaker would increase it by approximately 3dB:

$$dB = 10 \log_{10} (2) = 10 (0.301) = 3$$

However, in actuality, when sound level is measured, it is done in terms of pressure or voltage (through a microphone). Pressure or voltage is the square root of their power. Therefore, in describing a change in pressure or voltage, the formula for the decibel changes as follows:

$$dB = 20 \log_{10} (p2 / p1)$$

or

$$dB = 20 \log 10 (V1/V2)$$

where p = sound pressure and V = voltage.

In this equation, doubling the sound pressure would increase it by approximately 6dB:

$$dB = 20 \log_{10} (2) = 20 (0.301) = 6$$

Sound Reference and the Decibel Scale

As discussed above, the decibel scale is relative; the intensity of a particular sound is measured to a certain reference sound level. Three techniques of quantifying auditory stimuli are described in the ACNS guidelines for performing brainstem auditory EPs (BAEPs) (1). These are decibels peak-equivalent sound pressure level (dB pe SPL), decibels above normal hearing level (dB HL), and decibels above sensation level (dB SL). One way in which these techniques differ is with respect to their reference value.

dB pe SPL is a measure of the actual sound pressure delivered by the auditory stimulator. It is the unit used in calibrating auditory stimulators. The unit of pressure used in this measure is the micropascal, or $dyne^2/cm^2$. Sound pressure levels are compared to an arbitrary zero pressure level which is 20 micropascals, or 0.0002 $dyne^2/cm^2$.

dB HL is a measure comparing sound intensity to the hearing threshold of normal, healthy young adults. Therefore a sound level of 6 dB HL is twice as loud as the threshold of a population of normal subjects hearing the same sound. This measure is usually default in NIOM machines and most commonly used during NIOM.

dB SL is a measure using each patient as his or her own control. The reference point for this measure is the patient's own hearing threshold. This is an important measure in clinical BAEPs in dealing with a patient with a hearing deficit. By using dB SL, the stimulus intensity can be matched to each ear, so that the same perceived intensity is delivered to both sides.

NIOM machines should have the ability to provide stimuli in both dB HL and dB SL. dB pe SPL is impractical to use as a means of quantifying sound intensity in the operating room. It is imperative to know what measurement scales are available on one's equipment and how to select the appropriate measure so that the expected stimulus intensity is delivered.

Auditory Stimulators

The most common type of auditory stimulator used during NIOM is a piezoelectric transducer that delivers broadband clicks via a plastic tube and foam ear insert. These stimulators are commonly known as insert earphones. Traditional headphones are not recommended for intraoperative use as they are difficult to affix in such a manner that they do not become dislodged during surgery. It must be remembered that in using insert earphones, all BAEP waveform latencies will be delayed by about 1 ms. This occurs because of the time that it takes for the stimulus click to travel from the transducer through the tubing to the eardrum. Many NIOM machines have a feature that will automatically subtract this 1-ms delay if insert earphones are used. It behooves the operator to be aware of whether this feature is active when he or she is identifying BAEP waveform in the operating room.

NIOM auditory stimulators typically deliver a broadband click produced by a 100-μs electrical pulse to the transducer. The resultant click oscillates and can be up to 2 ms in duration. The polarity of the click should be selectable. Three types of polarity are available. The first, condensation, produces a sound wave that pushes the eardrum inward, away from the stimulator. Rarefaction produces a sound wave that pulls the eardrum outward, toward the stimulator. Alternating clicks, as the name implies, consist of alternating condensation and rarefaction stimuli.

The intensity of the auditory stimuli, as discussed above, should be selectable. The stimulator should be capable of producing a broadband click with an intensity of up to 120 dB pe SPL. Most NIOM machines use dB HL as the default method of measuring intensity. Therefore the auditory intensity should be selectable from 0 to 100 dB HL in 1-dB steps. Often NIOM machines will allow the technologist to set a preoperative threshold level for the patient, in which case the stimulus intensity will be expressed as dB SL.

The repetition rate for auditory clicks should be variable up to 200 Hz, although repetition rates in the range of 11 to 22 Hz are most common. Titration of the repetition rate to minimize the averaging time with acceptable degradation of signal fidelity is important, especially during surgery, where rapid assessment of the function of the auditory pathway is imperative. Conversely, deceasing the repetition rate can often improve the fidelity of intraoperative BAEPs in dealing with patients with preoperative deficits.

The availability of white noise masking is helpful in eliminating crossover of the auditory stimulus. Transmission of one-sided stimuli to the opposite ear by air or bone conduction can result in a BAEP that reflects activity in both ears. By delivering white noise at 60 dB SPL to the contralateral ear, this crossover component can be eliminated.

Amplification System

The Operational Amplifier

The operational amplifier (op-amp) is the basic building block of the amplification system of the NIOM machine. Its basic form is shown in Figure 6.3. It consists of two input poles and an output pole. It is a differential amplifier, meaning that its output depends on the nature of both of its inputs. One input, marked (–), is the inverting pole. It is also known as grid 1 (G1), the negative input, or the active input. The other pole, (+), is the noninverting pole, also known as grid 2 (G2), the positive input, or the reference input. The output signal consists of the difference between the input signals at the two poles (as seen in Figure 6.4). If the same signal is introduced at both the inverting and noninverting poles of the amplifier, no output signal will be seen. Signals introduced at the inverting pole

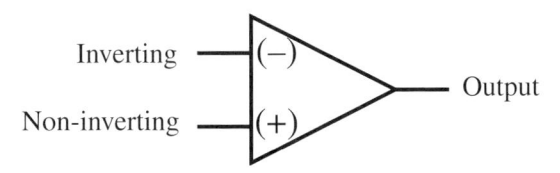

FIGURE 6.3 The electrical symbol for the operational amplifier. It consists of two input poles, one inverting (– ve), the other noninverting (+ ve). The output signal is the arithmetic difference between the two input signals.

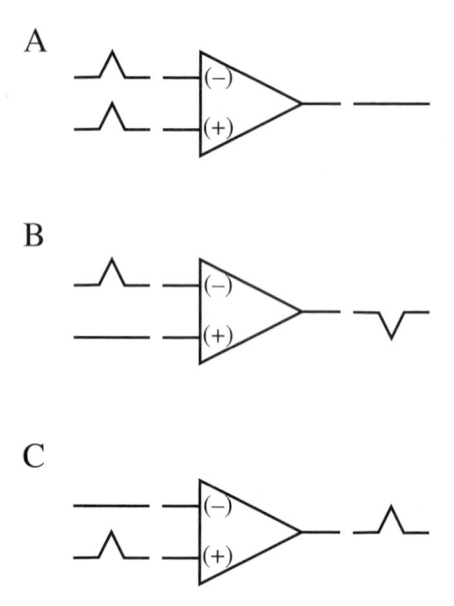

FIGURE 6.4 Examples of polarity convention in operational amplifiers. A. The same input signal is introduced at both inputs. The resulting output is a flat line. B. An upgoing signal is introduced at the inverting pole. The resulting output in downgoing. C. An upgoing signal is introduced at the noninverting pole. The resulting output is upgoing.

TABLE 6.1 Effect of Various Inputs on the Polarity of the Output Signal in an Op-Amp

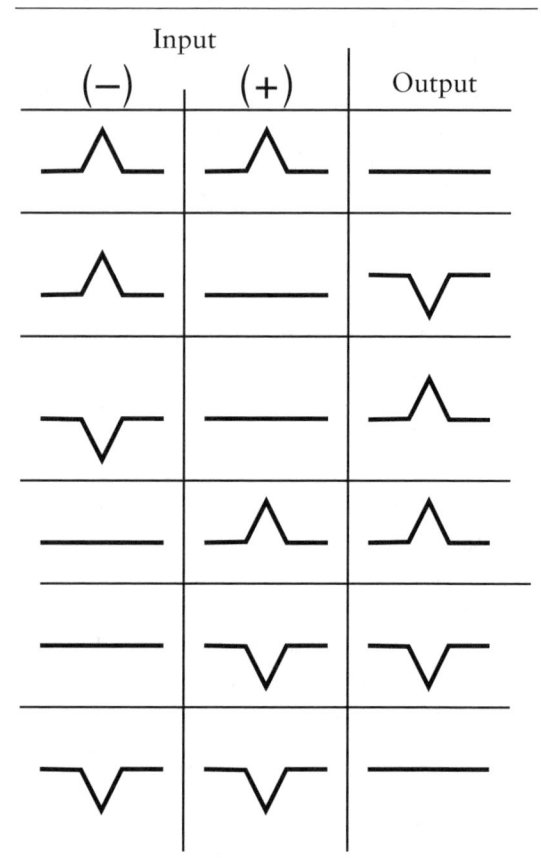

Input		Output
(−)	(+)	
∧	∧	—
∧	—	∨
∨	—	∧
—	∧	∧
—	∨	∨
∨	∨	—

are, as suggested by the name, inverted at the output. If an upgoing signal is placed at the inverting pole and no signal at the noninverting pole, the output will be a downgoing signal. Signals introduced at the noninverting pole have the same polarity at the output. If an upgoing signal is introduced at the noninverting pole and no signal at the inverting pole, the resulting output will be an upgoing signal (Table 6.1). In NIOM applications where near-field potentials are recorded, the electrode over the generator site is placed in the inverting pole of the op-amp. The input to the noninverting pole is placed at a site away from the generator, where no activity will be recorded. Therefore electrically negative signals introduced into the op-amp will be displayed as an upgoing signal at the output. This is why the normal convention for most NIOM modalities is "negative up." One exception to this during NIOM is the BAEP.

By convention, the BAEP is displayed "positive up." Some NIOM machines automatically invert the BAEP display so that a negative signal is downgoing and a positive signal is upgoing (positive up). In performing BAEPs on unfamiliar equipment, care must be taken to select the correct montages so as to ensure that the displayed waveforms are of the correct polarity.

Common Mode-Rejection Ratio

In an ideal op-amp, when the same signal is introduced at both input poles, there should be absolutely no signal at the output pole. In practice however, the op-amp's ability to do this is imperfect. There is always a stray signal that is seen at the output when a common signal is introduced at the input. This was more of a problem in the past, when vacuum tube amplifiers were used in neurodiagnostic equipment (this is where the terms G1 and G2 were introduced, as they referred to the metal grids seen in a vacuum tube amplifier). Today's solid-state amplifiers are much more efficient; however, they are still not perfect. The efficiency of an amplifier's ability to reject common input signals is expressed in the common mode-rejection ratio. According to ACNS guidelines, the common mode-rejection ratio of neurodiagnostic equipment should be at least 10,000:1 (or an 80-dB difference). For the purposes of this chapter, the specifics of how the common mode-rejection ratio is maximized are not important. A lot seems to be made of the common mode-rejection ratio; but for practical purposes, this ratio is within acceptable limits in all modern NIOM machines. Even the lowliest op-amp exceeds these common mode-rejection ratio specifications. It suffices to know that the higher the common mode-rejection ratio, the more efficient the amplification system is at discerning the differences between signals introduced at the input poles.

Input Impedance

The ACNS guidelines state that neurodiagnostic equipment's amplification system should have an input impedance of at least 100 Mohm (1). Again, all modern commercially available NIOM machines meet this specification. High input impedance is important, as it ensures that most of the recorded signal voltage will be across the inputs of the amplifier. This is how it works: The equivalent circuit of the patient amplifier interface in its simplest form is shown in Figure 6.5. The impedance of the patient and input impedance of the amplifier are in series. Since resistors in series act as a voltage dividers, the voltage recorded across the patient and the voltage recorded across the amplifier are proportional to their respective impedances. Assume that the impedance of the electrodes on the patient is 1 Kohm and the input impedance across the

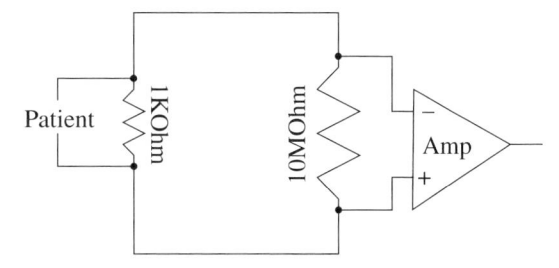

Voltage Divider Rule:
The voltage recorded across the patient and across the amplifier is proportional to their impedance. Vamp is 100,000 greater than Vpatient.

FIGURE 6.5 Simple representation of the patient, amplifier-equivalent circuit demonstrating the principle that as the impedance of both are in series, the voltage across each resistor in the circuit is proportional to its impedance.

amplifier is 100 MOhm. That means that the portion of the total signal voltage across the amplifier is 100,000 times greater than that across the patient. For all intents and purposes, all of the signal voltage is across the amplifier; only a minuscule amount (1×10^{-5}) is across the patient electrode. Therefore the output signal is a true representation of the input signal.

Amplification

The op-amp not only determines the morphology and polarity of its output signal, it also amplifies the signal so that it can be filtered, digitized, and displayed. The amplifier in an NIOM machine must be able to handle amplification of a wide variety of neurologic signals. EP signals are in the order of 0.1 – 5 μV, EEG signals are in the 10 to 100 μV range and EMG signals are in the millivolt range. So not only does an amplifier have to be sensitive enough to record very tiny signals, it has to be versatile enough to be able to amplify a wide range of signal types. It was not unusual in the not too distant past that in order to perform EPs, NCS, or EEG, separate pieces of equipment had to be brought into the operating room. Today, most NIOM equipment will perform all of these duties, not only separately, but also simultaneously.

Analog Filtering

After amplification, the first of a series of processes that separate the neurologic signal from electrical and biologic noise occurs. This first step is processing the signal through a series of analog filters. A raw recorded signal is composed of a wide spectrum of component frequencies. Ideally, only that part of the raw signal that contains neurologic signal should be processed. The frequency response that is introduced in signal processing can be limited by the use of filters. Typically for NIOM procedures, low-cut and high-cut filters are utilized to delineate a signal with a limited band of frequencies that will be further processed. A low-cut filter (otherwise known as a high-pass filter) will eliminate all component frequencies of the raw input signal lower than the set point. A high-cut (or low-pass) filter will eliminate all frequencies above its set point. Thus a bandpass of interest can be defined for each type of modality. Typically, for EEG, this is 1 to 70 Hz; for SEPs it is 30 to 3,000 Hz; for BAEPs, it is 10 to 3,000 Hz; and for EMGs, it is 10 to 32 kHz (Figure 6.6).

An ideal bandpass filter, also known as a brick-wall filter, should eliminate all frequencies outside of its low- and high-frequency set points (Figure 6.7). However, real filters do not behave in this manner. In fact, all filters have a roll-off, where frequency components outside of the bandpass are allowed to pass. The sharper the slope of this roll-off, the more like an ideal filter the bandpass filter acts. The roll-off slope can be quantified in the number of decibels per octave that the signal degrades. The higher the absolute roll-off, the more like an ideal the filter behaves.

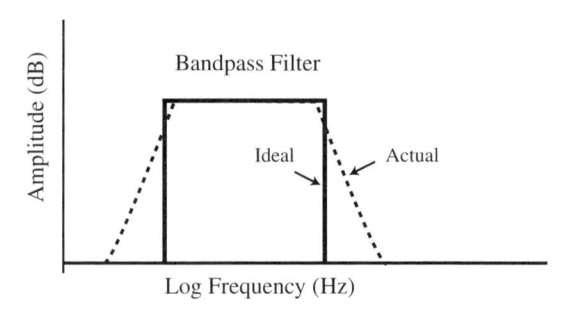

FIGURE 6.7 Amplitude-vs.-frequency plot showing characteristics of a bandpass filter. An ideal bandpass filter, or brick-wall filter, cuts off all frequencies outside of the selected endpoints of the filter. In reality, no analog filter behaves ideally; some portion of frequencies outside of the bandpass is allowed to pass.

In its simplest form, a low- or high-cut filter is an arrangement of resistors and capacitors or resistors and inductors. This simple filter with passive components is known as a first-order filter. It has a roll off of −6 dB per octave. This means that the signal strength will be cut in half each time the frequency doubles. Therefore, for a high-cut filter set at 3,000 Hz, about half the signal amplitude will be present at 6,000 Hz, one quarter at 12,000 Hz, etc. This is not an ideal situation. Analog filters with active components greatly improve the ability to exclude frequencies outside the bandpass. A second-order filter has a roll-off of −12 dB per octave. Third-order filters have a roll-off of −18 dB per octave, etc. The roll-off continues to improve with subsequent sophistication of filter design. The ACNS guidelines recommend that the low-cut filter have a roll-off of at least −12 dB per octave

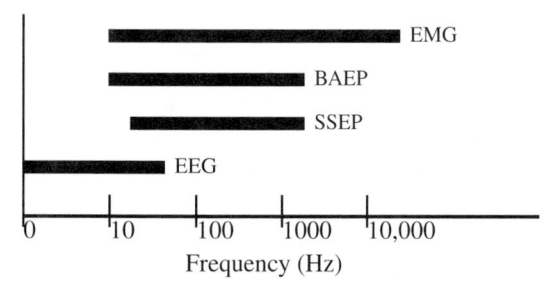

FIGURE 6.6 Representative bandpasses for electrically recorded biological activity, including EEG, SEP, BAEP, and EMG.

(second-order), and the high-cut filter have a roll-off of at least −24 dB per octave (fourth-order) (1).

The physical properties of an analog filter introduces an error at its set point, or cutoff frequency. Instead of the entire signal passing at the cutoff frequency, the signal is degraded whereby a small portion of the signal is lost. In fact, there is a decrease of −3 dB in the signal at the cutoff frequency (Figure 6.8). This error is reflected in the ACNS guidelines where analog filter settings are discussed. For example, the ACNS EEG guidelines state that the low-cut filter should not be higher than 1 Hz (−3 dB), and the high-cut filter should not be lower than 70 Hz (−3 dB) (1). The −3dB in parenthesis recognizes that the signal at the set points of the bandpass will be degraded by −3 dB.

When filter settings outside the recommended guidelines are used, distortions in the resultant waveforms can occur. Excessive use of low-cut filters (i.e., using a higher-than-recommended low-cut setting) will cause the resultant waveform to appear earlier. Excessive use of high-cut filters (i.e., using a lower-than-recommended high-cut setting) can cause a resultant waveform to appear later than normal. Excessive use of filtering or changing filter settings during an NIOM procedure can lead to confusion in waveform identification and can mask significant changes in neural function. Although waveforms can sometimes be "noisy," it is always better to preserve the fidelity of your recorded waveforms by judicious use of filtering, than to risk masking their true nature through overuse of analog filters.

Artifact Rejection

The next method of removing unwanted artifact from an NIOM EP recording is the use of automated artifact rejection. Artifact rejection causes signals over a certain voltage to be eliminated from subsequent processing. Therefore such signals will not be included in an EP average nor will they be displayed in a processed EEG trace. Artifact rejection is typically performed through a window discriminator, a device that compares the voltage of the incoming signal to a reference value (Figure 6.9A). If any portion of the input signal falls outside of the window, it is rejected (Figure 6.9B). It is important that the artifact rejection be user-controlled. Having the ability to adjust the size of the window in relation to the input signal is important in making the artifact-rejection feature efficient. Effective use of the window discriminator allows quicker acquisition of averaged responses. Therefore the user must be able to see both the raw input signal and the window in order to make this adjustment.

Central Computer System

Analog-to-Digital Conversion

The analog signal is then digitized for further processing, display, and storage. An analog-to-digital converter (ADC) is used for this process. There are several characteristics of the ADC that affects its ability to faithfully reproduce the analog signal. It must be understood, however, that the digitized waveform is a representation of the analog waveform, and

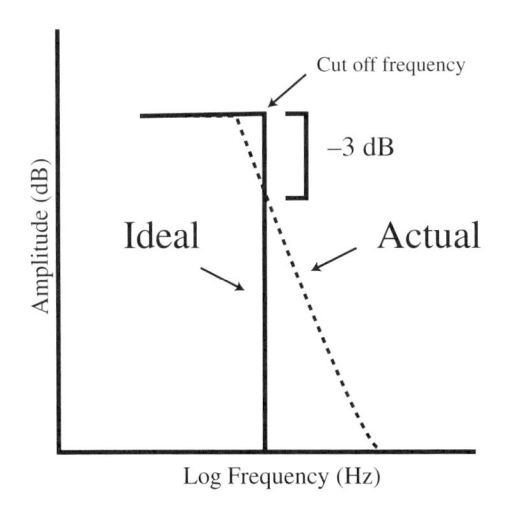

FIGURE 6.8 Diagram showing a decrease of −3 dB in the signal at the cutoff frequency. See text for details.

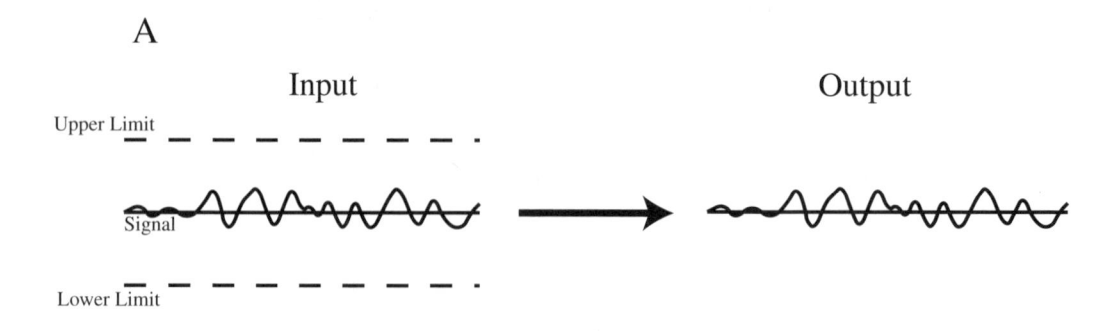

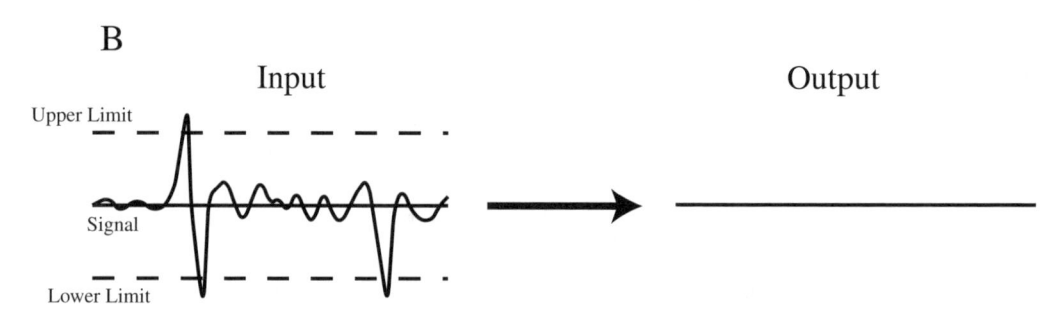

FIGURE 6.9 Characteristics of a window discriminator used in artifact rejection. A. If the input signal falls within the upper and lower limits of the window discriminator, it is allowed to pass. B. If however, the input signal is over either the upper or lower limits of the window discriminator, it is rejected from subsequent processing.

inherent in the digitization process is loss of information. Modern NIOM machines do a very good job of ADC, with very good fidelity in the digitized signal. Once the signal has been digitized, it can be manipulated to further reduce noise through signal averaging and digital filtering. It can easily be displayed, trended, printed, and stored for future analysis. The discussion that follows delves into the characteristics of the ADC, explaining how it works and how these characteristics come together to ensure faithful reproduction of the analog signal.

Sampling Frequency, Dwell Time, and Horizontal Resolution

Digitization of an analog signal involves several steps. First, a portion of the analog signal is isolated and held in memory. This analog signal may be an individual EP trial, a NCS waveform, or an epoch of EEG or EMG data. The analog signal is then "sampled" at a certain distinct points along its time base. This sampling is done at a fixed frequency, therefore a fixed number of data points along the waveform are examined. The voltage of the analog waveform at each sample point is recorded as a discrete number. This is digitization. What results is a series of number pairs representing the time of each sample and the voltage of the analog signal at that time. This digitized data can then be used to plot the waveform on a screen, be used for signal averaging and digital filtering in processed EEG waveforms, and stored for future analysis.

The fidelity of digital waveforms depends on how well the analog signal is sampled. The frequency with which the analog signal is sampled, or sampling frequency, must be high enough to ensure that enough data points are collected to faithfully represent the analog signal. The sampling frequency directly affects the horizontal resolution of the digitized waveform. The higher the sampling frequency, the more faithful the ADC representation of the analog signal will be. As seen in Figure 6.10, a sine wave is introduced into an ADC. In Figure 6.10A, the sampling frequency of the ADC is the same as the sine wave frequency. The resultant digitized waveform is a poor representation of the analog waveform; in this case, the digital waveform is a flat line.

If the sampling frequency of the ADC is increased to twice the frequency of the analog sine wave (Figure 6.10B), the digitized waveform is a better but not a faithful representation of the analog signal. As shown in Figure 6.10C and D, increasing the sampling frequency to four and eight times the analog sine wave frequency greatly improves the ability to faithfully represent the analog waveform digitally.

The theorem describing the minimum sampling frequency required for an ADC to faithfully represent an analog signal is known as the Nyquist theorem. It states that the sampling frequency of an ADC must be greater than twice that of the fastest-frequency component of a waveform. For example, the bandpass frequency of interest in a SEP waveform is 30 to 3,000 Hz. Therefore, to adequately represent the analog SEP waveform, the ADC must sample the waveform at greater than 6,000 Hz. That would mean that a sample would be taken every 0.00016 seconds, or every 0.16 ms, or 160 μs. This time between ADC samples is known as the dwell time. For EMG signals, where the upper end of the bandpass is in the range of 32,000 Hz, the sampling rate required would be in the 100-kHz range. Most modern NIOM machines have sampling frequencies in the megahertz range, so faithful ADC reproduction of neurologic signals is assured.

Bits and Vertical Resolution

Just as the sampling frequency (and dwell time) determines the horizontal or time reso-

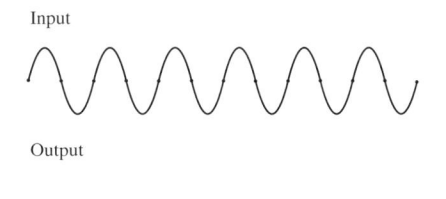

A: Sampling frequency = sine wave frequency
Input
Output

B: Sampling frequency = 2 x sine wave frequency
Input
Output

C: Sampling frequency = 4 x sine wave frequency
Input
Output

D: Sampling frequency = 8 x sine wave frequency
Input
Output

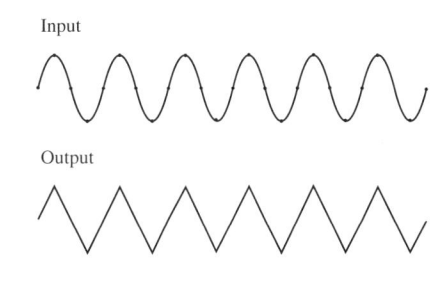

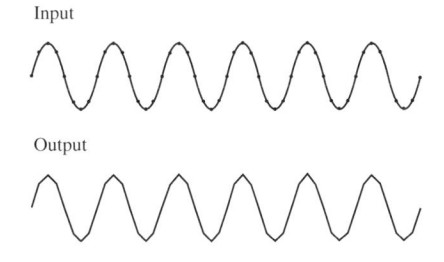

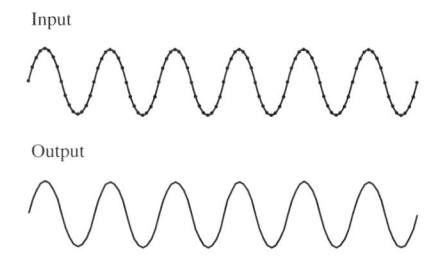

FIGURE 6.10 The effect of various sampling frequencies on the output of an ADC. If the sampling frequency is the same as the frequency of the analog signal, the digitized output is a straight line. As the sampling frequency of the ADC is increased, the fidelity of the digitized signal improves.

lution of an ADC, the number of bits available to the ADC determines the vertical, or amplitude, resolution of the digitized waveform. As discussed previously, the ADC converts the voltage of the analog waveform to discrete digital numeric data at each sample point. The number of vertical data points available determines how faithful the amplitude data are translated by the ADC. The number of vertical data points available for the full scale voltage of the analog waveform is expressed in bits. The number of vertical data points available per bit is expressed by the equation 2^n, where n = the number of bits available to the ADC. Therefore an eight-bit ADC would have 2^8 or 256 data points of vertical data resolution. Thus, when displaying a waveform that has a peak-to-peak voltage of 10 µV, an eight-bit ADC would in theory be able to resolve and display voltage changes of 0.04 µV. This is an ideal situation; in the real world, there is an error factor involved. A 12-bit ADC would have 2^{12} or 4,095 data points of vertical resolution, meaning that in theory it could resolve voltage changes of 0.002 µV for the same 10-µV signal. NIOM machines with inadequate vertical resolution were a factor back in the days when laboratories assembled their own neurodiagnostic equipment. However, most modern NIOM machines have at least 12-bit ADC.

The EP Waveform, Signal-to-Noise Ratio, and Signal Averaging

Signal-to-Noise Ratio

EP signals are tiny. When recorded from the scalp, they are buried in a myriad of electrical and biologic noise often several magnitudes larger than the signal of interest. EP signals are in the single-digit microvolt range. Ambient electrical (60 Hz) noise is 120 V at the source, but can be in the millivolt or volt range at or near the amplifier. EEG activity is in the 10-µV to 100-µV range; EMG and EKG activity is in the millivolt range. Bandpass filtering does not get rid of all this electrical and biologic noise. As seen in Figure 6.9, there is a lot of overlap in the component frequencies of EP, EEG, EMG, and 60-Hz electrical activity. A comparison of the amplitude of the EP signal to the amplitude of the background noise can be made. The signal-to-noise ratio (SNR) is just that, SNR = V_{signal}/V_{noise}. EP waveforms buried in background noise have low SNRs. EPs relatively free from background noise have greater SNRs. Filtering by itself, as discussed above, is limited in its ability to increase a waveform's SNR. Other techniques, the most important being signal averaging, are used to increase the ability to tease the EP out of background noise.

Signal Averaging

Signal averaging utilizes the principle that EPs are time-locked to their stimuli and all other background activity is random. If a sequence of EP trials is averaged together, the time-locked potential will be present in all trials while the random background activity will eventually cancel itself out. The caveat here is that all background activity must be random. This becomes a problem with 60-Hz noise. If the EP stimulus is synchronized to the 60-Hz signal, or some harmonic of 60 Hz, the 60-Hz signal will be included in the averaged waveform. Therefore it is imperative, in performing EP studies, that the stimulator be set at a repetition rate that is not a factor of 60 or its harmonics.

In Figure 6.11, an idealized EP waveform is presented with representations of five individual EP trials. Each EP trial contains the time-locked EP waveform and random background noise. As represented in Figure 6.12, a series of subsequent EP trials are averaged together. As the number of trials in the average increases, the EP waveform emerges from the background noise. Increasing the number of trials in the average further improves the signal until the background activity is negligible and the EP waveform is clear.

As subsequent EP trials are averaged, the SNR improves. The improvement in the SNR

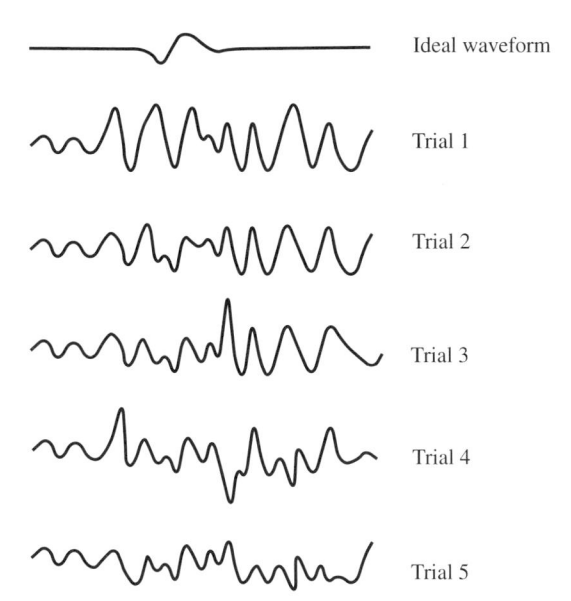

FIGURE 6.11 An ideal EP waveform as well as five representative individual trials. Each of the trials contains the idealized EP waveform as well as background biological and extraneous electrical noise. Signal averaging is used to separate the time-locked EP waveform from the background noise.

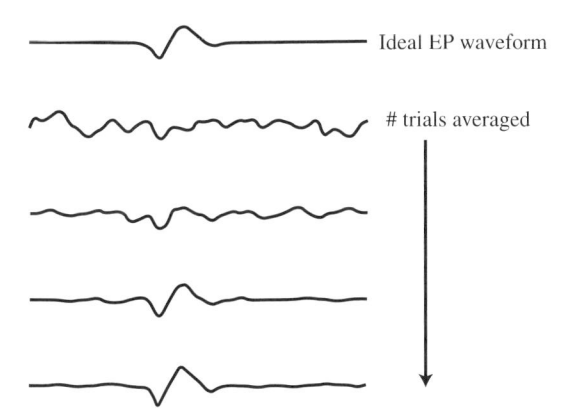

FIGURE 6.12 An idealized EP waveform as well as averaged waveforms with increasing number of trials. As the number of trials increases, random background noise is diminished until a true representation of the idealized waveform is obtained.

can be expressed mathematically, where improvement is equal to the square root of the number of trials averaged. For example, an EP waveform that contains the average of 16 sweeps would have a four time improvement in its SNR; 64 sweeps would improve the SNR by a factor of 8, or 256 sweeps by a factor of 16, or 1,024 sweeps by a factor of 32, etc. Early signal averagers and clinical EP machines had selections for number of averages that were squares of whole numbers for the simple reason that it was easy to calculate the SNR improvement.

Here is a sample problem that illustrates how SNRs are used in the laboratory: A 1-µV EP signal is buried in 5 µV of background noise. An appropriate SNR for this study is 5. How many averages would be necessary to accomplish this?

1. First calculate the starting SNR:

   $SNR = 1 \text{ µV} / 5 \text{ µV} = 0.2$

2. The target SNR is 5, which is 25 times greater than the present SNR.
3. The SNR must be improved by 25, which means that 25^2 or 625 trials will be needed to achieve the desired goal.

Digital Filtering and Smoothing

The digitized waveform can undergo digital filtering to eliminate the roll-off characteristic of analog filters. Digital filters act as the ideal brick-wall filter with no roll-off. In one common form of digital filtering, the digitized waveform undergoes a Fourier transform, where the amplitude of the waveform in individual frequency bands are determined. Waveform components in frequency bands outside of the selected bandpass are eliminated, and the digital waveform is reassembled from the remaining data.

Digital filters do not suffer from the phase shifting inherent in analog filters, therefore there is no temporal distortion of the resultant digitally filtered waveform.

Most EP equipment offers some form of smoothing involving software algorithms that appear to increase the SNR by eliminating a portion of high-frequency background activity. These algorithms vary; in their simplest form, however, they take a weighted average of the data points in the waveform and fit a curve to the data points that best represent this weighted average. In this way, stray high-frequency data are eliminated. Just as with other forms of digital filtering, phase shifts do not occur, but the amplitude and the morphology of the real waveforms do change. Digital filtering and smoothing, just like analog filtering, should be used carefully and their effects on the waveform understood.

Data Display, Trending, and Storage

After amplification, filtering, digitization, and signal processing, the final process of the NIOM machine is to display the resultant data in a manner that allows changes to be identified and tracked efficiently. NIOM machines all have the ability to display and trend data. In general, one should be able to see the live data, compare it to data previously recorded, set baseline data, be able to trend visual data to numerical data, and place time-locked comments to data sets.

For EEG and EMG data, a machine must have a clear and easy method of reviewing data on the fly. At best, the complete raw EEG and EMG data should be stored and a mechanism for reviewing data on the fly should be available. At the very least, several minutes of EEG and EMG data should be held in a buffer in order for transient events to be reviewed or replayed.

The NIOM machine should be capable of flagging epochs of EEG and EMG data, such as baseline data or data at critical periods. These flagged data should be easily accessible for comparison to current "live" data. A split-screen method of data presentation with stored data on one side of the screen and live data on the other is an excellent method of being able to compare EEG and EMG data of interest.

It is imperative that the NIOM machine be able to transmit data online and in real time to the supervising neurologist or neurophysiologist. The advent of wireless Internet connections makes this task easier than in previous years. One concern of data transmission is ensuring that that there is enough bandwidth to transmit raw EEG and EMG data accurately. Data transmission must adhere to Health Information Portability and Accountability Act (HIPAA) guidelines to protect patient confidentiality.

After completion of the case, a method for storing the data for review and archiving should be available. Although most personal computer–based machines have software for writing files to CDs or DVDs, it is much more convenient for NIOM software to be able to transfer data instead of using another stand-alone program. In addition, there should be a method of flagging which data have been reviewed and which have been archived to CDs or DVDs. Previous case data should be removed from the NIOM machine as soon as practible and stored with the patient's permanent record. This is important for two reasons. First, it ensures that there is sufficient room on the NIOM machine's hard drive for future studies. Second, it ensures that HIPAA-protected patient data are not residing on a hard drive that may be accessed by unauthorized persons.

EP, NCS, and tceMEP Data

EP displays should have the several features. The current average should be clearly displayed. Baseline waveforms for each trace in the montage should be easily set and prominently identified. It is a good idea to have a display that shows the current average and the baseline in a manner that allows the traces to be visually compared. A trend of previous averaged traces is helpful in visually determining changes in waveform morphology. It is also important that numeric data be displayed in such a way as to easily determine if significant changes from baseline have occurred. Time-locked comments linked to waveforms and numeric data reflect the function of the nervous system at the various stages of surgery and link changes in waveform morphology to what has occurred in the operative field.

A clear representation of the various stimulating and recording parameters should be available. Stimulating parameters should include rate, intensity, and pulse width. Recording parameters should include number of averages, gain, and bandpass information.

Data should be stored in such a way that individual averages, waveform trends, and numeric data can all be retrieved for any or all portions of the surgery.

EEG Data

Intraoperative EEG data consists of the raw signal and processed EEG data such as compressed spectral array (CSA) and density spectral array (DSA). The raw EEG data should be available at any time. Digital EEG technology allows the display montage to be changed at any time during the procedure to better localize changes. Unlike paper EEG, montages can be changed on the fly without losing the ability to go back and remontage stored data. The entire EEG recording should be stored for review. It is also helpful to be able to split the screen during recording and to compare the live EEG to the previously recorded EEG. Event markers with comments should be available, allowing the technologist to quickly search the record for significant events as well as to correlate changes in the EEG to events in the operative field.

The advent of CSA and DSA EEG allows the technologist to quickly identify major trends in frequency shifts and loss of amplitude or power. They are a good generalization of what is happening to the EEG but cannot replace vigilant interpretation of raw EEG data. They can miss subtle changes that may be clinically significant. All changes in processed EEG data have to be correlated with the raw EEG.

EMG Data

The NIOM machine should be able to display and capture multiple channels of free-running EMG data. At best, the live EMG record for the entire case should be stored, as is the case with EEG. If this is not possible, time- and event-marked epochs of EMG data should be stored for analysis. It is useful to have several seconds or minutes of EMG data in a buffer so as to be able to review the EMG data and store relevant epochs of activity. The ability to output audio EMG activity is helpful in providing feedback to the surgeon when he or she is irritating neural structures. Care must be taken in using audio output in the presence of electrocautery. Most NIOM machines have a method of muting the audio output when an electrocautery signal is detected.

Many NIOM machines have an autocapture function using a window discriminator. When the EMG signal is of greater amplitude than the threshold of the window, time-stamped EMG activity is captured on the screen and stored. This is very helpful when dealing with frequent EMG activity in multiple channels.

Summary

This chapter reviews the requirements of an NIOM machine to adequately record data in the operating room. The ACNS guidelines provide recommendations for the minimum features that must be present in these machines. Most commercially available machines meet these guidelines but differ in other features. The various features of most commercially available NIOM machines are compared in Table 6.2. It is recognized that NIOM machines are constantly being updated, and further changes will occur with time in each of these machines.

It is hoped that this chapter will help the reader to decipher the features of various NIOM machines and guide him or her in finding a system that will meet most needs. Once one understands what each part of the NIOM machine does and the reasons why certain features are important, one should be able to uti-

TABLE 6.2 Comparison of the Commonly Used NIOM Machines Currently Commercially Available

Manufacturer Model	Axon Eclipse	Cadwell Cascade	Nihon Kohden Neuromaster	Viasys Endeavor CR	XLTEK Protektor
# Channels	32	16 (32 Cascade Elite)	16 or 32	16	16
EP	Y	Y	Y	Y	Y
BAEP	Y	Y	Y	Y	Y
VEP	Y	Y	Y	Y	Y
EMG	Y	Y	Y	Y	Y
EEG	Y	Y	Y	Y	Y
Integrated tceMEP	Y	Y	N	N	N
Multimodality	Y	Y	Y	Y	Y
Storage	HD, CD, DVD	HD, CD, DVD	HD, CD, DVD	HD, CD, DVD	HD, CD, DVD
Amplifier					
ADC	N/A	16 bit, 25.6 KHz	16 bit, 5us/channel	N/A	16 bit, 60KHz
Input impedance	N/A	> 100 Mohm	> 100 Mohm	> 1000 MOhm	>100 MOhm
CMRR	> 100 dB	> 95 dB	>106 dB	110 dB	>110dB
Noise level	< 2 uV p-p	< 4uV p-p	< 3uV p-p	0.7 µV RMS	<0.1µV RMS
Sensitivity	N/A	0.01 µV–10 mV/div	0.05 µV–50 mV/div	10 µV–100 mV scale	0.1 µV–5 mV/div
Time base	N/A	1–1000 msec/div	1–6000 msec/div	N/A	0.5–500 msec/div
Filters					
Order/rolloff	N/A	2nd/12dB/octave	1st or 2nd/6 or 12 dB/octave	1st or 2nd/6 or 12 dB/octave	N/A
LFF	N/A	0.5–100 Hz	0.08 Hz–3 KHz	0.2–500 Hz	0.1–500 Hz
HFF	N/A	30–10 KHz	10 Hz–3 KHz	100–3000 Hz	30–15 KHz
Notch	50/60 Hz	50/60 Hz	50/60 Hz	50/60 Hz	50/60 Hz

Manufacturer	Axon	Cadwell	Nihon Kohden	Viasys	XLTEK
Model	Eclipse	Cascade	Neuromaster	Endeavor CR	Protektor
Estimated					
Number	16	16	6	4 high level, 1 low level	16
Rate	0.01–100 Hz	0.5–90 Hz	0.1–50 Hz	0.1–100 Hz	0.1–100 Hz
Interleave	Y	Y	Y	Y	Y
Intensity	0–100 mA (0–400 V)	0–100 mA	0–100 mA	0–100 mA (0–400 V)	0–100mA
Duration	0.1–500 msec	0.05–1 msec	0.05–1 msec	0.01–1 msec	0.05–1 msec
External Trigger	Y	N/A	Y	Y	Y
Auditory					
Signal Type	Tone/burst/click	Click	Tone/burst/click	Click	Click/pip/tone/noise
Intensity	N/A	−10–95 dB nHL	0–135 dB SPL	−21–103 db nHL	0–105 dB nHL
Polarity	N/A	Cond/rare/alt	Cond/rare/alt	Cond/rare/alt	Cond/rare/alt

N/A: Not available.

lize all the features of the equipment to their fullest, making NIOM more effective.

REFERENCES

1. American Clinical Neurophysiological Society. Guidelines 1–10. *Am J Electroneurodiagn Technol* 2006;46(3):198–305.
2. Moller AR, Janetta PJ. Preservation of facial function during removal of acoustic neuromas: Use of monopolar constant-voltage stimulation and EMG. *J Neurosurg* 1984;61:757–760.

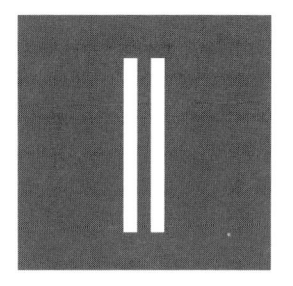

Clinical Methods

7 Vertebral Column Surgery

David B. MacDonald
Mohammad Al-Enazi
Zayed Al-Zayed

Surgery on the vertebral column risks spinal cord, nerve root, brachial plexus, and peripheral nerve injury. Although the overall incidence of major neurologic complications is only about 1%, the devastation of paraplegia strongly motivates efforts to monitor spinal cord integrity during these procedures (1). Consequently spine surgery was one of the first and remains one of the most frequent indications for neurophysiologic intraoperative monitoring (NIOM).

Two general characteristics tend to make these procedures ideal for monitoring: (a) most patients have monitorable evoked potentials (EPs) because they are neurologically intact and (b) the most commonly encountered injury mechanisms (ischemia, compression, traction) are reversible when detected quickly. Nevertheless, a few patients having antecedent neurologic pathology degrading their EPs can be challenging or even impossible to monitor. In addition, some injury mechanisms, such as contusion, may not be reversible, although it may be possible to minimize their effects if the cause is rapidly identified and corrected.

This chapter outlines the basic anatomy, pathology, clinical features, and surgery of common vertebral column disorders and then details NIOM techniques, interpretation, and technical issues. It emphasizes spinal cord monitoring; nerve root protection techniques that may also be relevant are addressed elsewhere in this book.

BASIC ANATOMY, PATHOLOGY, CLINICAL FEATURES, AND SURGERY

Vertebral Column Anatomy

The vertebral column consists of seven cervical, twelve thoracic, and five lumbar vertebrae, their interposed fibrocartilaginous discs, and connective tissues. It is normally straight in the coronal plane, but in the saggital plane it curves gently forward in the neck, backward in the thorax (normal kyphosis), and forward again in the lumbar spine. Each cylindrical vertebral body has a left and right pedicle projecting posterolaterally to the lateral transverse processes that articulate with neighboring transverse processes at facet joints. The left and right laminae project posteromedially from the transverse processes to join together as the midline spinous process. Longitudinal ligaments run down the ventral and dorsal surfaces of the vertebral bodies and discs; interspinous ligaments connect adjacent spinous processes, and the ligamentum flavum connects adjacent laminae.

Spinal Cord Anatomy

The vertical space between the vertebrae, their processes, and the ligaments forms the spinal canal containing the spinal cord, which normally ends at about the L1 vertebral level. Cervical and thoracic spinal nerve roots exit the spinal canal laterally through the foramina formed between adjacent pedicles. Lumbosacral roots pass downward as the cauda equina to exit through foramina below the spinal cord.

The corticospinal tracts important for voluntary movement descend from the cortex, decussate (cross the midline) in the caudal medulla, and then travel down the contralateral dorsolateral cord. Some of their axons form excitatory synapses on alpha motor neurons in the anterior horn gray matter, mostly contralateral to the originating hemisphere. A few corticospinal fibers descend without decussation through the ipsilateral ventral cord but are normally of minor importance. The axons of alpha motor neurons from each spinal cord segment coalesce to form motor roots (e.g., C5, L4), which eventually innervate muscles. Cervical and lumbosacral roots undergo complex interdigitation within the brachial and lumbosacral plexi, which rebranch into the various peripheral nerves supplying limb muscles. Consequently there is radicular overlap and anatomic variation of muscle innervation. Intraoperative monitoring of motor EPs (MEPs) can assess the corticospinal system from brain to muscle.

The dorsal columns contain sensory axons for position and vibration sense. These very long axons ascend the ipsilateral dorsal column to the gracile and cuneate nuclei at the cervicomedullary junction, where they finally synapse. The axons of the second-order sensory neurons then decussate as the internal arcuate fibers of the caudal medulla before ascending to the contralateral thalamus, where they synapse on third-order sensory neurons. These then project to somatosensory cortex. Intraoperative monitoring of somatosensory EPs (SEPs) can assess this system from peripheral nerve to brain.

The spinothalamic system conveying pain and temperature sensation and many other descending, ascending, and intrinsic spinal cord systems are unassessed by MEP/SEP techniques. F-wave, H-reflex, and bulbocavernosus reflex testing can provide information about segmental cord activity that may indirectly help assess long tract functions.

Spinal Cord Blood Supply

Radicular arteries from the aorta and its major branches in the neck and pelvis enter the spinal canal through the intervertebral foramina. With considerable variation, a few of these arteries branch to feed the longitudinal anterior spinal artery running down the anterior median fissure of the spinal cord and the left and right posterior spinal arteries running down the dorsal spinal cord. The anterior spinal artery supplies the ventral two-thirds of the cord including the anterior horns, central gray matter, ventral portions of the dorsal horns, and corticospinal tracts. The posterior spinal arteries supply the dorsal columns and superficial dorsal horn gray matter. A pial plexus of interconnecting arteries supplies the outer rim of the cord.

Vertebral Column Pathology

Scoliosis

Scoliosis consists of abnormal vertebral column curvature in the coronal plane. Cobb angle measured in spinal x-rays is an estimate of the degree of deformity. There is also a rotational deformity and there may be excessive kyphosis (kyphoscolsiosis). Following the shortest vertical path, the spinal cord adopts an ectopic and rotated position toward the concave side of the deformed spinal canal.

Most often scoliosis is idiopathic. Congenital scoliosis is also common, consisting of vertebral column malformation associated with hemivertebrae and other vertebral anomalies. Vertebral dysplasia due to neurofibromatosis or achondroplasia is another relatively common cause. Connective tissue disorders such as Turner's syndrome are less frequent causes. Several neurologic disorders are associated with scoliosis, including cerebral palsy, Arnold-Chiari malformation, Freidreich's ataxia, spinal cord tumor, neural tube defects, tethered cord, and neuromuscular disease. These are grouped together under the term "neuromuscular scoliosis."

Horizontal gaze palsy and progressive scoliosis (HGPPS) is a rare autosomal recessive disorder consisting of an inability to turn the eyes to either side along with progressive scoliosis (2). Although more frequent in regions where consanguinity is common (it comprises about 3% of the authors' scoliosis surgery series in Riyadh, Saudi Arabia), it has also been reported in Europe, Japan, and North America. The corticospinal and dorsal column systems are uncrossed (nondecussation) and NIOM techniques must accordingly be modified for accurate results (3).

Other Vertebral Column Disorders

Some other surgical spinal disorders that may require NIOM include cervical spondylosis, spinal fractures, vertebral column tumors, and ossification of the posterior longitudinal ligament (OPLL). Spondylosis is a degenerative process consisting of bony spur formation on the lips of adjacent vertebrae along with disc degeneration and prolapse. Spinal fractures normally result from substantial trauma unless there is a predisposing bone disease. Primary or metastatic vertebral column tumors may involve the vertebral bodies, their bony processes, and adjacent tissues. OPLL affects mostly Japanese patients and causes cervical spinal canal narrowing due to calcification and ossification of the posterior spinal ligament.

Clinical Features

Scoliosis

Idiopathic scoliosis usually presents as spinal deformity of a child or teenager noticed by the family or on routine medical examination. There may be associated back pain but usually no neurologic deficits. Only rarely, the disorder can be severe enough at presentation to have caused spinal cord compression with varying degrees of myelopathy. Severe thoracic scoliosis with rib cage deformity that impairs the movement of the chest wall may cause restrictive lung disease, but this is similarly rare with idiopathic scoliosis. Patients with congenital or dysplastic causes tend to present at an earlier age and are more likely to have preoperative neurologic or pulmonary complications.

Patients with neuromuscular scoliosis have neurologic pathology that may reduce the effectiveness of NIOM. In planning for and anticipating the results of monitoring, one should consider the nature and severity of the underlying neurologic disease. Cerebral disease such as cerebral palsy may interfere with MEP and cortical SEP monitoring. Posterior fossa disorders such as Arnold-Chiari malformation may cause EP abnormalities. Spinal cord disorders such as syringomyelia, diastamatomyelia, tethered cord syndrome, and spinal cord tumor, compression, or trauma may cause varying degrees of sensorimotor impairment and/or EP degradation that occasionally seems out of proportion to any clinical deficit. The chronic corticospinal and dorsal column pathway degeneration of Freidreich's ataxia can prevent effective NIOM. Pure motor system diseases like spinal muscular atrophy, polio, and muscular dystrophy interfere with muscle MEPs but do not affect SEPs. Peripheral neuropathies may interfere with both modalities.

HGPPS patients have no clinical sensorimotor deficits and, with techniques appropriately modified for their nondecussation, have easily monitored potentials (3). Because the patients naturally compensate for the gaze palsy by turning their heads, they, their families, and their physicians may not notice the abnormality unless it is specifically sought.

Other Vertebral Column Disorders

Cervical spondylosis presents in older patients with neck pain, radiculopathy, and sometimes myelopathy with segmental and long tract sensorimotor deficits. OPLL generally presents with cervical myelopathy. Vertebral column tumors cause pain, radiculopathy, and myelopathy when cord compression is present. Spinal fractures may or may not be associated with acute traumatic myelopathy, sometimes paraplegia or quadriplegia. Again, the nature and severity of antecedent neurologic deficits should be incorporated into the NIOM strategy and expectations.

Vertebral Column Surgeries

Diverse surgeries are performed on the spine. There must be a tangible risk of injury to justify spinal cord monitoring. Scoliosis surgeries, usually posterior spinal fusion and instrumentation (PSF), anterior spinal release, or both are the most frequent indications. Some others include anterior cervical discectomy and fusion, decompressive laminectomy for spondylotic myelopathy or ossification of the posterior longitudinal ligament, reduction and fixation of spinal fractures, and spinal tumor resections.

Scoliosis

Posterior spinal fusion and instrumentation for scoliosis correction basically involves straightening with bilateral metallic rods anchored to vertebral processes of the prone patient's exposed spine. The anchors consist of pedicle screws and sublaminar hooks or wires. A properly directed pedicle screw passes through the pedicle's center into the vertebral body without breaking through the pedicle wall into the spinal canal or foramina. Sublaminar hooks and wires enter the spinal canal. To straighten the spine, anchor pairs along the rod are strategically forced apart (distracted) or pushed together (compressed) along with any necessary rod rotation before rigidly fixing attachments. Laminae are then decorticated and cancellous bone fragments spread over them to promote subsequent osseous fusion.

Anterior spinal release may be necessary before PSF for patients with rigid and congenital scoliosis who have vertebral malformations. The procedure is performed endoscopically or through a thoracotomy with the patient in a lateral position. Intervertebral discs and malformed vertebrae are resected; associated radicular arteries are sacrificed. The PSF may immediately follow or take place in a subsequent surgery. Sometimes anterior fixation using metal screws, rods, or plates is performed without PSF.

The large forces applied to the spine can injure the spinal cord through compression, traction, or ischemia, which may be potentiated by the use of controlled hypotension (60 mmHg mean arterial pressure) intended to reduce blood loss. The insertion of sublaminar hooks or wires can cause cord contusion, compression, or ischemia. This is more likely with insertions on the deformity's concave side, where the spinal cord is located, or where the spinal canal is narrow. Misdirected pedicle screws can perforate through the pedicle wall and cause adjacent nerve root injury. Misdirected cervical or thoracic screws can compromise the spinal cord. During anterior release, acute spinal deformity following vertebrectomy or interference with critical radicular blood supply can cause compressive or ischemic cord injury.

Other Procedures

Anterior cervical discectomy and fusion is performed through neck dissection with the patient supine. Involved discs are exposed and resected along with any posterior bony spurs. Bone grafts to produce subsequent osseous fusion are tapped into the evacuated disc spaces. A metallic plate is screwed onto the anterior surfaces of adjacent vertebrae for fixation. Spinal cord complications can result from contusion, compression, or ischemia.

Posterior decompression is achieved through laminectomies. Various types of instrumentation are used to reduce and fix spinal fractures and subluxations. Spinal tumor surgery involves resection of tumor and associated bony structures through posterior, anterior, or combined approaches. This may include vertebral bodies, sometimes at multiple contiguous levels. Bone grafts, plates, and other devices are used for fixation and subsequent fusion. Any of these procedures can injure the spinal cord or nerve roots.

A special consideration for cervical surgeries is that positioning the patient with neck extension or flexion can cause cord injury through cord compression, particularly when there is already compressive cervical myelopathy.

Monitoring Techniques

Because motor deficit—paraplegia or quadriplegia—is the primary concern, it is illogical to rely on SEPs mediated through the dorsal columns. However, SEPs were the first applied modality because MEP technology was unavailable. Their application was based on the premise that spinal cord compromise threatening paralysis might affect the full transverse extent of the cord, thereby causing SEP deterioration due to dorsal column conduction block. Intervention to relieve cord compromise might then be undertaken to restore potentials and hopefully prevent injury. Indeed, SEP monitoring halves the risk of intraoperative cord damage and therefore remains a standard NIOM component today (1). However, due to the anatomic separation and distinct blood supplies of the corticospinal and dorsal column systems, discrete compromise of one or the other still occurs. Consequently, occasional motor compromise without SEP warning or SEP deterioration without motor compromise is unavoidable, and SEP monitoring alone is no longer sufficient now that MEPs are available. Conversely, MEP monitoring cannot predict dorsal column integrity; therefore the two modalities should be combined (4).

Somatic Evoked Potentials

No universally standardized SEP monitoring approach exists. The International Federation of Clinical Neurophysiology (IFCN) published guidelines in 1999 (5). The American Clinical Neurophysiology Society (ACNS) guidelines, last published in 1994, are undergoing revision, and an American Society of Neurophysiologic Monitoring (ASNM) position statement was published in 2005 (6,7).

Upper limb SEPs are advised for cervical spinal cord monitoring, although the legs are also at risk. Lower limb SEPs are advised for thoracic spinal cord monitoring, but two guidelines point out the value of including upper limb SEP systemic controls (5,7). It is good practice to monitor all four limbs for both levels. Median nerve stimulation is generally recommended for upper limb SEPs, but the ulnar nerve is suggested instead when surgery risks C7-C8 cord injury that might be missed by median SEPs. The tibial nerve at the ankle is recommended for lower limb SEPs, with the peroneal nerve at the knee as an alternate site. To avoid the chance that bilateral simultaneous lower limb testing might mask unilateral cord compromise, the testing of each side separately, using alternating stimulation and asynchronous parallel averaging, is unanimously recommended.

All three guidelines recommend scalp recordings of cortical potentials. They differ somewhat on montages, but all recommended derivations assume normal sensory decussation; derivations for detecting and monitoring patients with nondecussation are not addressed. Subcortical potentials and caudal or peripheral SEP controls are also recommended. None specifically base montage recommendations on derivation signal-to-noise ratio (SNR) and its profound effect on reproducibility and the rapidity of feedback. The

ASNM guidelines do point out the importance of rapid surgical feedback and suggest 300 to 500 sweep averages, but ACNS guidelines recommend time-consuming averages of 500 to 2,000 sweeps, and IFCN guidelines do not address this issue. IFCN and ACNS guidelines suggest the additional use of invasive spinal SEP monitoring.

Signal-to-Noise Ratio and Feedback Rapidity

By enhancing surgical correlation, rapid feedback helps determine the likely cause of a pathologic EP decrement, thereby guiding intervention. Furthermore, the likelihood of successful intervention probably increases with early detection. Surgical feedback occurs at intervals determined by SEP averaging time. For reliable interpretation, SEPs must be averaged to reproducibility, defined as less than 20% to 30% random trial-to-trial amplitude variation and convincing waveform superimposition in successive trials. Since SNR has a powerful nonlinear inverse relationship to the necessary averaging time, even modest gains substantially accelerate feedback, so that one should strive to maximize SNR and reject low-SNR techniques (8).

Cortical Potentials

Scalp cortical SEPs are noninvasive, relatively easy to obtain, and applicable to surgery at any neuraxis level. Consequently they are almost universally employed; only a few centers emphasizing invasive spinal SEPs omit them. Given this widespread reliance, methods to optimize cortical SEP SNRs should be used. Anesthesia is important in this regard. Traditional balanced anesthesia with halogenated gases and nitrous oxide produces marked dose-related depression of cortical SEPs and should not be used. Satisfactory results may be possible using less than 0.5 minimum alveolar concentration (MAC) halogenated gases and opioids without nitrous oxide. However, it currently appears that intravenous anesthesia such as propofol/opioid infusion is optimal because of less dose-related amplitude suppression, thus enhancing SNRs (5).

Cortical SEPs should be further optimized by derivation selection. Standard laboratory derivations are not necessarily appropriate for NIOM because the goals are different. In the laboratory, valid comparison to normative data requires standardized derivations; the primary interpretive criterion is latency, and SNR is not critical because there is time to average many sweeps. In the operating room, derivations need not be standardized because patients are their own controls, amplitude change is the primary criterion and SNR is critical. Therefore the highest SNR derivation should be selected for monitoring, and this can vary between patients and sides (8). The selection process is straightforward for upper limb SEPs, more complex for lower limb SEPs, and in either case should include decussation assessment.

Upper Limb Derivations

Following median or ulnar nerve stimulation in a patient with normal sensory decussation, a negative 'N20' peak generated by the contralateral primary sensory cortex for the hand occurs at the contralateral postcentral scalp and a positive 'P22' potential arises over the frontal scalp. With nondecussation, the N20 is ipsilateral instead because the ipsilateral hemisphere generates it. Stimulating one side while simultaneously recording from CPc and CPi (midway between 10 and 20 central and parietal sites, contralateral and ipsilateral to the stimulated nerve) assesses decussation (3) (Figure 7.1).

Thus, input 1 of the monitoring derivation should be CPc for normal decussation or CPi for nondecussation. A frontal input 2 (FPz or Fz) boosts signal amplitude because the inverted P22 adds to the N20. This makes CPc-FPz generally satisfactory for NIOM, and it is tempting to use it routinely. However, nondecussation produces an inverted P22 in CPc-FPz that will be inaccurately mistaken for

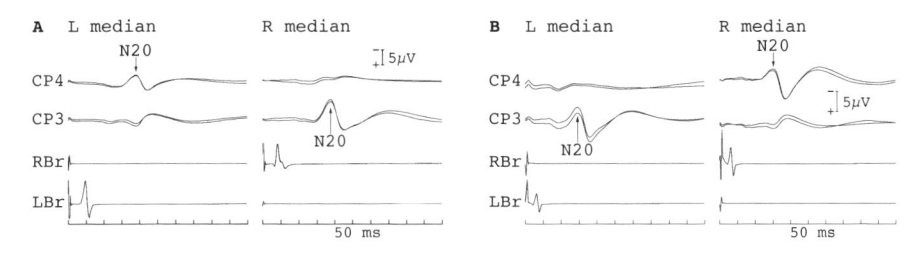

FIGURE 7.1 Median SEP decussation assessment. Mastoid reference; FPz can be used instead. RBr and LBr, right and left Brachial peripheral SEP traces. A. Normal decussation B. Nondecussation.

a small N20 unless decussation is assessed (Figure 7.2). Furthermore, frontal sites contain more anesthetic electroencephalographic (EEG) noise than centroparietal sites and, by overwhelming the amplitude advantage, this can reduce SNRs and slow feedback (8) (Figure 7.3). Because there is often substantially lower noise with CPc-CPi or CPc-CPz, these can thereby boost SNRs, thus accelerating feedback. The short interelectrode distance of CPc-CPz can further decrease noise, but in-phase cancellation when the N20 field reaches the midline may reduce signal amplitude. When this does not occur, it is often optimal.

In summary, the process for selecting the optimal upper limb cortical SEP monitoring derivation is to (a) assess decussation; (b) compare CPc-FPz, CPc-CPi, and CPc-CPz with normal decussation or CPi-FPz, CPi-CPc and CPi-CPz with nondecussation; and (c) use the derivation showing fastest reproducibility (highest SNR).

Lower Limb Derivations

Tibial nerve stimulation produces a positive 'P37' scalp potential generated by leg sensory cortex of the contralateral hemisphere with normal decussation and of the ipsilateral hemisphere with nondecussation. This potential's scalp field is highly variable (8–10). It is commonly maximal at CPz but may be maximal at Cz or Pz instead. With normal decussation, its field spreads over the scalp ipsilateral to the stimulated nerve while a simultaneous negative 'N37' potential usually arises over the contralateral scalp. The ipsilateral P37 field is sometimes so prominent that the maximum occurs at iCPi (intermediate centroparietal site CP1 or CP2, ipsilateral to the stimulated nerve) or even CPi rather than at the midline. In this case, the P37 may be small or virtually

FIGURE 7.2 Nondecussation and CPc-FPz. The median N20 arises over the hemisphere ipsilateral to the stimulated nerve. An inverted P22 (Inv. P22) from FPz masquerades as a small N20 in CPc-FPz, so that this derivation alone will miss nondecussation.

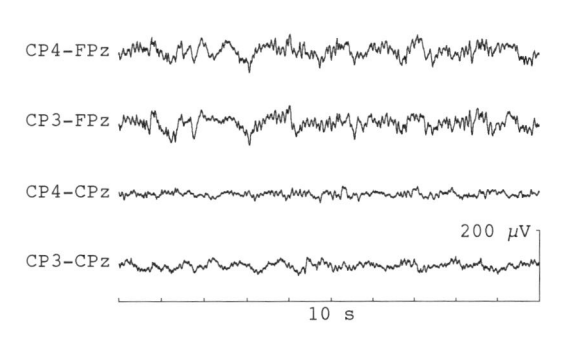

FIGURE 7.3 Frontal anesthetic EEG patterns. Higher EEG noise content in FPz derivations than centroparietal derivations reduces SEP signal-to-noise ratio.

absent at the midline. Occasionally, when the P37 maximum is at Cz, the N37 is ectopic at Pz. Furthermore, P37/N37 topography is most often different on each side. Finally, nondecussation reverses P37/N37 lateralization and cannot be detected by CPz-FPz alone (3). Simultaneously recording from CP4, CPz, and CP3 while stimulating one side assesses decussation (Figure 7.4).

To maximize SNRs, the monitoring derivation's input 1 should be the P37 maximum and input 2 the N37, usually CPc with normal decussation, CPi with nondecussation, and rarely Pz (8). Occasionally there is no apparent N37, and then an FPz input 2 may produce highest signal amplitude. However, by overwhelming this advantage, greater FPz noise often degrades SNR and slows feedback, so that FPz is infrequently used when the monitoring derivation is based on SNR (8). Note that Fz should not be used because it frequently contains anterior spread of the P37 field, causing in-phase signal cancellation, and it is likely also plagued by frontal EEG noise (10).

One must confront the marked topographic variability of lower limb cortical SEPs to provide consistently optimal monitoring. This presents the complex problem of identifying optimal derivations. A proven technique for the left tibial SEP follows (8,9):

1. A referential recording of FPz, Cz, CPz, Pz, CP4, CP2, CP1, and CP3-mastoid along with bilateral popliteal fossa recordings to confirm left stimulation is made in one panel and replicated. Simultaneously, a bipolar recording of Cz-CP4, CPz-CP4, Pz-CP4, CP1-CP4, CP3-CP4, Cz-FPz, CPz-FPz, Pz-FPz, CP1-FPz, CP3-FPz, and Cz-Pz is made and replicated in another panel.
2. The P37 and N37 are evaluated in the referential recording during acquisition. A predominantly ipsilateral scalp P37 field confirms decussation; there is usually also a confirmatory contralateral N37. Reversed lateralization identifies nondecussation.
3. If nondecussation is disclosed, the recording is repeated using Cz-CP3, CPz-CP3, Pz-CP3, CP2-CP3, CP4-CP3, Cz-FPz, CPz-FPz, Pz-FPz, CP2-FPz, CP4-FPz, and Cz-Pz bipolar traces. If nondecussation is known preoperatively, this montage is used in step 1.
4. The bipolar trace showing fastest reproducibility (usually but not always also having highest signal amplitude) is selected for monitoring. The optimal input 1 (P37 maximum) and input 2 (N37) are usually but not always evident in the referential recording.

In practice, both sides are simultaneously assessed using asynchronous parallel averaging and mirror-image bipolar montages (Figure 7.5). The procedure takes 5 to 10 minutes and is performed immediately after

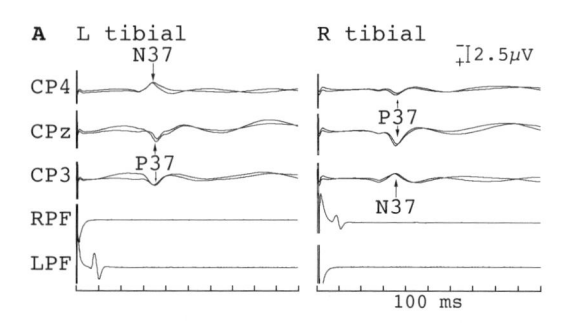

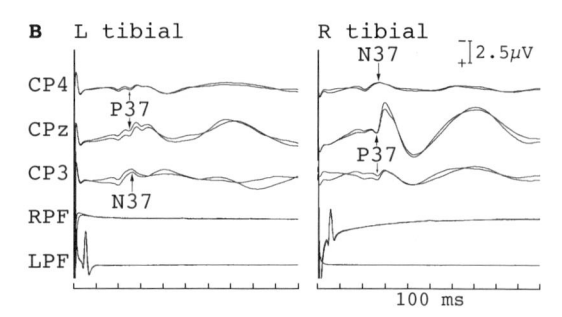

FIGURE 7.4 Tibial SEP decussation assessment. Mastoid reference. A. Normal decussation. B. Nondecussation. CPz-FPz alone will miss nondecussation.

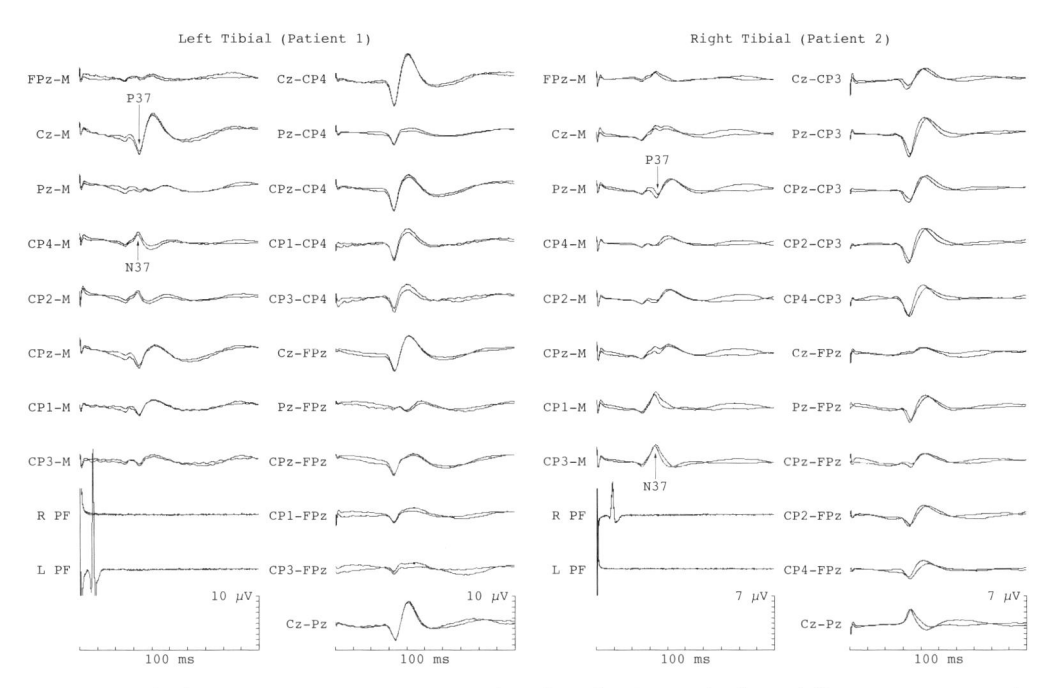

FIGURE 7.5 Tibial P37 optimization. M, mastoid. Left and right results from different patients are shown for illustrative purposes. The ipsilateral P37 field and contralateral N37 confirm decussation. Cz-CP4 was optimal on the left and Pz-CP3 on the right. Both had larger signal amplitude, less EEG noise and substantially greater signal-to-noise ratio than CPz-FPz.

induction using a multichannel averager with templates for normal decussation and nondecussation. It was developed with a simpler eight-channel averager using sequential tibial nerve stimulation to obtain a bilateral referential recording and then selective bipolar comparative recordings based on the referential results.

Table 7.1 lists the frequency of resulting optimal derivations. Note that commonly recommended routine monitoring derivations CPz-FPz, iCPi-FPz, and CPi-CPc are actually infrequently or rarely optimal.

This approach optimizes lower limb cortical SEP recording for each side of each patient. In addition, one can confidently attribute P37 absence to pathology without being concerned about spurious absence due to topographic variation. Most importantly, it produces a mean 2.1:1 SNR advantage over the traditional CPz-FPz derivation (8). The arithmetic of averaging translates this to a mean 4:1 acceleration of surgical feedback: the median sweep number to reproducibility is 128 for the optimized P37 and 512 for CPz-FPz (8). Furthermore, for any given sweep number, mean amplitude variation due to residual noise is substantially reduced, so that true amplitude change is more readily detected and the chance of misleading random amplitude fluctuation is diminished (8).

Although more complex than existing guidelines, the principles of patient-centered care justify the additional effort for superior results. If one chooses to apply only traditional FPz, CP4, CPz, and CP3 electrodes, some optimization can still be performed. Simultaneously recording CP4-, CPz-, and CP3-FPz will assess decussation. One could then compare CPz-CPc, CPi-CPc, CPz-FPz, and CPi-FPz for normal decussation or CPz-CPi, CPc-CPi, CPz-FPz, and CPi-FPz for nondecussation and select the best of these for monitoring. Of these derivations, CPz-CPc

TABLE 7.1 Optimal Tibial P37 Monitoring Derivations for 314 Tibial Nerves of 157 patients*

	Input 2 (− down)			
Input 1 (+ down)	CPc	FPz	CPi†	Pz
Cz	58	3	1	3
CPz	119	32	5	0
Pz	40	12	0	—
iCPi	35	1	—	0
CPi	5	0	—	0

*CPc and CPi, CP4 or CP3 contralateral and ipsilateral to the stimulated nerve; iCPi, CP2 or CP1 intermediate centroparietal sites, ipsilateral.
†Nondecussation.
Source: Combined data from MacDonald et al. (8,9).

will most often but not always be best because it combines the most common P37 and N37 maxima and has lower noise than FPz derivations. If one insists on routinely applying a single standard derivation, then CPz-CPc is the best overall choice, but decussation should still be evaluated because CPz-CPi would be needed for nondecussation.

In summary, the process for selecting the lower limb cortical SEP monitoring derivation is to (a) assess decussation, (b) compare derivations appropriate for the patient's decussation status, and (c) use the derivation showing fastest reproducibility (highest SNR). The full optimization described above accounts best for known topographic variability.

Subcortical Potentials

Subcortical SEP are noninvasive and show no significant topographic variability. Being generated in the cervicomedullary junction, they are applicable to spinal cord monitoring. Since this function is already served by cortical SEPs, the principal rationale for including subcortical SEPs is their lesser sensitivity to inhalation anesthesia. This was important when balanced inhalation anesthesia and suboptimal cortical SEP derivations were the rule, but it is not relevant to modern cortical SEP methodology, which should include appropriate anesthesia and derivation selection. In fact, in this context, the low SNR of subcortical potentials interferes with feedback rapidity, particularly for lower limb monitoring (8). Consequently these potentials are presently not universally applied to spine surgery NIOM.

Upper Limb

The upper limb subcortical P14-N18 complex is recorded with a scalp-noncephalic reference derivation. To avoid cortical N20/P22 contamination, the best input 1 is CPi for normal decussation or CPc for nondecussation. To avoid cervical cord potential contamination, EPc (Erb's point contralateral to the stimulated nerve) is commonly used for input 2. Some use the mastoids instead. Others prefer a C5S-FPz derivation that combines the cervical N13 and inverted P14 to boost signal amplitude. All these derivations are prone to high noise content from long interelectrode distance, electrocardiogram (ECG), frontal-dominant EEG fast activity, and sometimes electromyography (EMG). This tends to degrade SNRs and prolong averaging. Nevertheless, upper limb subcortical potentials are relatively quickly reproduced, but they can be considered optional when cortical SEPs are properly recorded and present.

Lower Limb

The tibial subcortical P31-N35 complex is recorded with a standard FPz-C5S or C2S derivation. Reversing the inputs produces an upgoing deflection that is sometimes incorrectly called cervical when FPz is actually the active electrode. Some prefer FPz-mastoid, which produces a slightly lower signal amplitude due to in-phase cancellation from some mastoid P31 activity. Owing to small signal (mean 1.1 µV) and high noise (mean 37 µV), the SNR of the P31 recorded with FPz-C5S is very low (mean 4.9 times lower than the optimized P37) (8). Thus, a median of 1,000 sweeps must be averaged for reproducibility,

2,000 sweeps are needed for about 24% of tibial nerves, and replication is not practically demonstrable for about 7% (8). Clearly this potential is too slow and inconsistent for reliably effective monitoring. It might be a useful fallback potential when the P37 is absent due to cerebral pathology and when it is depressed by inhalation anesthesia or suboptimally recorded, but it should not be standard (8).

Peripheral Potentials

Although not universally applied, peripheral SEPs enhance interpretation. The standard PF potential is satisfactory for lower limb monitoring. The traditional EP potential suffers from high noise content (particularly ECG). Instead, a brachial (Br) potential analogous to the PF and recorded medial to the biceps tendon just above the elbow is a better choice (4). Properly recorded peripheral SEPs require minimal averaging due to high SNRs that frequently make them visible in single sweeps (8). They provide a logical basis for determining supramaximal stimulus intensity. Moreover, they provide technical control and detect distal limb ischemia or pressure. When faced with cortical SEP decrement, simultaneous peripheral SEP loss immediately points to stimulus failure or distal limb problems, while preservation immediately excludes these factors.

Spinal Potentials

Spinal SEPs are ascending dorsal column volleys recorded with invasive epidural, subdural, or interspinous ligament electrodes. They are almost immune to anesthesia because they are purely conductive (5,6). The latter property may be valuable when cortical SEPs are pathologically absent, depressed by inhalation anesthesia, or suboptimally recorded – particularly since spinal SEPs are more rapidly reproduced than the P31. Despite a large experience with spinal SEPs in Japan and England, the technique is not widely used (11,12). This may be due to an avoidance of invasive electrodes to eliminate the small chance of hemorrhage or infection as well as to the evolution of modern noninvasive SEP methods.

Motor Evoked Potentials

No standardized MEP monitoring approach or guideline currently exists. Nevertheless, MEPs should be a standard component of spinal cord monitoring during vertebral column surgery, and future guidelines will certainly include them. The basic technique is discussed in Chapter 2, and MEP monitoring has recently been extensively reviewed (13). Transcranial electrical stimulation (TES) activates the corticospinal system, and recordings are made from the spinal cord (D wave) and/or peripheral muscle.

Spinal D Waves

Following single-pulse TES, a descending corticospinal tract volley known as the D (direct) wave can be monitored in the spinal epidural or subdural space. The bipolar recording electrode is inserted into the epidural space through a flavotomy after posterior spine exposure or threaded up the subdural space through lumbar puncture prior to opening.

The D wave has several advantages. It is relatively immune to anesthesia because no synapses are involved and it does not require omission of neuromuscular blockade. In addition, it has rapid reproducibility due to high SNR and high stability. Furthermore, there is excellent correlation to long-term motor outcome for intramedullary spinal cord tumor and cerebral tumor surgery.

On the other hand, there are several disadvantages in using the D wave for vertebral column surgery. The response is not clearly lateralized; excludes alpha motor neurons, which are more rapidly disabled by ischemia than tracts; and becomes too small to record at the lumbosacral cord where the corticospinal tracts end. In addition, the epidural technique cannot be used for anterior procedures or during opening and closure of posterior spine surgeries. Furthermore, there is always the concern about invasive electrode complications, although rare. Most importantly, epidural D waves can produce false results during scoliosis surgery: an up to 75% decrease – or increase – of D-wave amplitude has been found in a number of patients despite unchanged muscle MEPs and neurologic outcome (14). This might be due to an increase or decrease of the distance between the epidural electrode and the spinal cord, as its position within the spinal canal shifts after straightening. Subdural D waves possibly might not pose this problem.

Consequently, despite a large spine surgery D-wave monitoring experience in Japan and Australia, it seems unlikely that this technique will become a standard component of orthopedic NIOM (11,15). Note that it should be standard for intramedullary spinal cord tumor surgery (13).

Muscle Potentials

Pulse train TES that evokes muscle MEP through temporal summation at alpha motor neurons is a major advance, having important advantages for spine surgery. No averaging is required owing to very high SNRs, so that feedback can be instantaneous (although interrupted by SEPs). It incorporates alpha motor neurons and assesses the corticospinal system from brain to individual limbs or even specific muscles relevant to the level of surgery. There is excellent correlation with early postoperative motor outcome, and muscle MEPs are more sensitive for spinal cord compromise than SEPs during spine surgery. The technique makes unpredicted spinal cord motor injuries unlikely and will almost certainly further reduce the incidence of spinal cord complications.

Repetitive stimulation of the brain raises safety concerns; these are reviewed elsewhere (13,16,17). In short, the technique is sufficiently safe in expert hands using appropriate precautions. Bite injuries of the tongue or lips due to jaw muscle contractions are the most common adverse effect, having an estimated incidence of 0.3%; there has been one instance of jaw fracture and one of endotracheal tube rupture (13). Preventive soft bite blocks are mandatory. Seizures, cardiac arrhythmias, and scalp burns are very rare.

Muscle MEPs are even more sensitive to anesthesia than cortical SEPs. The main interference occurs at alpha motor neurons; anesthesia can obliterate muscle responses while having little effect on corticospinal volleys. Again, intravenous anesthesia such as propofol/opioid infusion appears optimal, but significant infusion increments or boluses can still reduce or obliterate muscle MEPs and may require increments of TES intensity and/or pulse number (13). Neuromuscular blockade is omitted after intubation or incomplete and tightly controlled.

Stimulating electrodes are commonly placed at 10 to 20 central scalp sites approximately overlying motor cortex. Sites 1 or 2 cm anterior may diminish TES artifact by increasing the distance from the scalp SEP recording electrodes through which TES current reaches the headbox. The authors use C+1-cm sites and name them M (motor) sites. For the same reason, CP scalp SEP recording sites that are slightly posterior to C' sites are preferred.

Published stimulus parameters use three to eight rectangular pulses and a 1- to 5-ms interpulse interval (IPI). There is evidence that an IPI of 4 ms may generally be optimal for leg muscle MEPs, and the authors find five pulses with 4 ms IPI to be a good starting point for spine surgery (18). Various stimulators are effective, including specialized devices from Digitimer (www.digitimer.com), Inomed (www.inomed.com), Axon Systems (www.axonsystems.com), and Cadwell (www.cadwell.com) as well as standard Nicolet Endeavor or Viking NIOM stimulators (www.viasyshealthcare.com) in constant-voltage mode (13). Stimulation is adjusted to clear suprathreshold responses of all targeted muscles or to the threshold of the last recruited muscle. Adjustments of pulse num-

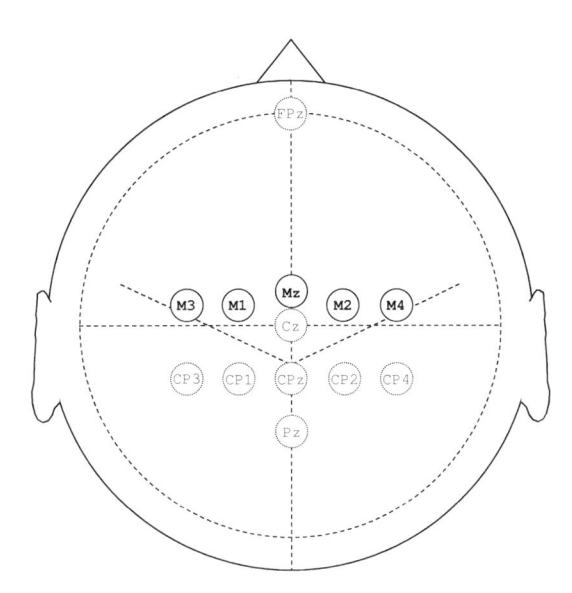

FIGURE 7.6 Scalp electrode sets. Solid circles designate the transcranial electric stimulation array and broken circles designate the scalp SEP recording set. [Modified from MacDonald (13), by permission of Springer.]

ber or IPI may be needed. Immediately preceding the test stimulus by one or more preconditioning stimuli facilitates the response and is a commonly used technique.

It is helpful to apply an array of TES electrodes such as M4, M2, Mz, M1, and M3 from which stimulus montages can be selected to optimize technique (Figure 7.6). Because TES preferentially activates brain underneath the anode, montages are given as anode-cathode. Vertex-frontal TES can evoke bilateral leg MEPs, but is not very efficient and is ineffective for arm MEPs. Coronal TES that is more efficient and evokes arm and leg MEPs is more commonly used. Inter-hemispheric M3/M4 TES is very efficient, but tends to produce a strong patient twitch and may increase the likelihood of bite injury (13). M1/M2 TES can be an effective alternative with fewer tendencies to these problems, but some patients require M3/M4 for monitoring. Because of asymmetric muscle responses maximal contralateral to the anode, M1-M2 or M3-M4 TES with right MEP recording is alternated with M2-M1 or M4-M3 TES and left MEP recording. This strategy is reversed for nondecussation because responses are then maximal ipsilateral to the anode instead (3). Because hemispheric M3-Mz and M4-Mz TES produces predominantly unilateral corticospinal activation, these montages are used for decussation assessment (Figure 7.7). The authors do not recommend them for monitoring spine surgery because they are less efficient for leg MEPs (13).

Thus, a way to optimize TES montages is to (a) assess decussation with M3-Mz and M4-Mz, (b) Compare M1/M2 and M3/M4 montages appropriate for the patient's decussation status, and (c) favor M1/M2 montages if effective or use M3/M4 montages if needed (Figure 7.8).

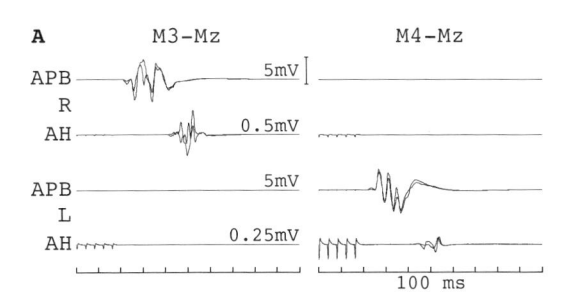

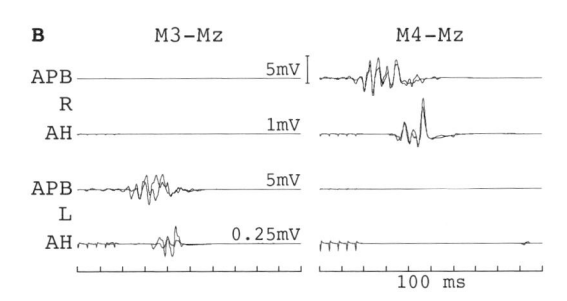

FIGURE 7.7 Muscle MEP decussation assessment. APB = abductor pollicis brevis; AH = abductor hallucis. A. Normal decussation. B. Nondecussation.

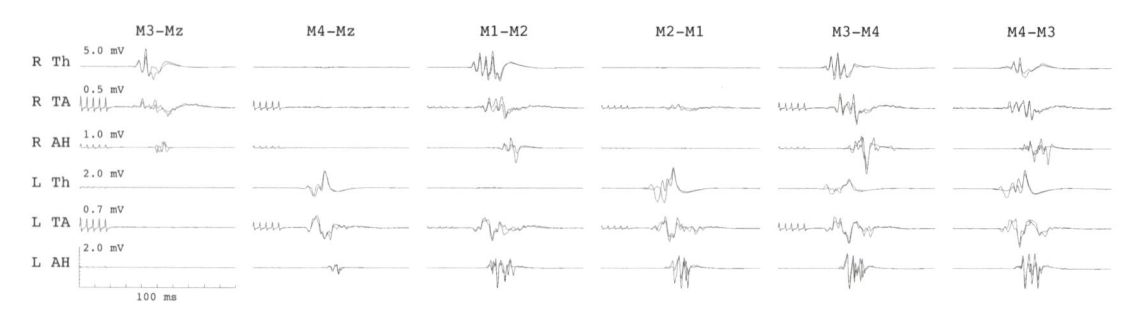

FIGURE 7.8 Transcranial electric stimulation montage selection. Th = thenar; TA = tibialis anterior; AH = abductor hallucis. Nicolet Endeavor stimulator, 5 pulse trains, 4 ms IPI, 300 V. Hemispheric M3-Mz and M4-Mz stimuli confirmed motor decussation by showing anode-contralateral muscle MEP. Interhemispheric M3/M4 stimulation produced largest bilateral responses, maximal contralateral to the anode. M1/M2 stimuli produced sufficiently large leg MEP with less bilateral activation. M1-M2 and M2-M1 were selected for monitoring right and left MEP. Some patients require M3/M4. [From MacDonald (13), by permission of Springer.]

INTERPRETATION AND WARNING CRITERIA

Interpretation means to "set forth the meaning of." Reliable NIOM interpretation requires appropriate training and experience in order to properly synthesize the relevant neurophysiologic, systemic, technical, and surgical factors.

Fundamental Considerations

The wholly empiric traditional EP warning criteria of a more than 50% decrease of amplitude or 10% increase in latency need qualification. Latency prolongation is an illogical criterion because it is the hallmark of demyelination, a chronic process that is not expected during spine surgery. Rather, acute axonal conduction block or neuronal failure underlies intraoperative pathologic SEP or MEP decrement and predominantly reduce potential amplitude. Thus, amplitude is the primary intraoperative consideration.

It is important to keep in mind that each successive SEP provides only an estimate of true potential amplitude distorted by residual noise that causes random trial-to-trial variation of this estimate. Poor reproducibility (greater than 30% amplitude variation, unconvincing trace superimposition) compromises the identification of true amplitude change because large deviations of estimated amplitude can be due to chance alone; then it is best to rely on potential disappearance. Good reproducibility (20% to 30% variation, convincing superimposition) is essential to reliably identify true greater than 50% SEP amplitude decrements. With excellent reproducibility (less than 20% variation, nearly exact superimposition), lesser degrees of true SEP amplitude decrement can be detected and may be significant (4). The issue is whether there is an amplitude decrement that clearly exceeds random variation. Note that pathologic SEP decrements tend to underestimate the degree of sensory pathway conduction block due to central amplification.

Muscle MEPs have no significant noise distortion but show substantial trial-to-trial variation due to inherent fluctuations of alpha motor neuron excitability (13). They also exhibit high sensitivity, so that pathologic decrements tend to overestimate the degree of corticospinal system compromise. Because of these properties, only disappearance or possibly marked attenuation amounting to virtual disappearance of a previously consistent muscle MEP is generally accepted as significant (13). This is not an excessively late warning during spine surgery because reappearance commonly follows intervention. Although there is supportive evidence for more sensitive criteria –such as a threshold elevation greater than 100 V MEPs or transformation from long-duration polyphasic to short-duration biphasic potentials—these approaches are presently controversial.(13)

Systemic Factors

Systemic factors cause cortical SEP and/or muscle MEP alterations in virtually every surgery. Mild hypothermia prolongs latency but has less effect on amplitude; intentional deep hypothermia obliterates both potentials but is not used during spine surgery. Anesthetic increments can reduce amplitude, but even with stable anesthesia there is often unexplained progressive "potential fade" manifest by falling cortical SEP amplitudes and muscle MEP fading and/or increasing stimulus requirements (13,19). Modest blood pressure fluctuation does not normally cause EP changes because autoregulation maintains constant blood flow within the spinal cord and brain, but blood pressure and potential amplitude may rise and fall together with anesthesia that alters both. Systemic effects vary from minor to greater than 50% cortical SEP amplitude reduction, which occurs in at least 10% of spine surgeries, as well as striking muscle MEP reduction, threshold elevation, or even loss (4) (Figure 7.9). This undermines the traditional comparison to "baseline," which incorrectly assumes a stable systemic state. Consequently, a different approach is needed for these systemically sensitive potentials in order to avoid false alarms.

Systemic effects are generalized and tend to be gradual. Thus they produce approximately parallel four-limb EP changes that are reliably identified by upper limb controls during thoracic procedures (4). During cervical surgery, when four-limb EP decrement could be due to spinal cord compromise, gradual changes evolving over many minutes or hours

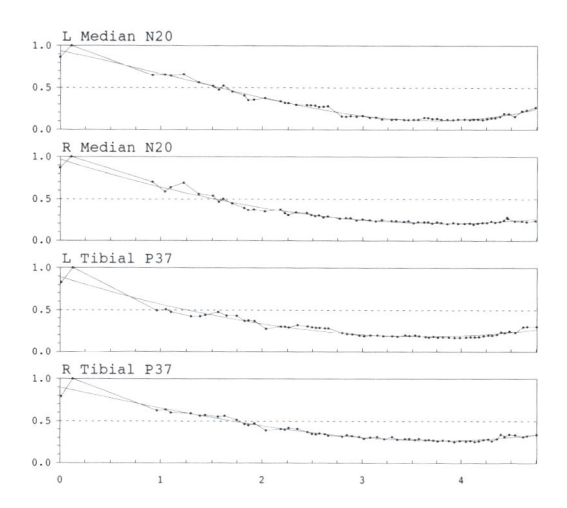

FIGURE 7.9 Unusually marked cortical somatosensory EP fade during scoliosis surgery. Plotted amplitudes are normalized to the largest observed values (1.0). Note the gradual generalized and approximately parallel amplitude reductions, making valid baseline determinations impossible. There was no injury.

are likely to be systemic. Large anesthetic boluses that can produce relatively abrupt generalized EP decrements should be avoided. Similarly, administration or potentiation of neuromuscular blockade can cause generalized muscle MEP loss (13).

Technical Factors

Technical problems must also be identified. Peripheral SEP loss immediately points to the possibility of stimulus failure, which can then be rectified without surgical alarm. Similarly, simultaneous arm and leg MEP loss during thoracic procedures and loss of cranial muscle contractions or MEPs during cervical surgery suggests TES failure. Elevated TES or scalp SEP electrode impedance occasionally causes spurious potential reduction, identified by rechecking impedance. Amplifier saturation (flat line) of variable duration following electrosurgery or even TES can cause spurious EP reduction or loss. Resuming monitoring only after raw traces such as EEG from scalp

SEP derivations show amplifier recovery prevents this problem.

Pathologic EP Decrements

After excluding systemic and technical factors, an abrupt focal EP decrement is the hallmark of pathologic compromise (4,13). These events typically occur within seconds or minutes, depending on the recording time resolution. In properly designed recordings, they are visually obvious, so that their interpretation does not really benefit from quantification.

Distal Nerve Disturbances

Distal limb ischemia or pressure can cause EP decrement of the affected limb due to peripheral nerve conduction block and is readily identified by peripheral SEP loss. Resolution of these conditions might help to prevent peripheral nerve injury.

Proximal Nerve or Plexus Disturbances

Proximal nerve or plexus conduction block occasionally causes EP decrement of the affected limb without affecting peripheral SEPs. This occurs frequently enough in the arms during spine surgery due to extreme shoulder positions that routine upper limb monitoring may also help prevent postoperative neuropathy or brachial plexopathy (4). Proximal nerve and plexus lesions have not yet been described in the legs.

Radiculopathy

Due to radicular overlap, these NIOM methods do not reliably identify isolated root conduction block or injury (13). Dermatomal SEP monitoring might identify individual sensory root dysfunction but is controversial and must increase complexity and slow feedback. A discrete motor root injury may not be apparent in muscle MEPs, but sometimes does produce a visually obvious abrupt step reduction of MEP amplitude when the injured root supplies part of the recorded muscle's innervation (13). It is therefore reasonable to monitor MEPs from several arm muscles spanning C4 through T1 roots during cervical surgery or from multiple leg muscles during lumbosacral surgery. There is evidence that concomitant EMG and pedicle screw stimulation may enhance lumbar nerve root protection.

Spinal Cord Compromise

Thoracic spinal cord compromise produces abrupt bilateral or unilateral leg MEP loss and/or tibial cortical SEP amplitude decrement; an initially unilateral decrement can become bilateral but may remain asymmetric (4,13). Frequently there is no indication of impending MEP loss and the potential simply disappears in the next trial. Occasionally there is a retrospectively appreciable amplitude reduction immediately before, but muscle MEP instability makes it difficult to ascertain its significance until disappearance occurs. Four patterns of EP decrement are seen: (a) MEP only, (b) MEP followed by SEP, (c) simultaneous MEP/SEP, and (d) SEP only (rare). So far SEP followed by MEP decrement has not been reported but might be possible. These patterns confirm higher MEP than SEP sensitivity for cord compromise.

Cervical cord compromise produces the same patterns but affecting both arm and leg potentials, depending on the level of involvement. Focal EP decrements can be seen to spread and such patterns further indicate pathologic change because systemic effects cannot explain them (Figure 7.10).

Rapid surgical feedback assists interpretation by implicating the current or last surgical maneuver as the most likely cause of cord compromise. Undoing of this maneuver (e.g., releasing instrumentation, removing the last inserted hook, etc.) is frequently followed by EP restoration and no postoperative deficit, suggesting cord injury prevention. Because hypotension (mean arterial pressure less than 60 mmHg) can cause ischemia of a compromised spinal cord already having marginal perfusion, restoring blood pressure may be followed by potential restoration. Even without hypotension, raising mean arterial blood

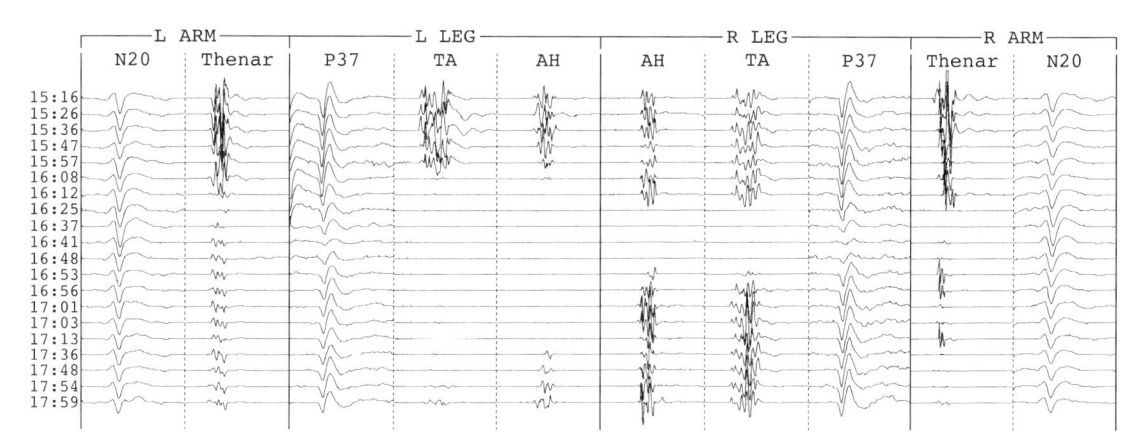

FIGURE 7.10 Evolving focal EP decrements. TA = tibialis anterior; AH = abductor hallucis. Traces are selected from the intraoperative record that had faster time resolution. The patient had nondecussation requiring reversed montages for monitoring. There was isolated left leg MEP loss at 16:08 immediately after T1 hook placement. Raising blood pressure had no beneficial effect. At 16:25 there was generalized MEP loss, and by 16:37 bilateral tibial SEP decrement. The hook was finally removed, followed by potential reappearance. Left leg muscle MEPs did not reappear until closure, and there was mild transient postoperative left leg weakness. The pattern suggests asymmetric high thoracic evolving to bilateral low cervical cord compromise and cannot be explained by systemic factors. [From MacDonald (13), by permission of Springer.]

pressure above 80 mmHg can sometimes appear to be effective and is a reasonable additional intervention. High-dose steroid administration may be considered but is not proven to improve outcome.

Occurrences suggesting injury prevention should not be classified as false positive. Test condition analysis is inappropriate because intervention based on the test's result influences the condition (outcome). This analysis can only be valid for the final EP results before patient awakening. Pathologic EP decrements persisting to the end of monitoring regularly predict clinical deficits that are congruent to the affected modality and limbs but not necessarily complete or permanent (13).

TECHNICAL CONSIDERATIONS

Preparation

Preparation begins with the monitoring request. The diagnosis and proposed surgical procedure indicate the structures at risk. The patient's neurologic status should be incorporated into monitoring expectations. Ideally, each patient would have a preoperative consultation including neurologic examination and EP studies, but this is not essential for neurologically intact patients. When resources permit, it is worthwhile doing this at least for those patients known to have neurologic impairment. Already absent SEPs are highly unlikely to be monitorable and the effort of attempting to do so can be avoided. However, some patients with impaired muscle strength and absent muscle MEPs to transcranial magnetic stimulation have monitorable TES MEPs. Patients with complete paraplegia or quadriplegia are an exception and should not undergo attempted MEP monitoring. Scoliosis patients with horizontal gaze palsy should have preoperative SEP and transcranial magnetic MEP decussation assessment whenever possible.

Relative contraindications for TES must be noted, including epilepsy, cortical lesions, defects in the skull, raised intracranial pressure, cardiac disease, intracranial electrodes, vascular clips, shunts, cardiac pacemakers, or other implanted biomedical devices (16). Because these are not proven to increase TES hazards, they must be carefully weighed against the risk of omitting MEPs, and a number of patients with these conditions have undergone uneventful TES MEP monitoring (13,17).

Patients should be informed about monitoring procedures and all material hoped-for benefits and possible adverse effects including bite injury and the rarer possibilities of intraoperative seizure, cardiac arrhythmia, movement-induced injury, skin burns at electrode sites, and potential complications of any invasive electrodes to be used. Informed consent should be obtained.

Monitoring equipment should be assembled. The recording instrument should have NIOM software and at least 8 channels; 16 or more channels are preferable. An integrated or external stimulator suitable for TES must be available. The necessary electrodes and supplies should be gathered. EEG cup electrode scalp sets can be prebraided to save time during application. Packaged sterile needle electrodes for scalp recording cannot be prebraided, but commercially available paired needles are convenient for distal stimulation and recording.

Procedure

Hands should be washed and gloved for patient preparation (17). The head must be accurately measured. Recording leads destined for the same recording derivation must be tightly braided or paired to reduce extraneous electrical artifact. Impedances must be checked and should at least be less than 5 kOhms; a 2-kOhm limit is preferable to ensure balanced impedance values.

The application of surface electrodes before the patient's call to surgery minimizes impact on operating room and anesthesia time. Proper skin preparation with light abrasion regularly produces low impedance. A few patients unable to tolerate preparation while awake need postinduction application. Prebraided EEG cup scalp electrode sets for SEP recording and TES are effective and securely attached with collodion. Standard adhesive ECG discs are effective for shoulder ground and limb SEP stimulation and recording sites. Their snap-on reusable leads can be prebraided and labeled for rapid connection. Patients with unusually thick or edematous ankles may require needles for tibial nerve stimulation. Stimulating bar electrodes can cause pressure necrosis and are discouraged (17). Surface electrodes are suitable for muscle MEPs, but paired subdermal needles inserted after induction are widely preferred.

The routine application of all electrodes in the operating room after induction is a common alternative. The quickness of needle electrodes minimizes preparation time, which becomes an issue in this setting. Spiral needles fix securely in the scalp; straight needles are more difficult to secure here but are readily fixed with tape elsewhere.

Although surface electrodes are more time-consuming and require skill in the use of collodion, they have excellent recording and safety profiles. Needle electrodes pose a greater risk of accidental electrosurgery-induced skin burns, infectious complications, needle-stick events, and broken tips lodged under the skin (17). They are generally discouraged for neurophysiologic testing but are convenient for NIOM. Both are effective and monitoring teams should decide which best matches their circumstances and patients' needs.

The anesthesiologist should be consulted for assistance in obtaining optimal monitoring. Ideally this will involve intravenous anesthesia if possible. Neuromuscular blockade may be necessary for intubation but should be short-acting to avoid interfering with initial muscle MEP recordings. A courteous reminder to place a soft bite block may be needed.

The first traces after induction should identify optimal derivations and assess decussation if not already done. The authors begin with tibial cortical SEP optimization that simultaneously assesses sensory decussation. Then initial upper limb SEP can be obtained without needing to reassess decussation. The first MEP should be recorded bilaterally to M3-Mz and then M4-Mz TES to assess motor decussation if not already known. Then right and left MEP are obtained to M1/M2 or if necessary, M3/M4 stimuli according to the patient's decussation status. Muscle MEPs may initially be absent if inhalation agents have been used for induction or there is residual neuromuscular blockade; one may need to wait until a favorable state for MEP recording to be established.

Initial baselines are set after determining optimal technique. During cervical procedures, this should be accomplished prior to patient positioning. The anesthesiologist's collaboration in quickly establishing a suitable systemic state for SEP/MEP recording is particularly important for these patients. One or more EP sets should be obtained after positioning. Monitoring is suspended during the electrosurgery of opening and then resumed.

Baselines are reset after opening, and then sequential EP sets (upper and lower limb SEPs, right and left MEPs) are acquired as rapidly as permitted by the averaging time needed for SEP reproducibility. Spinal cord ischemia causes muscle MEP loss within 2 minutes and is an important injury mechanism during spine surgery (4,13). Therefore set acquisition within about 2 minutes without compromising reproducibility should be the goal (4,8). SNR-based SEP optimization allows this in the majority of patients (Figure 7.11). Pathological EP decrements commonly arise within this time frame (Figure 7.12). The routine use of lower SNR derivations such as CPz-FPz and FPz-C5S will very often exceed 2 minutes acquisition time or impair accuracy if averaging is cut short of reproducibility (8).

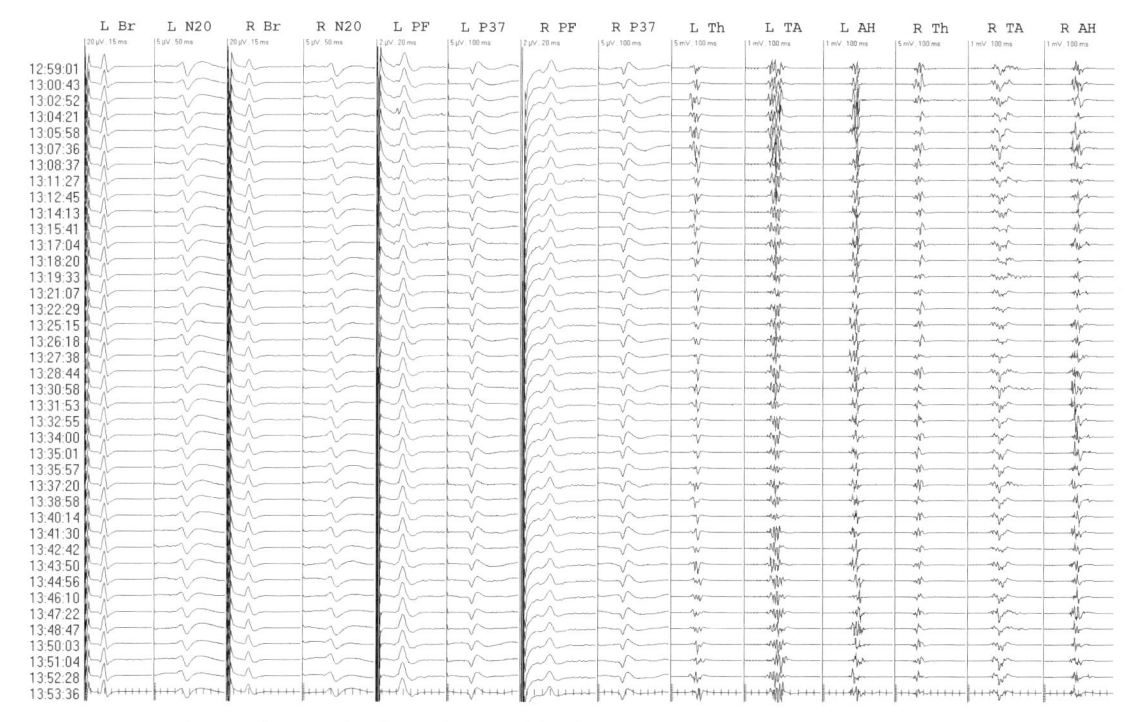

FIGURE 7.11 A typical example of rapid surgical feedback made possible through SNR-based SEP optimization. The average feedback interval was 1.4 minutes. Br = median brachial peripheral SEP; Th = thenar; TA = tibialis anterior; AH = abductor hallucis.

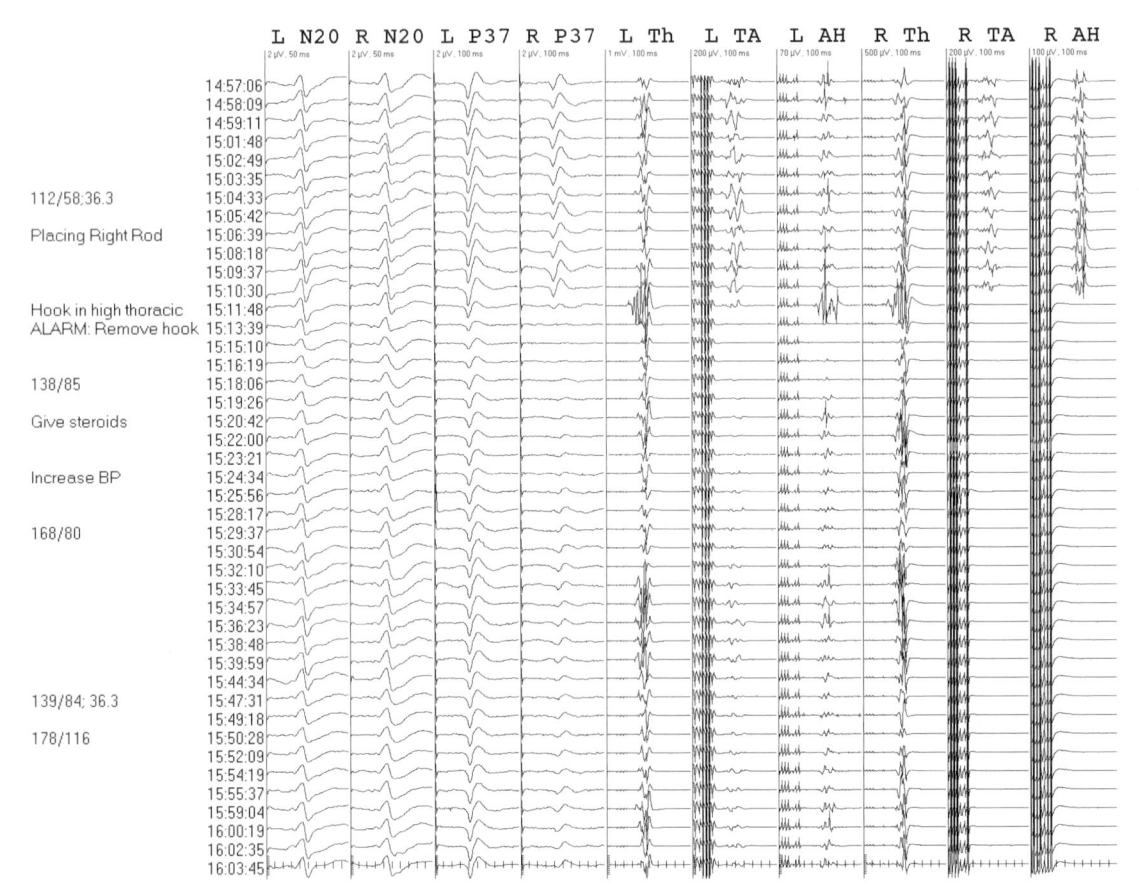

FIGURE 7.12 Typically abrupt focal decrements. Th = thenar; TA = tibialis anterior; AH = abductor hallucis. The average feedback interval was 1.5 minutes. There was no sign of trouble at 15:10:30 while a high thoracic sublaminar hook was being inserted, but 1 minute and 18 seconds later there was right leg MEP loss and marked tibial SEP decrement. One minute and 9 seconds after that, decrements were bilateral. The hook was removed and potentials started reappearing in a few minutes. Left leg potentials showed full SEP and partial MEP recovery; there was no clinical deficit of this limb. Right leg potentials showed partial SEP recovery and persistent MEP absence; there was moderate postoperative leg weakness and dorsal column sensory deficit but preserved ambulation and eventual complete clinical recovery. This suggested probable spinal cord contusion. [From MacDonald (13), by permission of Springer.]

Baselines can be reset if systemic potential fading is observed. Maintaining the presence of fading muscle MEP may require intensity and/or pulse number increments, more facilitation with repetitive preconditioning pulse trains, and sometimes a switch from M1/M2 to M3/M4 (13).

Patient twitching with TES normally does not interfere with spine surgery; surgeons quickly become accustomed to it and need not be warned before stimulation (4). Anterior cervical surgery is an exception, because neck muscle contractions may interfere and careful stimulus timing and communication may be required (13).

Documentation should be thorough. Anesthesia, blood pressure, temperature, TES parameter or other technical changes, surgical maneuvers, and communications with anesthesiology and surgery teams must be noted. The surgeon need not be informed about systemic changes unless they begin to prevent effective monitoring, in which case the anesthesiologist must also be consulted for help. Technical problems must be corrected without surgical alarm. The likely meaning of and possible interventions for pathologic decrements must be brought to surgical attention immediately; a competent intraoperative neurophysiologist should be responsible for this call and the surgeon's response and interventions should be documented.

Every effort must be made to avoid false warnings or reassurance. These can adversely affect the patient's surgical result or neurologic outcome and seriously undermine the surgeon's confidence (17). Such events should be rare with good technique.

Postprocedure

Monitoring is normally discontinued at closure. Rarely, a patient is kept under sedation postoperatively; then the possibility of extended intensive care unit monitoring can be considered. Unless sedation is very deep, TES may be too painful to apply in this circumstance.

Hands should be washed and gloved for disassembly (17). Collodion-fixed electrodes are removed with acetone. Neither of these flammable substances should be in open use during electrosurgery (17). EEG cup electrodes are bagged for later cleaning and disinfecting (17). Needle electrodes are handled by the stem, not recapped, and disposed of in a sharps container (17). Adhesive and invasive electrodes are disposed of in the appropriate biomedical hazard waste container. Any sign of skin burn or injury apart from minor abrasion from skin preparation should prompt an investigation to rectify the cause (17). Subdermal broken needle tips must be brought to the surgeon's attention for subsequent surgical removal.

The monitoring instrument and its cables and boxes are cleaned with disinfectant. Standard maintenance procedures must be followed, including inspection and leakage current testing at least every 6 months, at any sign of malfunction, and after any repair (17).

The patient's outcome should be correlated with NIOM results. Any discrepancies should be thoroughly evaluated, and this may include postoperative EP studies. It is important that monitoring, surgical, and anesthesiology teams understand the relationship of their NIOM results to patient outcome.

CONCLUSIONS

Vertebral column surgeries risk spinal cord, nerve root, brachial plexus, and peripheral nerve injury. SEP monitoring halves the risk of spinal cord injury, but the possibility of discrete corticospinal or dorsal column compromise makes the addition of muscle MEP monitoring important. Modern techniques—including intravenous anesthesia, SNR-based SEP derivation selection, and decussation assessment—optimize recording for each patient. These methods provide four-limb EP surgical feedback within 2-minute intervals for the majority of patients to enhance surgical correlation and the prevention of injury. Systemically sensitive cortical SEPs and muscle MEPs do not conform well to percentage of baseline amplitude criteria. Instead, gradual, generalized EP changes are systemic, while abrupt focal decrements clearly exceeding trial-to-trial variation identify pathologic change. The addition of TES muscle MEP monitoring will almost certainly further reduce the risk of spinal cord injury because of its greater sensitivity and motor specificity.

REFERENCES

1. Nuwer MR, Dawson EG, Carlson LG, et al. Somatosensory EP spinal cord monitoring reduces neurologic deficits after scoliosis surgery: results of a large multicenter survey. *Electroencephalogr Clin Neurophysiol* 1995; 96:6–11.

2. Bosley TM, Salih MA, Jen JC, et al. Neurologic features of horizontal gaze palsy and progressive scoliosis with mutations in ROBO3. *Neurology* 2005;64:1196–1203.
3. MacDonald DB, Streletz L, Al-Zayed Z, et al. Intraoperative neurophysiologic discovery of uncrossed sensory and motor pathways in a patient with horizontal gaze palsy and scoliosis. *Clin Neurophysiol* 2004;115:576–582.
4. MacDonald DB, Al-Zayed Z, Khodeir I, Stigsby B. Monitoring scoliosis surgery with combined transcranial electric motor and cortical somatosensory EP from the lower and upper extremities. *Spine* 2003;28:194–203.
5. Burke D, Nuwer MR, Daube J, et al. Intraoperative monitoring. The International Federation of Clinical Neurophysiology. *Electroencephalogr Clin Neurophysiol Suppl* 1999;52:133–148.
6. American Electroencephalographic Society. Guideline eleven: guidelines for intraoperative monitoring of sensory EP. *J Clin Neurophysiol* 1994;11:77–87.
7. Toleikis JR. American Society of Neurophysiological Monitoring. Intraoperative monitoring using somatosensory EP. A position statement by the American Society of Neurophysiological Monitoring. *J Clin Monit Comput* 2005;19:241–258.
8. MacDonald DB, Al Zayed Z, Stigsby B. Tibial somatosensory EP intraoperative monitoring: recommendations based on signal to noise ratio analysis of popliteal fossa, optimized P37, standard P37 and P31 potentials. *Clin Neurophysiol* 2005;116:1858–1869.
9. MacDonald DB, Stigsby B, Al-Zayed Z. A comparison between derivation optimization and Cz'-FPz for posterior tibial P37 somatosensory EP intraoperative monitoring. *Clin Neurophysiol* 2004;115:1925–1930.
10. MacDonald DB. Individually optimizing posterior tibial somatosensory EP P37 scalp derivations for intraoperative monitoring. *J Clin Neurophysiol* 2001;18:364–371.
11. Iwasaki H, Tamaki T, Yoshida M, et al. Efficacy and limitations of current methods of intraoperative spinal cord monitoring. *J Orthop Sci* 2003;8:635–642.
12. Forbes HJ, Allen PW, Waller CS, et al. Spinal cord monitoring in scoliosis surgery. Experience with 1168 cases. *J Bone Joint Surg Br* 1991;73:487–491.
13. MacDonald DB. Intraoperative motor EP monitoring: overview and update. *J Clin Monit.* 2006; EPub ahead of print July 11, 2006.
14. Ulkatan S, Neuwirth M, Bitan F, et al. Monitoring of scoliosis surgery with epidurally recorded motor EP (D wave) revealed false results. *Clin Neurophysiol* 2006;117:2093–2101.
15. Burke D, Hicks RG. Surgical monitoring of motor pathways. *J Clin Neurophysiol* 1998;15:194–205.
16. MacDonald DB. Safety of intraoperative transcranial electric stimulation motor EP monitoring. *J Clin Neurophysiol* 2002;19:416–429.
17. MacDonald DB, Deletis V. Safety issues during surgical monitoring. In: Nuwer MR, ed, *Intraoperative Monitoring of Neural Function: Handbook of Clinical Neurophysiology.* 2008 (in press).
18. Deletis V, Rodi Z, Amassian VE. Neurophysiological mechanisms underlying motor EP in anesthetized humans. Part 2. Relationship between epidurally and muscle recorded MEP in man. *Clin Neurophysiol* 2001;112:445–452.
19. Lyon R, Feiner J, Lieberman JA. Progressive suppression of motor EP during general anesthesia: the phenomenon of "anesthetic fade." *J Neurosurg Anesthesiol* 2005;17:13–19.

8 Spinal Cord Surgery

Thoru Yamada
Marjorie Tucker
Aatif M. Husain

The neurophysiologic intraoperative monitoring (NIOM) of spinal cord function has been used for spinal fusion and instrumentation surgeries by orthopedic surgeons, surgeries of thoracic and thoracoabdominal aorta and cardiac surgeries requiring cardiopulmonary bypass by cardiothoracic surgeons, coarctation repair by vascular surgeons, and surgeries of intramedullary and extramedullary tumors and arteriovenous malformations (AVMs) of the spinal cord by neurosurgeons. This chapter focuses on NIOM in the latter procedures.

Most surgeries on the spinal cord are for the resection of tumors. During surgery, spinal cord injury may occur either by direct physical damage or by ischemic insult to the spinal cord. In orthopedic procedures the risk of physical damage is more likely, and ischemia often occurs in cardiac and vascular surgery ischemia; however, both can occur in neurosurgical procedures.

Historically, the standard for NIOM of spinal cord function has been the monitoring of somatosensory evoked potentials (SEPs). However, SEPs evaluate primarily posterior spinal cord function, and false-negative findings (i.e., anterior spinal cord damage and paraplegia occurring without being detected by SEPs) have been reported.(1,2) More recently, transcranial electrical motor evoked potentials (MEPs) evaluating the anterior spinal cord and motor pathways have become available.

There are several methods for SEP and MEP monitoring. Which method is chosen depends on the type of surgery and the preference of the neurophysiologist. Each method has advantages and disadvantages. The NIOM laboratory should be able to perform any alternative method if one method does not work. Since SEPs and MEPs are complementary and combining them extends the coverage of spinal cord functions, both types of monitoring should be performed whenever possible. Using both types of NIOM will also help in cases when one modality fails to yield measurable or consistent responses.

BASIC ANATOMY OF THE SPINAL CORD

Spinal Cord Anatomy

The spinal cord is protected by multiple vertebrae, passing through the vertebral foramina of 7 cervical, 12 thoracic, 5 lumbar, and 5 sacral vertebrae. The spinal cord is the downward extension of the medulla oblongata and ends at the conus medullaris at the level of the T12 spine. From the conus, a bundle of nerve fiber called the cauda equina extends down to the coccyx and ends as the filum terminale. The dura and arachnoid (subarachnoid space) mater extend down to the level of S2 vertebra.

There are 31 pairs of spinal nerves: 8 cervical, 12 thoracic, 5 lumbar, 5 sacral, and 1 coccygeal. Each spinal nerve passes through an intervertebral foramen between two vertebrae. In the cervical spine, the C1 spinal nerve passes above the C1 vertebra and the C8 spinal nerve passes below the C7 vertebra (i.e., between the C7 and T1 vertebrae). In the thoracic, lumbar, and sacral spine, each spinal nerve is numbered in accordance with the number of the vertebra just above it. For example, the T1 spinal nerve passes below the T1 vertebra and the L5 lumbar spinal nerve passes below the L5 vertebra. The nerves of the upper cervical spinal lie horizontally; further caudally, however, the spinal nerves assume an increasingly oblique and downward direction as they proceed to their foramina to exit the spinal canal.

The C7 spine level is identified by a protruded spinous process at the lower part of the neck when the neck is flexed. The T12 spine level is identified by the lowest rib, while the L4 spine level corresponds with the horizontal line between the left and right upper borders of iliac crest.

Fiber Tracts of the Spinal Cord

The spinal cord consists of gray matter, which occupies the central portion of spinal cord, and white matter surrounding the gray matter. The gray matter is made up of collections of cell bodies, dendrites, axons, and axon terminals; the white matter consists of axons of longitudinally running nerve fiber tracts. Only the anatomic structures relevant to spinal cord NIOM are discussed here.

The spinal cord comprises two major pathways. One is an afferent (sensory) pathway, which carries information from the peripheral receptors to the brain, and the other is an efferent (motor) pathway, which conveys messages from the brain to the periphery. The afferent pathway starts from peripheral receptors, ascends in the sensory nerve fibers, and enters the spinal cord via the dorsal root. In the spinal cord, the sensory fibers carrying temperature and pain (superficial sensation) via unmyelinated or small myelinated fibers cross to the opposite side and ascend in the spinothalamic tract, which is located in the anterior and lateral aspect of the spinal cord. The sensory fibers carrying position and vibration sensation via large myelinated fibers enter the dorsal column, which occupies the posterior portion of the spinal cord. These fibers then ascend on the same side to the brainstem. The dorsal column consists of two fasciculi: the fasciculus gracilis carries fibers from the lower limb and the fasciculus cuneatus carries fibers from the upper limb. The fasciculus gracilis and fasciculus cuneatus reach the brainstem and synapse on the gracilis nucleus and cuneatus nucleus. The fiber tract then crosses to the opposite side, forming the medial lemniscus. There the spinothalamic tract carrying superficial sensation and the fasciculi gracilis and cuneatus carrying deep sensation join together and ascend through the brainstem contralateral to side that is stimulated. Eventually the fiber tracts reach the thalamus and synapse on the ventral posterolateral (VPL) nucleus. From here the sensory fibers pass through the posterior limb of internal capsule and reach the sensory cortex at the postcentral gyrus. The sensory cortex representing the upper limb is located on the lateral convexity of the hemisphere, and the lower limb is represented at the vertex and mesial aspect of the hemisphere.

It is important to note that SEPs elicited by electrical stimulation are primarily mediated by the dorsal column pathway and posterior spinal cord, not the spinothalamic tract or anterior spinal cord. An abnormal SEP, therefore, is seen primarily in patients with impaired proprioception but not in those with impaired pain and temperature sensation.

The main efferent pathway is the corticospinal tract, which starts from the motor cortex at the precentral gyrus. It descends via the posterior limb of the internal capsule to the pyramidal decussation of the brainstem, where a major part of tract crosses to the opposite side. The tract continues to descend in the lateral aspect of the spinal cord and finally reaches the anterior horn cells. After synapsing on the anterior horn cells, the motor fibers exit the spinal cord via ventral roots and end at the motor points of muscle fibers.

Arteries of the Spinal Cord

The spinal cord is supplied by one anterior and two posterior spinal arteries. For details on vascular supply of the spinal cord, the reader is referred to the Chapter 15. An overview is presented here.

The anterior spinal artery runs the entire length of spinal cord in the midline. It is supplied by the subclavian and vertebral arteries superiorly. In the cervical and upper thoracic region, it is supplied by one or two radicular arteries. In the lower thoracic to upper lumbar region, it receives blood supply from the arteria radicularis magna (ARM), also known as the artery of Adamkiewicz. This large artery is responsible for supplying much of the lower part of the spinal cord. Branches of the ARM also synapse with the posterior spinal arteries.

The posterior spinal arteries are paired arteries that travel in parallel on the posterolateral aspect of the entire length of the spinal cord. They receive blood supply from the vertebral arteries with contributions from posterior radicular arteries. In the cervical region, the radicular arteries arise from deep cervical and subclavian arteries. At thoracic, lumbar, and sacral regions, posterior radicular arteries arise from posterior intercostal, lumbar, and lateral sacral arteries.

SPINAL CORD TUMORS

Most surgeries on the spinal cord are for resection of tumors. Approximately 2% to 4% of all primary central nervous system tumors occur in the spinal cord. This section offers a brief overview of these tumors—their presentation, diagnosis, and surgical management.

Classification

Spinal cord tumors are most often classified based on their location. Extradural tumors arise outside the dura mater, most often from the vertebral bodies. Intradural extramedullary tumors arise from within the dura mater but outside the spinal cord. Finally, intramedullary tumors arise from within the spinal cord. A classification of these tumors is presented in Table 8.1.

TABLE 8.1 Classification System for Spinal Cord Tumors

Extradural		Intradural, Extramedullary	Intramedullary
Malignant	Benign		
Osteosarcoma	Osteoid osteoma	Meningioma	Astrocytoma
Chondrosarcoma	Osteoblastoma	Schwannoma	Ependymoma
Leiomyosarcoma	Osteochondroma	Neurofibroma	Oligodendroglioma
Ewing's sarcoma	Chondroblastoma	Metastases	Ganglioglioma
Chordoma	Giant cell tumor	Lipoma	Neuroblastoma
Multiple myeloma/ solitary plasmacytoma	Hemangioma		Hemangioblastoma
	Aneurysmal bone cysts		Vascular lesions
Metastases			Metastases

Extradural Tumors

Extradural tumors can arise either from the bone or soft tissues surrounding the spinal cord, or they may be metastatic (3). Primary tumors of the bone and soft tissue are rare and can be malignant. Osteosarcomas arise from bony structures and may be seen in patients with Paget's disease. Chondrosarcomas are tumors of cartilage and usually originate in the vertebral body. Leiomyosarcomas arise from mesenchymal elements such as muscle cells. Ewing's sarcomas can arise in the bone or soft tissue and are small, round, blue-cell tumors. Chordomas arise from remnants of the notochord and occur most often near the clivus, cervical spine, and lumbosacral region. Multiple myeloma or a solitary plasmacytoma can occur in the spine; these are malignancies of plasma cells. Metastatic tumors can also involve the spine. Any malignant tumor can metastasize to the spine, but the commonest primaries are prostate, breast, and lung.

A variety of benign lesions can also occur in the extradural space. Osteoid osteomas are small lesions (less than 2 cm in diameter) that typically arise from spongy bone and occur in the posterior aspect of vertebral bodies. Osteoblastomas are similar to osteoid osteomas but are larger (greater than 2 cm) and consequently more likely to produce neurologic symptoms. Osteochondromas consists of healthy bone with a cartilaginous cap and occur most often in the cervical spine. Chondroblastomas are tumors of immature cartilage and only rarely occur in the spine. Giant-cell tumors are very vascular and usually affect the vertebral body; they have a high recurrence rate after resection. Vertebral hemangiomas are nonneoplastic lesions consisting of thin-walled blood vessels and are often incidental findings. Aneurysmal bone cysts are nonneoplastic expansile blood-filled cysts commonly located along the posterior aspect of the thoracolumbar spine; they cause symptoms by their local expansion.

Intradural Extramedullary Tumors

Intradural extramedullary tumors make up the majority of intradural spinal cord tumors (4). Meningiomas and nerve sheath tumors are the commonest types. Meningiomas arise from arachnoid cells and are adherent to the dura mater. They occur most often in the thoracic spine. Rarely, meningiomas can be extradural, but in these situations they almost always have an intradural extension. Schwannomas and neurofibromas are nerve sheath tumors. They typically arise from spinal nerve roots before they leave the dural sac. Occasionally they extend beyond the dural sheath, making them dumbbell-shaped. Schwannomas are usually solitary lesions, whereas neurofibromas are often multiple and seen in neurofibromatosis type I. Intradural, extramedullary metastatic tumors are rare and are often the result of drop lesions of systemic or intracranial neoplasms. They occur most often in the thoracic spine. Other types of intradural, extramedullary tumors are rare and typically located in the cauda equina; they are not discussed further.

Intramedullary Tumors

Intramedullary tumors are seen more often in children than in adults. Astrocytomas are the commonest type of intramedullary tumor and are most often located in the cervicothoracic region. Pilocytic astrocytomas are low-grade, well-circumscribed neoplasms that are amenable to near complete resection. Fibrillary astrocytomas are more likely to be high-grade neoplasms; they are diffuse lesions. They cannot be resected in their entirety. Intramedullary ependymomas are more common in adults than children and can occur anywhere in the spinal cord. There is a discrete plane between the ependymoma and adjacent spinal cord, allowing for easier surgical dissection. Oligodendrogliomas are infiltrating tumors located mostly in the thoracic spine and are often associated with a syrinx. They frequently have leptomeningeal metastases and total resection is not possible. Gangliogliomas contain neurons and glial cells and are most often located in the cervicothoracic region. They can often be removed in total. Neuroblastomas contain neuroblasts, ganglion cells, and Schwann cells and are located mostly in the cervical spine. Lipomas consist of fatty tissue mixed with neuronal and connective tissue and are seen mostly in the cervicothoracic region. They are infiltrating tumors and treatment is aimed at debulking rather than complete removal. Hemangioblastomas are highly vascular tumors whose feeding arteries and draining veins can be seen on magnetic resonance imaging (MRI). They are most often present in the cervicothoracic region and are associated with von Hippel–Lindau syndrome. Complete resection of these tumors is possible. Vascular lesions of the spinal cord are considered AVMs and not true neoplasms. Those with small dominant vessels are called capillary hemangiomas, whereas those with larger vessels are called cavernous hemangiomas. They are most commonly seen in the cervicothoracic region, but multiple lesions are not infrequent. Complete surgical resection is possible, although endovascular treatment is also sometimes considered. Intramedullary metastases are uncommon; when they occur, the primary is most likely to be lung. These are rarely treated surgically.

Clinical Presentations

Spinal cord tumors can be silent for many years. Onset is usually insidious, the most frequent complaint being back and neck pain. The pain is usually worse in the horizontal position and has a diffuse aching character rather than a radiating one. Many patients, especially those with a thoracic lesion, have a spinal deformity.

Paresthesias are also common and are often asymmetric. Motor complaints occur after sensory symptoms. This may be manifest as clumsiness and falling in adults and as motor regression in children. Spasticity, hyperreflexia, and Babinski signs will also be present. Flexor spasms can also occur, causing considerable pain. Sphincter dysfunction occurs late in the course of disease progression. The presentation is highly dependent on the location of the tumor. A tumor located in the posterior spinal cord is much more likely to causes dorsal column dysfunction prior to weakness, whereas the opposite is true for a more anteriorly located lesion.

In most cases of spinal cord tumors, progression of symptoms is insidious owing to gradually worsening compression of neural structures. Sudden worsening often implies a vascular compromise and is often not reversible. When symptoms are slowly progressive, treatment outcome is likely to be much better than when the worsening is acute.

Diagnostic Evaluation

The diagnostic study of choice for spinal cord tumors is MRI. This must be obtained with and without a contrast agent (gadolinium). The T1 sequences are useful in showing solid parts of the tumor, whereas T2 sequences demonstrate the cerebrospinal fluid (CSF) and cystic components of the tumor. Although MRI cannot make histologic diagnoses, the characteristic appearance of lesions allow a reasonably accurate classification.

Myelography and computed tomography (CT) myelography were the "gold standard" in imaging spinal cord lesions prior to MRI. These tests are now reserved for exceptional situations in which an MRI cannot be obtained. Lesions of the bone may be better visualized by CT scans. Plain x-rays can be helpful if the tumor causes lytic bone lesions. Angiography may be helpful with hemangioblastomas and hemangiomas.

Surgery

Surgery for spinal cord tumors is preformed with the patient in the prone position, although some surgeons prefer a flexed crouch position. The incision is usually limited to two vertebral levels over the focal point of the tumor. Dissection is carried to the lamina and then either a laminectomy or hemilaminectomy is performed, depending on the location of the tumor. Extradural tumors can be removed or debulked without opening the dura mater.

Intradural tumors can often be seen even prior to opening the dura mater. A longitudinal incision is used to open the dura mater over the site of the tumor. For extramedullary tumors, the arachnoid mater over the tumor is opened and the tumor is entered. Intracapsular debulking of the tumor is achieved with blunt dissection or with alternative techniques such as the cavitronic ultrasound surgical aspirator (CUSA) or the carbon dioxide (CO_2) laser. Once the tumor is debulked, the capsule collapses and can be removed from the dura mater.

Intramedullary tumors can be localized in the surgical field with ultrasound. These tumors are usually approached through a midline incision of the spinal cord between the dorsal columns (myelotomy). For more laterally placed lesions, the approach can be through the dorsal root entry zone. The myelotomy may cause significant changes in the NIOM, as discussed below. Dissection of the tumor depends on its suspected pathology. Astrocytomas are dissected from inside out until the cord–tumor interface is reached. Ependymomas are dissected from one pole to the other, as a cleavage plane can be found in these tumors. Lipomas are well demarcated but tightly adherent to the spinal cord; consequently complete resection is not possible. Dissection of these tumors can be aided with a CUSA or CO_2 laser. The spinal cord is then reapproximated with sutures.

Once the tumor is removed and hemostasis is achieved, if the dura mater was opened, it is sutured in a watertight fashion. The thecal sac is reexpanded with fluid to prevent hemorrhage. The paraspinal muscles, fascia, and skin are then approximated and closed in layers.

MODALITIES AND METHODS OF NIOM

Somatic Evoked Potentials

There are several methods for SEP monitoring. The most commonly used method is scalp SEP recording after stimulation of peripheral nerves—for example, ulnar or median nerve stimulation for the upper limb and tibial or peroneal nerve stimulation for the lower limb. This is the gold standard for SEP monitoring and is been discussed elsewhere in this chapter. Here alternative methods are be described.

Peripheral Nerve Stimulation with Recording from the Spinal Cord

After stimulation of a peripheral nerve in the lower extremity, a spinal potential can be recorded from a pair of electrodes embedded in a soft, flexible wire placed in the epidural space of the high thoracic or cervical spinal cord. The waveform becomes smaller and more polyphasic the more rostral the level of recording (5) (Figure 8.1). The onset latency of the waveform is dependent on the location of the recording electrodes. In general, the onset latency in adults at the low cervical or high thoracic spine is about 25 to 30 ms with stimulation in the lower extremity.

There are several advantages to this recording method. Because the response is robust, less averaging is required than scalp-recorded SEPs. This response is affected little by anesthetics, since it is oligosynaptic. Finally, the waveform can be recorded at multiple levels, which allows determination of the segmental level of damage if multiple electrodes are used.

Spinal Cord Stimulation and Spinal Cord Recording

Two sets of epidural electrodes are placed both rostral and caudal to the surgical site. Either pair of electrodes can be the recording or stimulating site. A single stimulus usually yields a robust response consisting of two negative peaks (NI, NII) with a latency of less than 7 ms (5) (Figure 8.2).

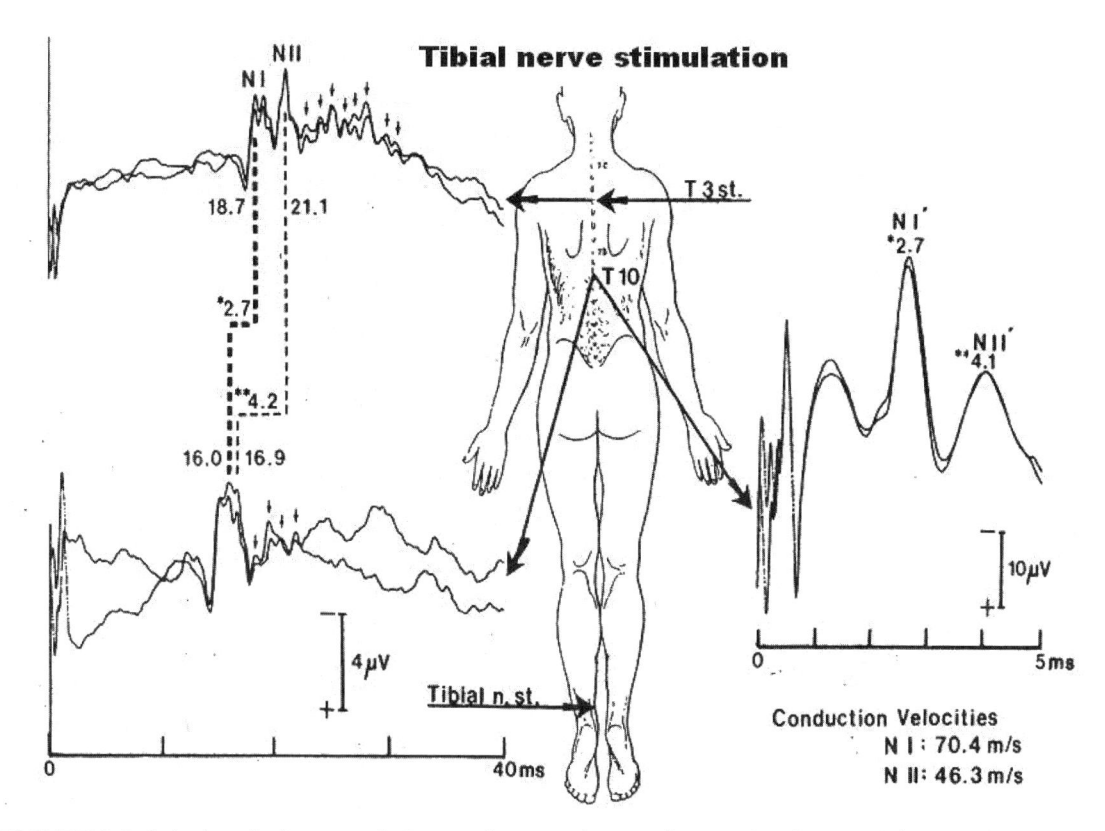

FIGURE 8.1 Spinal evoked potential (SpEp) after stimulation of a peripheral nerve (left) and after stimulation of the spinal cord (right). After stimulation of tibial nerve, SpEps are recorded at the T10 and T3 spinal levels. Note greater polyspike waves with the higher level of recording. After stimulation of the spinal cord at T3 spine, SpEps recorded at the T10 spine showed W-shaped waveform consisting of NI and NII potentials. Reversing the stimulating and recording electrodes will record a similar waveform. [Reproduced with permission from Machida et al. (5).]

Among the advantages of this method is that the stimulus intensity required is much lower, usually less than 5 mA, compared to peripheral nerve stimulation, where 20 to 40 mA is used. It is not dependent on peripheral nerve function and can be applied to the patient who has a peripheral neuropathy or whose peripheral nerves cannot be adequately stimulated. Additionally, in this technique no averaging is required, and it is not affected by anesthetics.

Spinal Cord Stimulation and Scalp Recording

Instead of stimulating peripheral nerves, essentially the same waveform but with a much shorter latency can be recorded from the scalp after stimulation of the caudal spinal cord via an epidural electrode (Figure 8.2). The stimulus intensity is less than 10 mA, and usually less than 50 responses need to be averaged, which is much less than required for peripheral nerve stimulation.

The advantage of this method is that it is not dependent on peripheral nerve conduction and can be used for patients with a peripheral neuropathy or those whose peripheral nerves are not accessible. It has a shorter acquisition time compared to the usual method of obtaining SEPs. Additionally it can be used for monitoring cervical cord function, while spinal cord stimulation and recording are primarily

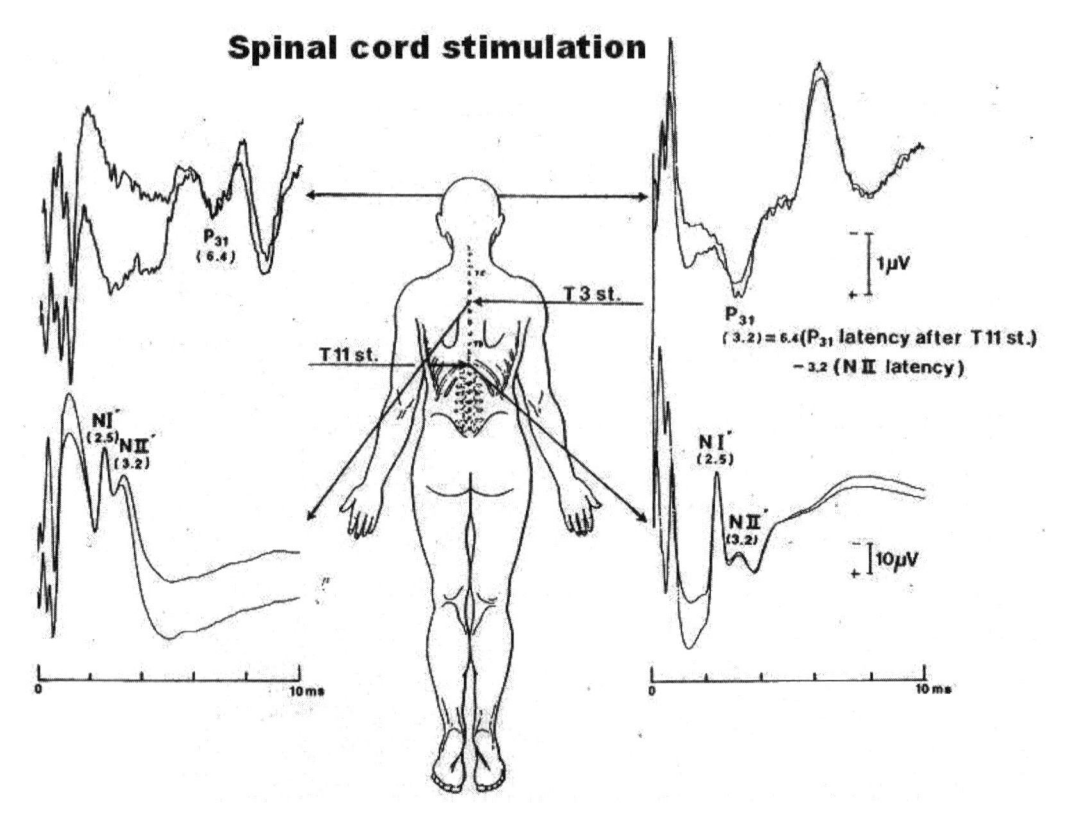

FIGURE 8.2 Scalp-recorded SEPs and SpEps after stimulation of the spinal cord. With stimulation of the spinal cord at the T3 spine level (right), the scalp-recorded far-field potential of P31 showed an expectedly shorter latency than the response to stimulation at the T3 spine level (left). SpEps, either by T11 stimulation with T3 recording or vice versa, showed similar waveforms with the same NI and NII latencies. [Reproduced with permission from Machida et al. (5).]

used for surgeries of the thoracic or lumbar spinal cord.

Disadvantages of Epidural Spinal Cord Stimulation and Recording

Although there are many advantages of epidural spinal cord stimulation and recording, there are some disadvantages as well, which limit their use. The main disadvantage is the insecurity of electrode placement; the electrodes can easily be dislodged. Unless the patient is paralyzed, even a low-intensity stimulus will cause vigorous paraspinal muscle twitches that could interfere with the operative procedure. The epidural electrodes can easily be applied when the spine is exposed, as in some neurosurgical procedures; however, for others, such as those with an endovascular approach, the epidural electrodes must be inserted percutaneously. Insertion of electrodes in the epidural space, although uncommon, poses the potential risk of injuring the spinal cord.

Motor Evoked Potentials

In order to evaluate the anterior spinal cord or motor function, it is necessary to monitor descending motor pathways. This also can be done by several methods. The stimuli can be applied transcranially by electrical or magnetic stimulation or to the spinal cord via epidural electrodes. The recording may be from the spinal cord, peripheral nerves, or muscles. Although transcranial magnetic stimulation is effective and painless in an awake subject, it is not suitable for NIOM because it is highly sensitive to the orientation of the stimulating coil as well as to anesthetics. Transcranial magnetic stimulation is not used for NIOM and is not discussed here. The most commonly used method is transcranial electric stimulation (TES) and recording compound muscle action potentials (CMAPs) from muscles. This is described further on. In this section, other methods of MEP recording are described.

Transcranial Electric Stimulation and Recording from the Spinal Cord

The potential is recorded from the caudal spinal cord via an epidural electrode and consists of a bi- or triphasic sharp discharge, called a D (direct) wave, followed by a series of polyphasic waves, called I (indirect) waves (5,6) (Figure 8.3). Stimulation is delivered to the scalp with an anode at the vertex and the cathode 6 to 7 cm anterior or lateral to the vertex. The stimulus intensity is usually 400 to 500 V of 50 to 100 μs duration, which gives approximately 400 to 600 mA in current intensity. The D wave results from direct stimulation of corticospinal neurons, whereas I waves are generated by transsynaptic activation of corticospinal neurons. D waves are resistant to inhalation anesthetics but I waves are extremely sensitive.

Since the D wave's amplitude is robust (15 to 25 μV at high-thoracic and 5 to 10 μV at low-thoracic levels), a single stimulus usually yields a measurable response, but 15 to 25 sweeps may be averaged for a better-defined response. The major advantage of this method is that neuromuscular blocking agents and inhalation anesthetics can be used without affecting the response.

Spinal Cord Stimulation and Recording from Muscles or Nerves

A low-intensity stimulus (less than 10 mA) applied to the rostral thoracic spinal cord via epidural electrodes can elicit CMAPs from lower extremity muscles and nerve action potentials (NAPs) from the tibial and peroneal nerves (7,8) (Figure 8.4). CMAPs are robust responses and no averaging is necessary to elicit a measurable response. NAPs can be recorded by averaging 10 to 25 sweeps. The advantage of both techniques is their insensitivity to anesthetics. The use of paralytic agents, however, attenuates or abolishes the CMAPs but not the NAPs. However, both CMAPs and NAPs elicited in this manner are likely not to reflect motor function of the spinal cord. Rather, they are antidromic sensory responses or mixed motor and sensory responses. Regardless, this method monitors at least certain functions of the spinal cord and can be useful in some cases when anesthetics or neuromuscular blocking agents cause problems in eliciting measurable responses.

Common NIOM Paradigm for Spinal Cord Surgery

NIOM during spinal cord surgery usually involves SEP and MEP monitoring. SEPs are usually obtained with peripheral nerve stimulation and recorded with scalp electrodes. Stimulation for MEPs is at the scalp with

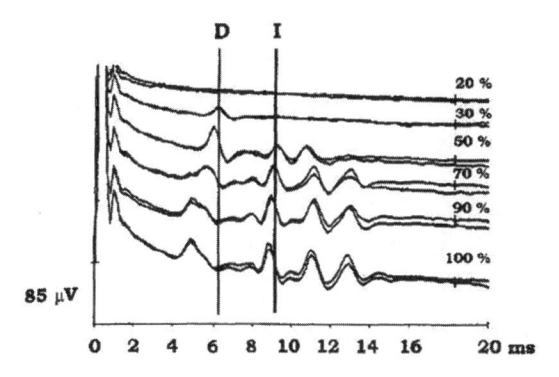

FIGURE 8.3 D and I waves recorded from the spinal cord via epidural electrodes after TES. Stimulus intensity 100% = 750 V. Note that only the D wave is elicited by a weak stimulus and the latency shortens with the greater stimulus intensity. [Reproduced with permission from Deletis (6).]

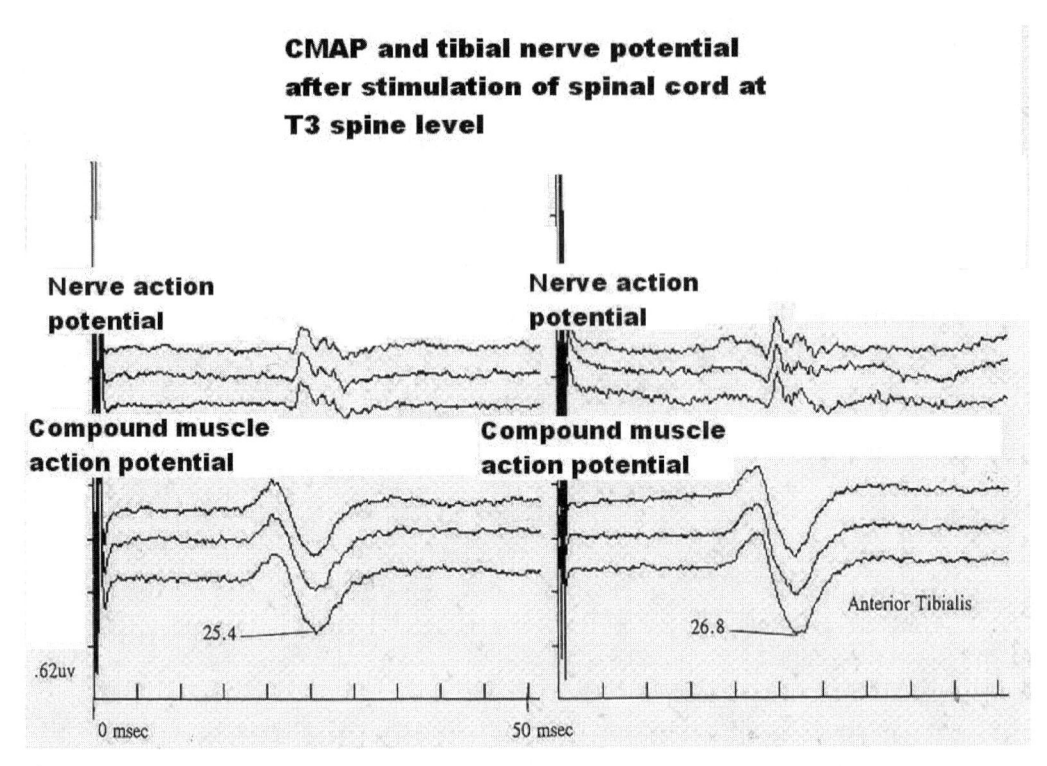

FIGURE 8.4 Simultaneously recorded tibial NAPs (upper three tracings) and anterior tibialis CMAP (lower three tracings) after stimulation of the spinal cord via epidural electrodes placed at the T2 spine level.

CMAP recordings from muscles. At times, the recording of D waves may be useful as well. The methodology used in obtaining these responses in the authors' practice is discussed below.

Somatic Evoked Potentials

SEP recording montages may differ depending on the preference of the laboratory. Subcortical far-field potentials (P14-N18 for upper and P31-N34 for lower extremities) are important to record, as they are affected little by anesthesia and consequently are a more consistent and reliable potential than the cortical potentials (N20 for upper and P37 (P40) for lower extremities). These far-field potentials can be recorded from any scalp electrode (the exact scalp location is not critical for far-field potential recordings because of a wide field distribution) using a noncephalic reference. Instead of using a distant reference, which may be prone to contamination by the electrocardiogram (ECG) or other physiologic or nonphysiologic artifacts, ear reference recordings are technically much easier and yield cleaner far-field potentials.

Commonly used montages for upper and lower extremity SEPs are presented in Tables 8.2 and 8.3. The authors primarily focus on and follow far-field potentials (P14 for upper and P31 for lower extremities) of the SEPs (Figure 8.5). Channels 1 and 2 are redundant, but recording both helps in cases where one does not work. Channel 3 records only the cortical potential and is the least useful, but this may help in case the far-field recording fails. Monitoring peripheral potentials (channel 4) is important because this assures the appropriate delivery of stimulus. One average requires about 500 to 1,000 responses, which usually takes several min-

TABLE 8.2 A Typical Montage Used for Upper Extremity SEPs

Channel	Montage	Waveform(s) recorded
1	CP3/4 (i)—A1 + A2	P14—N20
2	CP3/4 (c)—A1 + A2	P14—N18
3	CP3/4 (c)—CP3/4 (i)	N20
4	Erb (i)—Erb (c)	Erb potential

(i) = ipsilateral to side of stimulation; (c) = contralateral to side of stimulation.

TABLE 8.3 A typical Montage Used for Lower Extremity SEPs

Channel	Montage	Waveform(s) recorded
1	CPz—A1+A2	P31—P37
2	CP1/2 (i) - A1+A2	P31—P37
3	CPz—Fpz	P37
4	Popliteal fossa	Popliteal fossa potential

(i) = ipsilateral to side of stimulation.

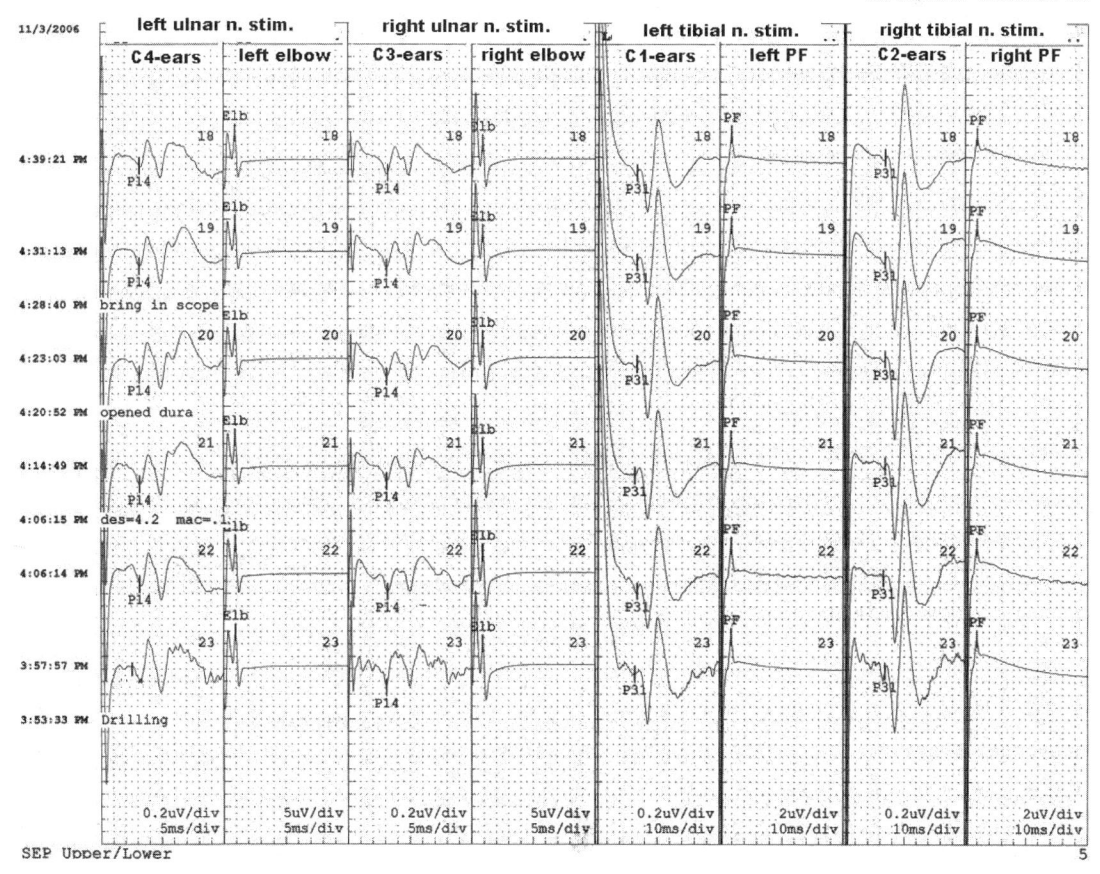

FIGURE 8.5 Typical examples of 16-channel recording of left/right ulnar and tibial nerve SEPs based on Tables 8.2 and 8.3 montages arrangement (only 8 channels are shown here). Each stimulus was delivered sequentially starting with the left and right ulnar nerves and then left and right tibial nerves with a slight latency delay (50 ms each). Note that the P14 of the ulnar and P31 of the tibial nerve SEPs are registered only with an ear reference but not with a F7 reference.

utes with a stimulus rate of 5 to 7 Hz. A caveat to this monitoring method is when total intravenous anesthesia (TIVA) is used. In this situation, cortical responses are robust and easily reproducible, making subcortical responses less important.

When surgery is performed on the caudal part of the cervical spinal cord or lower, tibial nerve SEPs are continuously averaged. Median nerve SEPs can serve as controls in such cases and are performed after several tibial nerve SEP averages. However, if the pathology is in the rostral cervical spinal cord, median or ulnar nerve SEPs should be used primarily. Ulnar nerve SEPs, though harder to obtain, provide more coverage of the cervical spinal cord. In such surgeries, tibial nerve SEPs should be obtained as redundant information at periodic intervals.

Motor Evoked Potentials

The stimulating electrodes for MEPs are placed 2 cm anterior to C3 (C3'), C4 (C4'), Cz, (Cz'), C1, C2, and Fz. These may be surface disc, needle, or corkscrew electrodes. Low electrode impedance for both recording and stimulating electrodes is important, which minimizes the stimulus artifact and decrease the stimulus intensity required to elicit reliable responses (Figure 8.6).

The stimulating electrodes must be covered with a nonconductor to avoid delivering accidental shock to the operating room personnel (especially the anesthesiologist), other instruments, or surgical devices. Using C3' and C4' stimulus sites usually elicits MEPs in both upper and lower extremities, although Cz'-Fz or C1-C2 may be used for lower

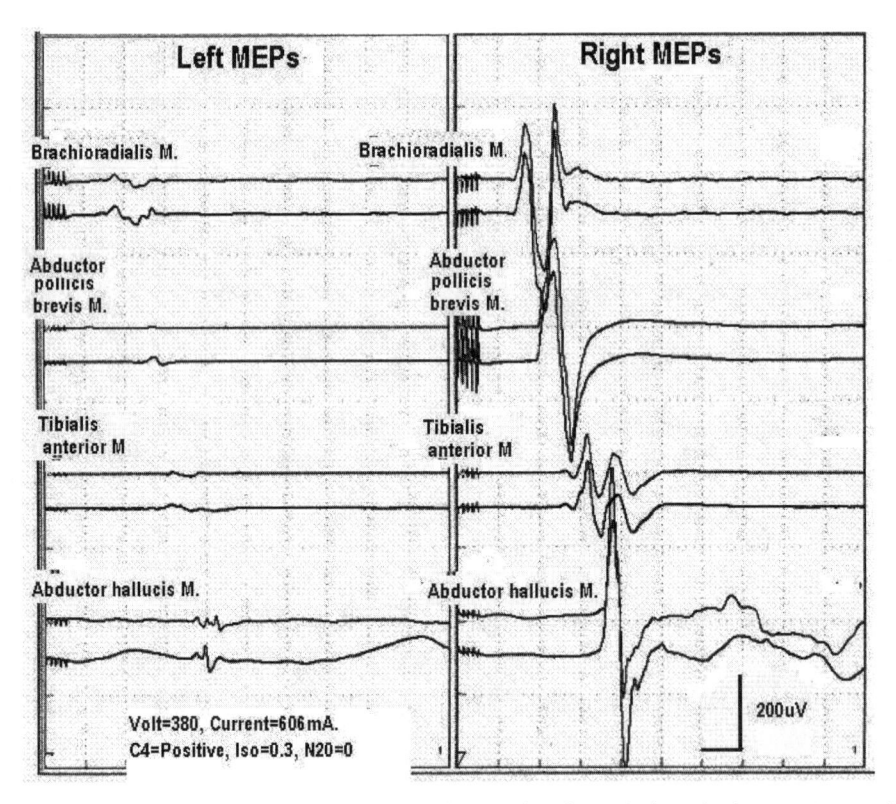

FIGURE 8.6 MEPs from left/right abductor pollicis brevis, brachioradialis, tibialis anterior, and abductor hallucis muscles after TES. Stimulating electrodes were placed at C3 and C4. In this case MEPs were recorded bilaterally with either-side stimulation. In this figure greater amplitude is noted in the right-sided muscles with stimulation of the left hemisphere by anodal electrode at C3.

extremity MEPs. The best sites for the stimulation of upper and lower MEP recordings are variable; in some cases changing the stimulus sites may improve responses and decrease the stimulus artifact. Unlike peripheral nerve stimulation, in which the cathode acts as the stimulus site, in TES the anode is the site for excitation. Therefore if the anode is on the left side of the scalp, this primarily activates the left hemisphere, resulting in activation of right limb muscles.

The TES to elicit MEPs requires the stimulating device to be capable of delivering high voltage (up to 1,000 V) and multipulse stimulation (as with the Digitimer). Multipulse stimulation is more effective in yielding a robust and consistent MEP than single-pulse stimulation due to temporal summation. Usually a train of three to five stimuli with an interstimulus interval of 1 to 3 ms is used. The stimulus intensity and duration parameters have been noted above.

Whether MEPs are best recorded from muscle (CMAPs), spinal cord (D and I waves), or both is still in dispute. Generally the spinal cord recording is more popular in Europe, Japan, and Australia, but in the United States most laboratories use CMAP recordings. Combining CMAP and D-wave MEP recordings has been shown to be of particular utility in spinal cord surgery, as discussed further on (9). Commonly used muscles for recording CMAPs include the brachioradialis and abductor pollicis brevis muscles in the upper limb and anterior tibialis and abductor hallucis brevis muscles in the lower limb. Small muscles generally produce robust MEPs because of their rich innervation by corticospinal fibers.

Ideally the first trial of MEP recording is done shortly after the patient is anesthetized and before the start of electrocautery use. However, sometimes the effect of neuromuscular blocking drugs used during induction may prevent obtaining CMAP MEPs until later. Once the electrocautery starts, it is almost impossible to get a good MEP baseline. Warning the surgeon and surrounding personnel before delivering a MEP stimulus is important, so that sudden patient movements will not disrupt the surgery. The first MEP stimulus should start with 0 V to verify that the stimulus correctly triggers the sweep. The stimulus intensity is then increased to 100 V, which should give about 100 mA or greater current intensity. If the current delivered is extremely low, the impedance of the stimulating electrodes should be checked. If no response is elicited, the intensity is increased in 50- to 100-V increments until an adequate MEP is obtained. MEPs should be performed every 2 to 5 minutes. Even more frequent trials can be obtained during dissection of the spinal cord lesion.

If D waves are to be recorded, an epidural electrode must be placed caudal to the tumor. This can be placed percutaneously by the surgeon, anesthesiologist, or neurophysiologist. Alternatively, once the laminectomy has been performed, the surgeon can place the electrode caudal to the surgical site and suture it in place. When D waves are to be recorded, only a single TES is needed. However, the stimulus intensity should be increased as described above until a reliable response is recorded.

It is best to alternate between SEPs and MEPs; however, some surgeons prefer to tell the NIOM technologist when to stimulate for MEPs. This should be clarified with the surgeon prior to the surgery.

ANESTHETIC CONSIDERATIONS

Anesthesia can be beneficial as well as detrimental for NIOM during spinal cord surgery. When the patient is anesthetized, a higher stimulus intensity can be used than in an awake state. Anesthetics also reduce movement and muscle artifacts, yielding better and "cleaner" responses than recorded in an awake state. However, anesthesia also changes SEP and MEP waveforms considerably, and the responses under anesthesia are quite different from those obtained while the patient is awake. All inhalation agents attenuate or abolish CMAP MEPs and prolong the latencies. CMAP MEPs are more sensitive to anesthesia than SEPs.

Inhalation Anesthesia

The common inhalation anesthetics are nitrous oxide (N_2O), halothane, desflurane, isoflurane, etc. The relative potency of inhalation agents is described by the minimal alveolar concentration (MAC), which is the anesthetic concentration needed to prevent movement to a painful or surgical stimulus in 50% of patients. The actual concentration needed to obtain one MAC varies among anesthetics. For example, the MAC for isoflurane is 1.3% and that for halothane is 0.7%. The short-latency oligosynaptic SEP components are more resistance than long-latency polysynaptic components. Thus, short-latency far-field evoked potentials (P14 and P31 for the upper and lower extremities, respectively) are affected little with inhalation anesthesia. Often one can obtain consistent and well-defined far-field SEPs with isoflurane greater than 1% with 50% to 60% N_2O. However, CMAP MEPs usually cannot be recorded with isoflurane greater than 0.5%. D waves are little affected by inhalation anesthetics.

Total Intravenous Anesthesia

TIVA has recently become increasingly popular for NIOM. TIVA includes barbiturates, opioids (morphine, alfentanil, sufentanil, remifentanil, etc.), propofol, etomidate, and ketamine. The effect of barbiturates on evoked potentials is similar to that of halogenated agents. Propofol has a short duration of action and little effect on SEPs and MEPs unless a very high dose is used. Both ketamine and etomidate may enhance evoked potential responses by heightening synaptic function at a low dose. However, both may induce seizures, especially in patients with a history of seizures. Most often, when both SEPs and MEPs must be recorded, TIVA with propofol and an opioid is used.

Neuromuscular Blocking Drugs

Neuromuscular blocking drugs (pancuronium, vecuronium, atracurium, etc.) are often used in combination with intravenous or inhalation anesthetics. "Balanced anesthesia" includes narcotics for analgesia plus a neuromuscular blocking drug with a relatively weak anesthetic, such as N_2O.

The neuromuscular blocking drugs do not affect SEPs. However, they eliminate muscle twitches in association with stimulation of a mixed nerve. Therefore they may give the erroneous impression that an adequate stimulus was not delivered to the nerve. The NIOM technologist should document the degree of paralysis if neuromuscular blocking drug are used. Their use is detrimental for CMAP MEPs, but the latter can be recorded if there are two twitches in a train-of-four repetitive stimulation. D waves are not affected by neuromuscular blocking drugs. If it is necessary for the patient to have complete neuromuscular blockade, D waves should be used for monitoring the MEPs.

WARNING CRITERIA

The warning criteria for SEPs have arbitrarily been accepted as greater than 50% reduction of amplitude and/or a 10% prolongation of latency of a given component. There is little consensus regarding the warning criteria for CMAP MEPs. Some consider a greater than 50% amplitude reduction of CMAPs as significant; however, because of their variability, others consider only a complete or near complete loss of response as significant. In some situations, abrupt loss or marked attenuation of CMAP MEPs can occur right after recording a robust response. The reason for this marked fluctuation of amplitude is not known but may be involve the spontaneous fluctuation of excitability of the anterior horn cells. The loss or attenuation of CMAP MEPs, therefore, must be verified before deciding that the change is "real."

Warning criteria for D waves may be more reliable than those for CMAP MEPs, as D waves are less sensitive to systemic and anesthetic changes; therefore marked fluctuations in amplitude are uncommon. When corticospinal tract fibers are damaged, there is an incremental decrease in the D-wave amplitude, and a decrease of 50% is considered significant (9). Drops of 30% to 50% are considered minor warning signs, and the surgeon may chose to pause the surgery transiently when this occurs. A drop of 50% or more, however, should discourage the surgeon from further dissection. A sudden drop in D-wave amplitude indicates vascular compromise and is often irreversible.

Combining CMAP and D-wave MEP monitoring has been noted to be particularly useful in spinal cord surgery by some investigators (9–11). Preservation of both CMAP and D-wave MEPs during surgery is consistent with no lower extremity weakness postoperatively. Loss of CMAP MEPs with preservation of D waves (amplitude greater than 50% of baseline) suggests transient postoperative paraparesis. Loss of both CMAP and D-wave MEPs will result in persistent weakness of the lower extremities. Thus, if there is loss of the CMAP MEPs and D waves are not being recorded during removal of a spinal cord tumor, the surgeon will likely stop dissecting the tumor and perform an incomplete resection. If, however, D waves are being recorded and their amplitude is maintained when CMAP MEPs are lost, the surgeon can continue dissection, thereby allowing a more complete resection. A postoperative paraplegia will likely occur but will be transient. It should be cautioned that this methodology has been tested in only a few centers.

After the NIOM team has alerted the surgeons of changes in responses, the surgeons must decide if they want to modify the surgical procedure, continue with the case, or wait until the responses recover. Data from a combination of SEP, CMAP, and D-wave MEP monitoring can help them considerably in making their decision. In some cases, either only SEPs or MEPs can be recorded or responses are small and "noisy." In such cases the surgeon must be made aware that recordings are suboptimal and may not be reliable.

When a posterior myelotomy is necessary, as in surgery for intramedullary tumors, the injury to the spinal cord is mostly mechanical and inflicted preferentially to the dorsal columns. With a posterior myelotomy, it is expected that SEPs transmitted through the dorsal columns will become impaired (Figure 8.7A, B, and C). Under those circumstances, the corticospinal tracts are spared from injury, and MEPs may be preserved. In such cases, MEPs should be followed more closely.

Excision of extramedullary tumors—such as meningiomas, nerve sheath tumors, and metastases—often requires some traction of the spinal cord. Overzealous retraction of the spinal cord can result in a unilateral mechanical injury. Such an injury to the spinal cord can occur wherever the traction is applied. Depending on the location of the traction, changes in SEPs or MEPs may be noted.

To facilitate exposure and tumor resection, especially if the tumor is ventral, the surgeon may resort to nerve root sectioning. Sacrificing a nerve root in the thoracic spinal cord is usually not associated with any significant neurologic deficit, since many of the nerves overlap in their dermatomal distribution. However, radicular arteries that supply the spinal cord travel within the dural sheaths of the nerve roots. Thus when a nerve is sacrificed in the neural foramen, the radicular artery is also sacrificed. If this radicular artery is a major contributor to spinal cord blood supply, such as the ARM, or if several roots are sacrificed, spinal cord ischemia and infarc-

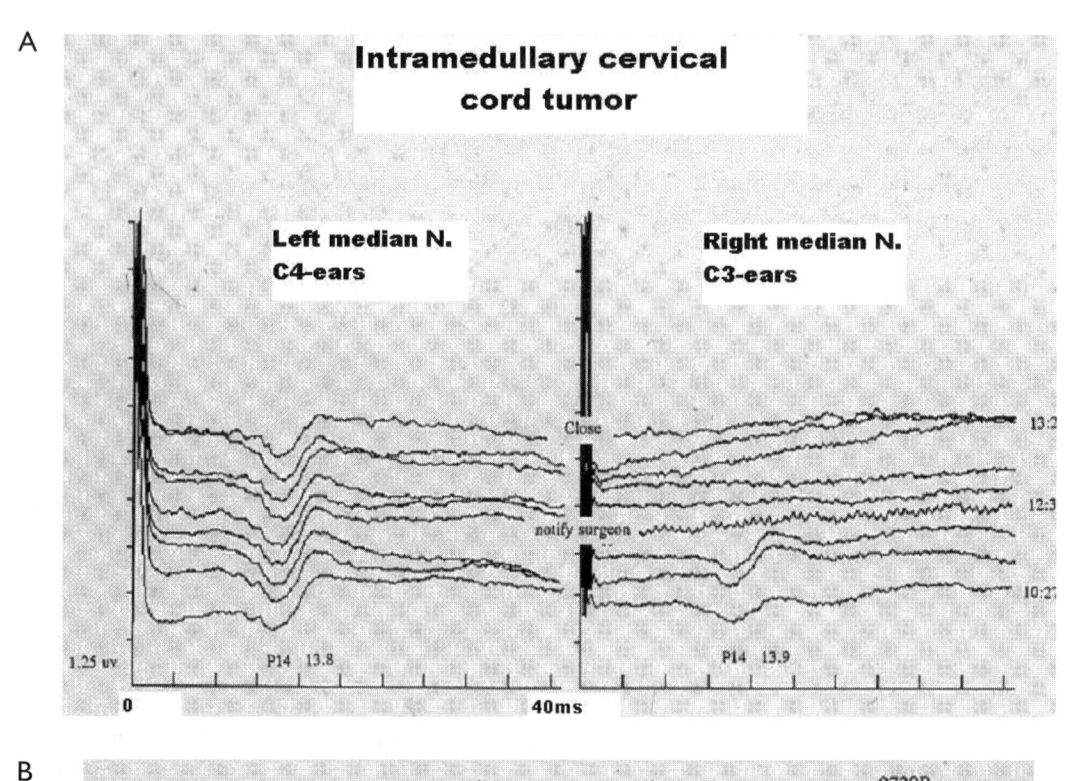

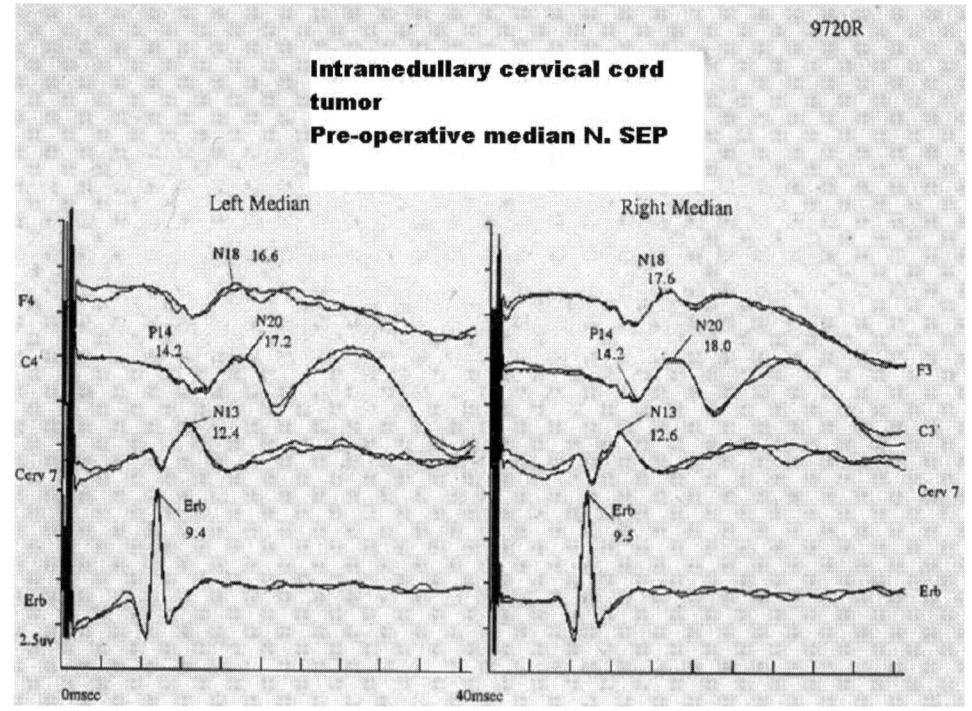

FIGURE 8.7 A. Median nerve SEP monitoring during surgery for intramedullary cervical spinal cord tumor. After a midline myelotomy, there was sudden lost of SEP to right-side stimulation. B. The preoperative median nerve SEP was normal. C. The postoperative SEP showed absence of the P14 and subsequent peaks to right-side stimulation. Postoperatively, the patient had severe loss of proprioceptive sensation of the right arm.

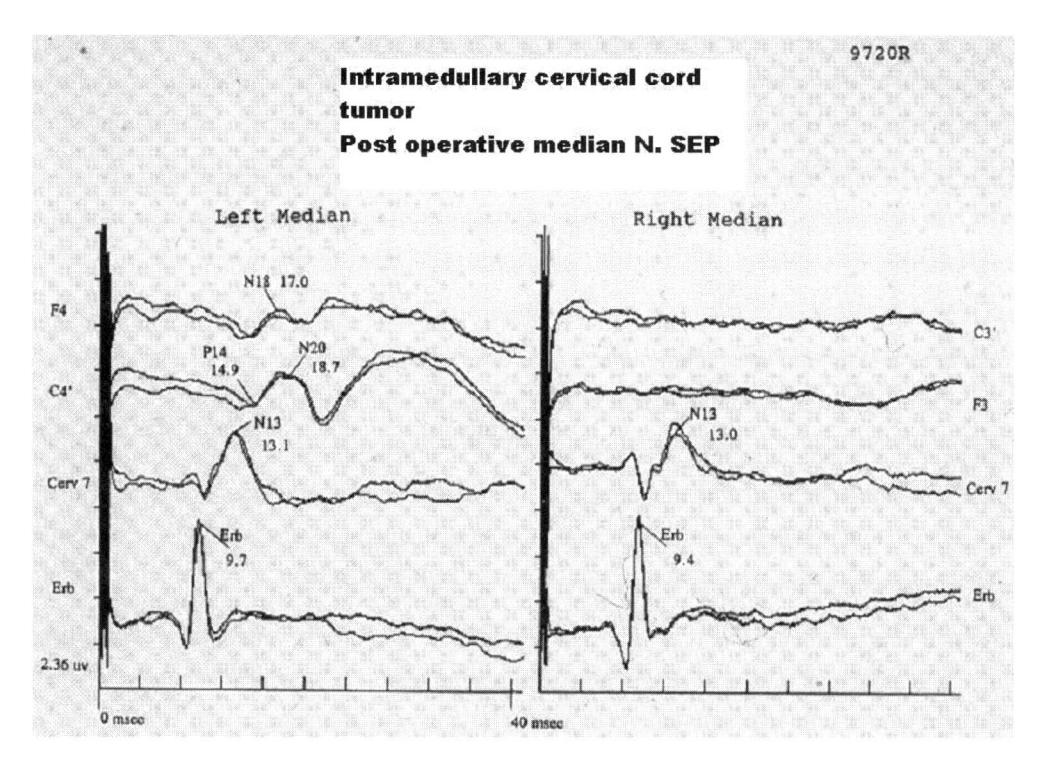

C

**Intramedullary cervical cord tumor
Post operative median N. SEP**

[Figure: Left Median and Right Median SEP traces with labels F4, C4', Cerv 7, Erb (left) and C3', F3, Cerv 7, Erb (right); waveform markers N18 17.0, P14 14.9, N20 18.7, N13 13.1, Erb 9.7 (left) and N13 13.0, Erb 9.4 (right); 2.36 uV; 0 msec to 40 msec; 9720R]

tion can occur. The thoracic spinal cord is most vulnerable to ischemic damage because this region is considered a watershed zone with relatively sparse collaterals. This type of ischemia would affect the MEPs more significantly than the SEPs, as the ventral spinal cord would be affected more. Sectioning of nerve roots is therefore ill advised.

UTILITY OF NIOM

There is a growing body of literature suggesting that NIOM can reduce morbidity in spinal cord surgeries. Until recently, most data were for SEP monitoring. In one series, 20 patients were monitored with SEPs; 6 of these developed postoperative deficits. In one patient, baseline SEPs were not obtained in the limb that developed weakness. In all the others, SEP changes occurred during dissection, warning of postoperative complications (12). In another series of 30 patients undergoing spinal cord surgery for pain syndrome, intramedullary tumors, and syringomyelia, changes in subcortical SEP waveforms suggested damage to the spinal cord; as a result, the surgical procedures in several cases were modified (13). There are no reports in which SEP monitoring did not detect impending spinal cord damage. However, in other types of surgeries on the spine, preservation of SEPs has been noted despite the occurrence of postoperative paraplegia; this most likely happens with spinal cord surgery as well.

In the last decade, the utility of MEP monitoring has been reported. It should be noted that SEP monitoring is almost always performed in addition to MEP monitoring. In a series of 28 patients who underwent CMAP MEP monitoring after TES, significant changes were noted in 13 patients; 12 of these had persistent postoperative paraparesis (14). In another series of 32 patients, D-wave MEP monitoring was possible in 19 (15). A decrease in D-wave amplitude of greater than 50% was seen in 3 patients; all 3 had postoperative paraplegia, which eventually recovered in 2. Postoperative weakness was not noted in any of the patients who had a decrease in D-wave amplitude of less than 50%. Of the 13 patients in this series in whom MEP monitoring was not possible, 5 had postoperative weakness.

The most convincing data on the utility of NIOM come from a recent historical control study (16). In this study, outcomes of 50 patients who underwent NIOM with SEPs, CMAPs, and D-wave MEPs were compared to matched controls who had previously had surgery without NIOM. The investigators used the SEP and MEP interpretation criteria described earlier. The patients who had NIOM were less likely to experience a deterioration in neurologic status as compared to controls.

TECHNICAL CONSIDERATIONS

Preparation

One of the main responsibilities of the NIOM technologist is to communicate with the patient and his or her family about the NIOM and how this will be achieved. The patient should be assured that NIOM usually does not hurt, but if acetone and/or collodion is used to attach the electrodes, there may be a strong associated odor.

Many patients presenting for spinal cord surgery will have neurologic deficits caused by the spinal cord lesion. These deficits, such as lower extremity weakness, should be assessed, as they may affect MEP NIOM. Other medical problems, such as a peripheral neuropathy and orthopedic problems, should also be noted, as they may affect SEP monitoring. The technologist should also determine if there are any relative contraindications for MEP monitoring, such as the presence of a cardiac pacemaker, other implantable devices, seizures, etc. This information must be conveyed to the neurophysiologist, and, with the surgeon's input, the neurophysiologist and technologist should decide which modalities of monitoring are most appropriate for the scheduled surgery.

Preoperative baseline SEP studies should be obtained whenever possible. Because the preoperative baseline studies are done in the awake state, the patient may not able to tolerate the sufficient stimulus intensity or may be unable to relax to yield "clean" responses. It is not uncommon to obtain well-defined responses during surgery when preoperative baseline responses were poorly reproducible. If baseline responses are not present, the NIOM team should be prepared to perform the more unusual types of monitoring discussed previously.

The NIOM technologist should also ensure that he or she has all the necessary electrodes for the surgery. If an epidural electrode will be used to record D waves, arrangements must be made with the surgeon, anesthesiologist, or neurophysiologist about implanting it. Almost any modern NIOM machine can be used for these surgeries; however, having at least a 16 channels available is important. This will allow performing upper and lower limb SEPs and CMAP MEPs from all four extremities, as well as D waves if necessary. The NIOM machine should be capable of delivering a high-intensity TES; if it is not, a separate machine for this purpose should be used, such as the Digitimer.

Procedure

Electrode application on the day of the surgery can be done in the preoperative holding area. Needle electrodes should not be applied when the patient is awake. Instead, once the patient is anesthetized, these electrodes can easily be inserted. In special situations where the patient is extremely frightened or cognitively impaired, all the electrodes should be applied after the patient has been anesthetized.

There are many types of recording and stimulating electrodes available in today's market. Whichever electrodes are chosen, it is important to maintain consistency in application and placement. Skin preparation should be done with a light sandpaper or skin preparation product such as Nu Prep or Lemon Prep. This should be done for surface and self-adhesive electrodes. Placement of scalp electrodes should be based on the international 10-20 system. It is also wise to place redundant electrodes in case some electrodes do not work or become disconnected. If the epidural electrode is to be inserted percutaneously, it should be done before the patient is draped. Alternatively, if it will be placed after the laminectomy, it should be made available to the scrub nurse to pass to the surgeon at the appropriate time.

It is ideal if the first sets of SEPs and MEPs are obtained before the patient is draped and covered in the sterile field. This will establish the integrity of the recorded system and allows adjustment of stimulating or recording electrodes if necessary. This is an important step, as once the patient is draped, it is virtually impossible to change or reapply the electrodes. These steps will ensure successful recording after the patient is placed under the sterile field.

The first operative baseline studies are done after the patient is in a stable anesthetic state. This is the "true" baseline response and the one to which any changes in the operating room must be compared. This baseline is likely to be different than the preoperative baseline study obtained in the outpatient laboratory, as the patient was awake during the latter study. Under anesthesia, unlike the SEPs recorded in the awake state, middle- and long-latency components are abolished and only the short-latency components are preserved. In some cases, especially with high doses of inhalation anesthetics, even the first cortical potential (N20 for upper and P37 for lower SEPs) may not be present.

For surgeries involving the upper cervical spine, median or ulnar nerve SEPs and CMAP MEPs from all four extremities should be monitored. For lower spinal cord lesions, tibial nerve SEPs and CMAP MEPs should be obtained. For lower spinal cord surgeries, median SEPs should also be obtained and serve as a control. Recording D waves from an epidural electrode should also be considered. Alternating between SEP and MEP monitoring is useful except if a posterior myelotomy is performed; this renders SEP monitoring impossible; thus MEP monitoring becomes more important. During tumor or lesion dissection, frequent MEPs should be obtained. The surgeon should always be warned prior to the delivery of a MEP stimulus so that sudden patient movement does not disrupt the surgery.

A crucial role of the NIOM technologist is to recognize and troubleshoot artifacts. The operating room is an electrically hostile environment. There can be several types of interference and artifacts causing problems for NIOM. The blood warmers, warming blankets, electrocautery, CUSA, x-ray machine, surgical microscope, and anesthesia machine may give off very high frequency noise. The technologist should be able to identify the different types of artifact and adjust accordingly. Sometimes it can be as simple as regelling an electrode or unplugging the device that is causing the problem. Operating room equipment should never be unplugged without first conferring with the circulating nurse. At other times, the artifact can be recalcitrant and difficult to eliminate. Troubleshooting can best be accomplished by using a systematic and organized approach.

If a significant change in responses is observed, the NIOM team must determine the source, so that appropriate corrective steps can be taken. The first step is to make certain that the change is reliable and consistent, not just a one-time instance. At least two sets of responses should be obtained to verify change. If the change is verified and cannot be attributed to systemic processes or artifact, it must be localized to the brain, cervical spinal cord, or peripheral nervous system. The significance of the change should be interpreted by the neurophysiologist, and the surgeon should be alerted.

Several steps must be taken to troubleshoot a decrement in NIOM responses. The first thing to check is the original incoming raw data. If one channel has a lot of artifact, it may be due to a high impedance or loss of an electrode. If all channels are affected, there could be loss of the ground electrode or introduction of an external interference. With newer equipment, the technologist can monitor original data continuously throughout the procedure together with averaged responses. It helps to determine whether the incoming raw EEG data are intermittently contaminated by the external physical or electrical interference. Next, an impedance check must be performed. Thereafter, the stimulators should be checked to ensure that adequate stimulation is being given. The right and left stimulators can be switched as a test. If the problem moves to the other side, the stimulator cable is most likely at fault. Finally, sources of external interference should be sought. A new instrument can cause electrical noise, a patient under very light anesthesia will have EMG contaminating the average, an unexpected bolus of medicine given by the anesthesiologist may cause a drop in amplitude of the response, and changes in temperature and blood pressure can also have significant effects.

Occasionally situations are encountered in which 60-Hz or other high-frequency external interference or large stimulus artifact cannot be eliminated. Recording parameters such as frequency bandwidth, averaging number, or stimulus rate can be changed to help eliminate the artifact. The high-frequency filter may be reduced to 500 Hz or less and the low filter may be increased to 20 to 50 Hz. With a filter setting change, waveform latency and amplitude may change. Use of a 60-Hz filter can produce "60-Hz ringing," which consists of rhythmic waves after the stimulus artifact, mimicking the "reproducible evoked response." If the external interference is extremely large and most trials are rejected, it may be necessary to decrease the sensitivity or change the rejection threshold.

Postprocedure

NIOM for most spinal cord surgeries continues until the surgical wound is closed. Electrodes are removed at the end of the case. Needle electrodes are removed slowly, so as to not to cause injury. Disposable electrodes are discarded in an appropriate container. Any reusable electrodes, such as surface disk electrodes, are placed in a plastic bag, later to be cleaned and disinfected according to laboratory protocol. If possible, the NIOM technologist should examine the patient after his or her recovery from anesthesia to document adequate movement and sensation in the limbs.

All the documentation is completed with a copy of all the waveforms and log of events printed for the report. In addition to the recording parameters, all alerts issued to the surgeon should be well documented, along with any changes that occurred owing to the alerts. The neurophysiologist should create a report documenting all these findings.

CONCLUSIONS

Spinal cord surgery can be associated with high neurologic morbidity, paraparesis being the most significant complication. NIOM offers surgeons a technique that can help reduce the incidence of postoperative paraparesis. Unlike other types of spinal surgery, surgery on the spinal cord itself is likely to result in selective damage to various fiber tracts, making multimodality monitoring essential. Advances in MEP monitoring have helped reduce morbidity and may be more specific in predicting impending permanent postoperative paraparesis. NIOM for spinal cord surgery should include at least SEP and CMAP MEP monitoring and preferably D-wave monitoring as well.

REFERENCES

1. Lesser RP, Raudzens P, Luders H, et al. Postoperative neurological deficits may occur despite unchanged intraoperative somatosensory evoked potentials. *Ann Neurol* 1986;19:22–25.
2. Zornow MH, Grafe MR, Tybor C, Swenson MR. Preservation of evoked potentials in a case of anterior spinal artery syndrome. *Electroencephalogr Clin Neurophysiol* 1990; 77:137–139.
3. Sansur CA, Pouratian N, Dumont AS, et al. Part II: spinal-cord neoplasms: primary tumours of the bony spine and adjacent soft tissues. *Lancet Oncol* 2007;8:137–147.
4. Traul DE, Shaffrey ME, Schiff D. Part I: spinal-cord neoplasms: intradural neoplasms. *Lancet Oncol* 2007;8:35–45.
5. Machida M, Weinstein SL, Yamada T, Kimura J. Spinal cord monitoring. Electrophysiological measures of sensory and motor function during spinal surgery. *Spine* 1985;10: 407–413.
6. Deletis V. Intraoperative neurophysiology and methodologies used to monitor the functional integrity of the motor system. In: Deletis V, Shils J, eds. *Neurophysiology in Neurosurgery: A Modern Intraoperative Approach*. San Diego, CA: Academic Press, 2002:25–51.
7. Erwin CW, Erwin AC. Up and down the spinal cord: intraoperative monitoring of sensory and motor spinal cord pathways. *J Clin Neurophysiol* 1993;10:425–436.
8. Owen JH. The application of intraoperative monitoring during surgery for spinal deformity. *Spine* 1999;24:2649–2662.
9. Kothbauer K, Deletis V, Epstein FJ. Intraoperative spinal cord monitoring for intramedullary surgery: an essential adjunct. *Pediatr Neurosurg* 1997;26:247–254.
10. Deletis V. Neuromonitoring. In: McLone DG, ed. *Pediatric Neurosurgery: Surgery of the Developing Nervous System*. Philadelphia: Saunders, 2001:1204–1213.
11. Sala F, Lanteri P, Bricolo A. Motor evoked potential monitoring for spinal cord and brain stem surgery. *Adv Tech Stand Neurosurg* 2004;29:133–169.
12. Kearse LA Jr, Lopez-Bresnahan M, McPeck K, Tambe V. Loss of somatosensory evoked potentials during intramedullary spinal cord surgery predicts postoperative neurologic deficits in motor function [corrected]. *J Clin Anesth* 1993;5:392–398.
13. Prestor B, Golob P. Intra-operative spinal cord neuromonitoring in patients operated on for intramedullary tumors and syringomyelia. *Neurol Res* 1999;21:125–129.
14. Quinones-Hinojosa A, Lyon R, Zada G, et al. Changes in transcranial motor evoked potentials during intramedullary spinal cord tumor resection correlate with postoperative motor function. *Neurosurgery* 2005;56:982–993; discussion 982–993.
15. Morota N, Deletis V, Constantini S, et al. The role of motor evoked potentials during surgery for intramedullary spinal cord tumors. *Neurosurgery* 1997;41:1327–1336.
16. Sala F, Palandri G, Basso E, et al. Motor evoked potential monitoring improves outcome after surgery for intramedullary spinal cord tumors: a historical control study. *Neurosurgery* 2006;58:1129–1143; discussion 1129–1143.

9 Lumbosacral Surgery

Neil R. Holland

The adult spinal cord ends opposite the lower border of the L1 vertebra; below that, the spinal canal contains only individual lumbosacral nerve roots descending toward their respective neural foraminae, collectively known as the cauda equina. Nerve roots can be injured during lumbosacral surgery by probing, drilling, misplaced hardware, or stretching during correction of spinal deformity. There is a 10% risk of new postoperative neurologic deficit from nerve root injury during spinal fusion for degenerative lumbosacral spine disease, 10-fold greater than the risk of spinal cord injury from scoliosis surgery. The most common deficit is a new foot drop from surgical injury to the L5 nerve root, although findings can include any pattern of dermatomal numbness, radicular weakness, and/or sphincter dysfunction. Nerve root injuries are more frequent during revision than primary surgery and in cases where multiple levels are fused (1). Obviously, the purpose of neurophysiologic intraoperative monitoring (NIOM) with electromyography (EMG) during these lumbosacral spine cases is to detect early and potentially reversible surgical nerve root irritation, alert the surgeon, and thus prevent more significant injury and postoperative deficit.

NERVE ROOT MONITORING USING FREE-RUNNING EMG

Background

Mixed nerve somatosensory evoked potentials (SEPs) and transcranial electrical motor evoked potentials (MEPs) are the NIOM techniques most often used for spinal cord monitoring, but they are not sensitive for detecting nerve root injuries. SEPs represent the summation of neural signals that enter the spinal cord through multiple segments, and because of central amplification, they can remain completely unchanged after an individual nerve root lesion. MEPs recorded from an epidural electrode will obviously not be affected by a more caudal nerve root injury. MEPs recorded from a single distal limb muscle throughout surgery will not detect nerve root injuries affecting other myotomes. There have been numerous well-documented cases of patients with acute radiculopathy from spine surgery despite normal SEP and MEP monitoring. Dermatomal somatosensory evoked potentials (DSEPs) can detect individual nerve root injuries but are technically difficult to resolve in the operating room; moreover, they need to be averaged many times, resulting a slow turnaround time, and they test only dorsal root (sensory) function.

For these reasons EMG has become the neurophysiologic technique most often used to monitor nerve root function during lumbosacral spine surgery. EMG is more sensitive than SEPs and DSEPs for detecting nerve root dysfunction, provides immediate results without averaging, and can be monitored from multiple channels (i.e., multiple myotomes and nerve roots) simultaneously, giving instantaneous feedback to the surgeon during critical phases of the procedure.

Technique

Continuous free-running EMG is monitored from muscles innervated by nerve roots considered to be at risk for injury during surgery. Blunt mechanical trauma to nerve roots causes a depolarization that will be conducted down the nerve, across the neuromuscular junction, and evoke identifiable motor unit potentials in the monitored muscle (Figure 9.1). Minor nerve root manipulation will result in a short burst of motor unit potentials (Figure 9.2A). More severe mechanical nerve root injury or retraction will cause prolonged trains of high-frequency motor unit potentials, often referred to as neurotonic discharges (Figure 9.2B and C). Repetitive grouped motor unit potentials, myokymic discharges, are seen less frequently and usually indicate very severe nerve injury (Figure 9.2D). These are the very same EMG abnormalities seen in the diagnostic laboratory in cases of spontaneous motor nerve hyperexcitability (Isaac's syndrome). Identification of this abnormal EMG activity can be used to alert the surgeon of inadvertent trauma to nerve roots, allowing evasive action in an

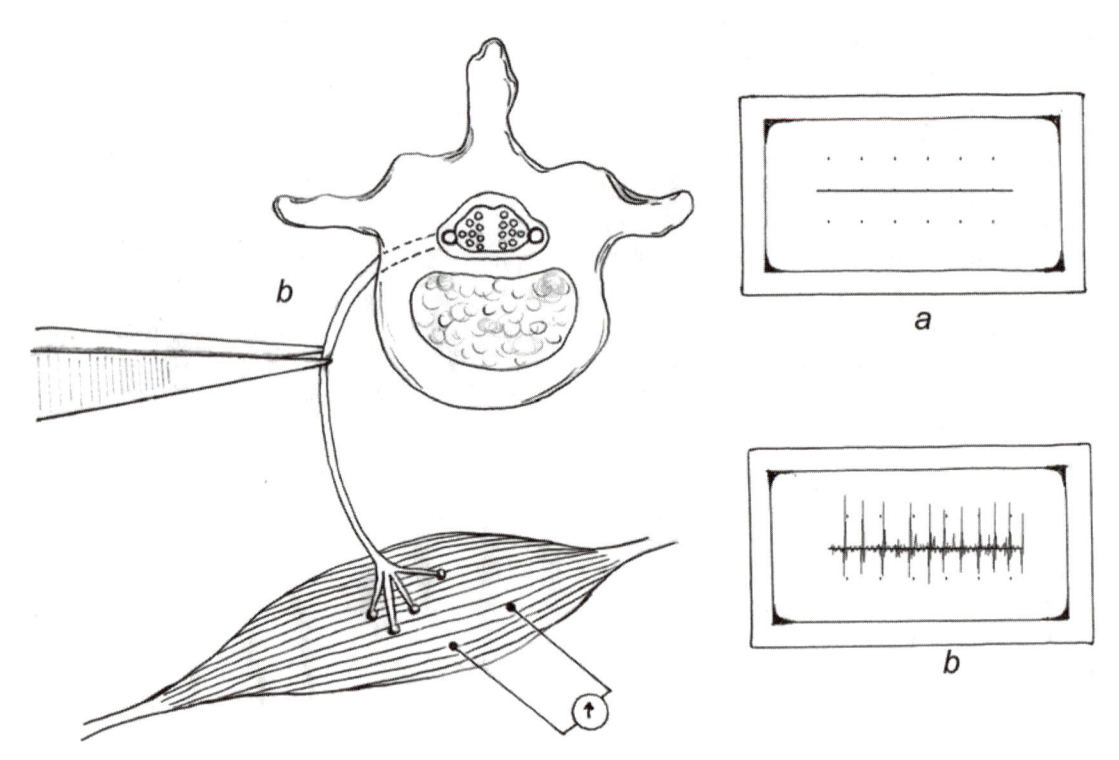

FIGURE 9.1 Free-running EMG activity for nerve root monitoring. A. EMG monitoring should be quiescent under normal conditions. B. Blunt mechanical nerve root irritation activates the motor nerve fibers, is transmitted down the nerve and across the neuromuscular junction, and evokes recordable motor unit potentials in the monitored muscle.

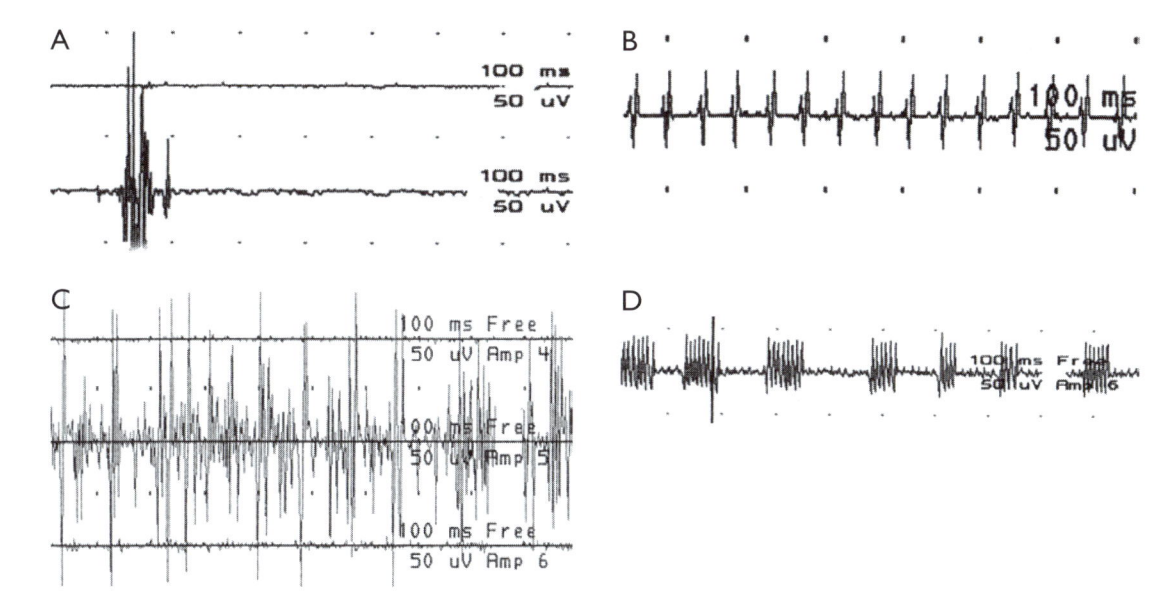

FIGURE 9.2 EMG activity from nerve root irritation or injury. A. Minor nerve root manipulation evokes a short burst of motor unit potentials. B and C. More severe blunt mechanical nerve root injury or retraction evokes prolonged trains of high-frequency motor unit potentials, known as neurotonic discharges. D. Rarely, myokymic discharges can be seen, but usually only after very severe nerve injury. In each case the time base shown is 100 ms/div and the display sensitivity is 50 μV/div.

effort to prevent more severe or irreversible injury. The loudspeaker on the EMG machine can be used to provide the surgeon with an instantaneous audible warning of potential nerve root injury. Limb muscles can be used to monitor spinal levels down to the S2 nerve roots. The anal and/or urethral sphincter muscles should be monitored in cases where the conus medullaris or lower sacral nerve root are felt to be at particular risk for iatrogenic injury (Table 9.1).

Outcome Data

Significant EMG activity occurs in 80% of monitored lumbosacral spine surgeries, although less that 10% of these develop a new persistent postoperative neurologic deficit (Table 9.2). In other words, EMG monitoring has a high sensitivity for detecting mechanical nerve root manipulation but a low specificity and positive predictive value for postoperative nerve root injury. SEP monitoring has a lower sensitivity, but a higher specificity and positive predictive value (2) (Table 9.3). However, sensitivity is preferable to specificity for NIOM, as it is more important to detect a mild degree of nerve root irritation and alert the surgeon in time to take evasive action, than it is to correctly predict an irreversible postoperative deficit.

TABLE 9.1 Muscles Suitable for Intraoperative Electromyographic Monitoring of Thoracolumbosacral Nerve Root Segments during Lumbar Fusion

Nerve roots at risk	Appropriate muscle for EMG monitoring
T7–12	External oblique and rectus abdominus
L1–2	Iliacus
L2–4	Vastus medialis
L4–5	Tibialis anterior
S1–2	Medial gastrocnemius
S3–5	Anal and urethral sphincter

TABLE 9.2 Intraoperative EMG Activity vs. Postoperative Outcome in 213 Monitored Lumbar Spine Cases

Postoperative symptoms	EMG activity	No EMG activity
Improved, 177	133 (75%)	44 (25%)
No change, 21	17 (81%)	4 (19%)
Worse, 14	14 (100%)	0 (0%)

From Gunnarson et al. (2).

Although there are many published anecdotal case reports touting the benefits of intraoperative EMG monitoring during lumbar spine surgery, there is a paucity of prospective outcome data. Some studies have shown reduced incidence of postoperative C5 radiculopathy after cervical decompression using EMG monitoring from the deltoid muscle, and cases detected during surgery with EMG monitoring were felt to have been milder, with a more rapid recovery because the surgeon was alerted immediately (3,4) (Table 9.4). These data can probably be extrapolated to nerve root monitoring during lumbar spine surgery. Monitored patients undergoing complex lumbosacral procedures for spinal cord tumors and tethered cord syndrome show abnormal EMG activity confined to the sphincter muscles in 33% cases (28% anal and 5% urethral sphincter), underscoring the importance of recording sphincter EMG in these cases (5).

Precautions

Although EMG monitoring is sensitive for blunt mechanical irritation and injury to motor nerves, it may remain quiescent during sharp nerve transection. Furthermore, even after acute nerve transection the distal nerve stump can still be activated by mechanical irritation and electrical stimulation, and the presence of these ongoing evoked EMG responses may be mistakenly interpreted as evidence of nerve root continuity. Mechanical trauma is less likely to evoke neurotonic discharges from abnormal motor nerves, and EMG monitoring may miss additional intraoperative injury to nerve roots already partially injured by preexisting lumbosacral radiculopathy.

Neurotonic discharges must be differentiated from other EMG findings that can occur during surgery without nerve injury to avoid false alarms. Spontaneous fibrillation potentials may be seen throughout surgery in patients with preexisting radiculopathy and denervation. They can be distinguished from neurotonic discharges because they occur continuously (even before critical phases of surgery) and fire regularly at slow rates (less than 15 Hz). Unlike neurotonic discharges, fibrillations are action potentials of single muscle fibers and not motor units, so they are simple triphasic or biphasic spikes (Figure 9.3A). Voluntary motor unit potentials can be seen under conditions of light anesthesia. These are semirhythmic motor unit potentials that usu-

TABLE 9.3 Sensitivity and Specificity of EMG vs. SEP Monitoring for Detecting 14 New Postoperative Deficits in 213 Monitored Lumbar Spine Cases

	Sensitivity	Specificity	Positive predictive value	Negative predictive value
EMG monitoring (neurotonic discharges)	14/14 or 100%	23.7%	0.085	1.0
SEP monitoring (>50% change in amplitude)	4*/14 or 28.6%	94.7%	0.286	0.947

*All 4 patients with abnormal SEP also had abnormal EMG monitoring.
From Gunnarson et al. (2).

TABLE 9.4 Incidence of Postoperative C5 Radiculopathy after Cervical Laminectomy for Cervical Myelopathy with and without Intraoperative EMG Monitoring from the Deltoid Muscle

Study	EMG monitoring	No EMG monitoring
Jimenez, 2005 (3)	1/116 (0.9%)	4/55 (7.3%)
Fan, 2002 (4)	2/68 (2.9%)	6/132 (4.5%)

ally occur simultaneously in muscles from multiple bilateral myotomes (Figure 9.3B). Electrocautery artifact is easy to recognize but precludes concurrent EMG monitoring (Figure 9.3C). Needle electrode movement artifact can be mistaken for EMG activity when the surgeon is working close to the recording electrode (Figure 9.3D). Neurotonic discharges may occur without mechanical injury—for example, during cold-water irrigation within the surgical field. Finally, EMG cannot be monitored in the presence of total pharmacologic neuromuscular blockade because nerve activation from mechanical irritation must be transmitted across the neuromuscular junction in order to evoke identifiable myogenic responses.

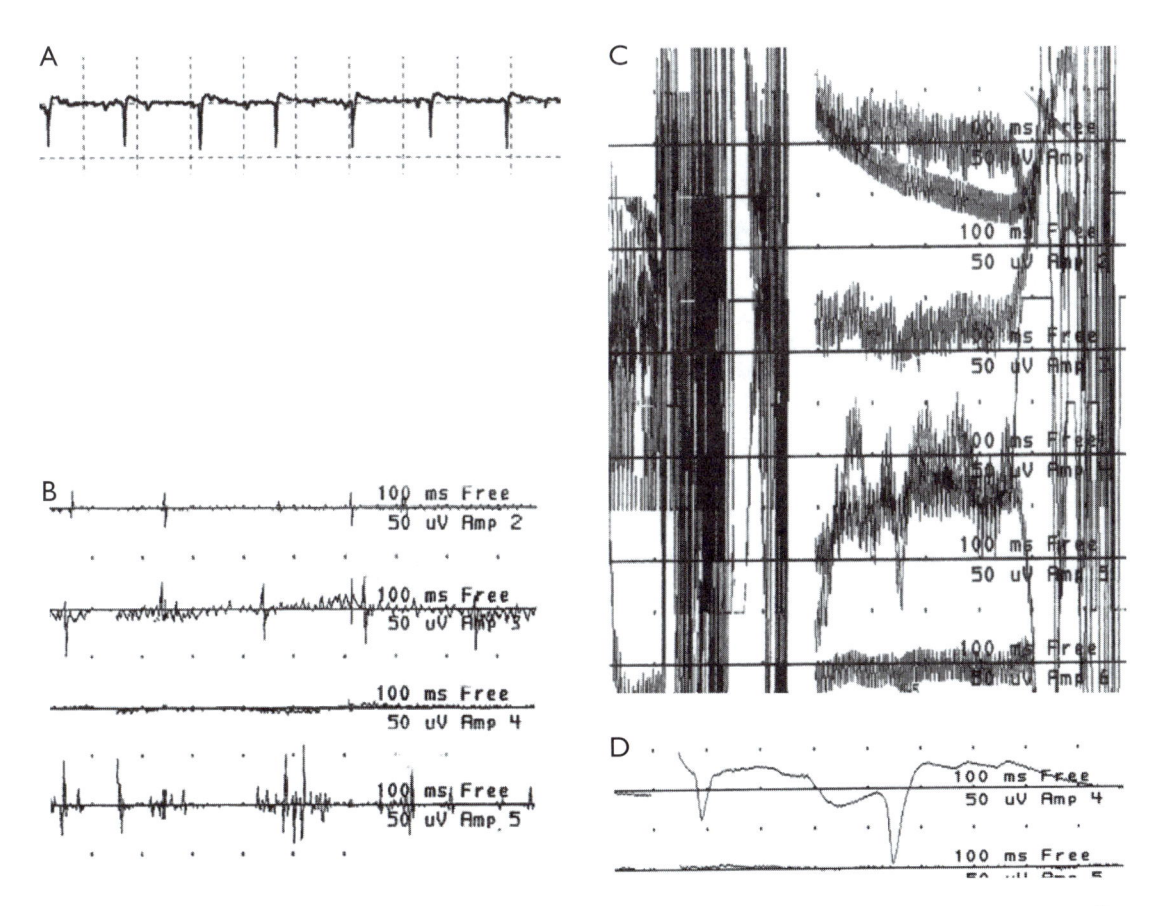

FIGURE 9.3 Other EMG findings that can occur during surgery without nerve injury. A. Spontaneous fibrillation potentials may been seen throughout surgery in patients with preexisting radiculopathy and denervation. B. Voluntary motor unit potentials can be seen under conditions of light anesthesia. C. Electrocautery artifact. D. Needle electrode movement artifact. In each case the time base shown is 100ms/div and the display sensitivity is 50 µV/div..

STIMULUS-TRIGGERED EMG MONITORING TO VERIFY CORRECT PLACEMENT OF PEDICLE SCREWS

Background

Many spinal instrumentation systems use pedicle screws as a point of fixation. Holes are drilled blindly through the narrow pedicles into the vertebral body to facilitate pedicle screw placement. Cadaver studies have shown that as many as 20% of screws are misdirected, lying outside the bony pedicle wall (Figure 9.4). Clinical studies have detected postoperative symptoms from irritation or injury to the adjacent nerve roots by misplaced pedicle screws in 5% to 10% cases. Intraoperative fluoroscopy and radiographs have been used in an attempt to verify correct pedicle screw placement during surgery but are not always reliable, perhaps because of limited available projections. Computed tomography is more definitive, but of course is not available in real time in the operating room. Direct inspection and palpation of the medial wall of the instrumented pedicle by the surgeon is the "gold standard" test for misplaced screws during surgery, but doing this for every screw may necessitate unnecessary laminectomies and excessive operative times.

Fortunately, stimulus-triggered EMG can be used to quickly verify correct pedicle screw placement in real time during surgery. Holes or screws that are correctly positioned within the pedicle wall are separated from the adjacent nerve roots by a cortical bony layer with high impedance to the passage of electrical current. (Figure 9.5B). However, a hole or screw that has perforated the bony pedicle wall will lie directly against adjacent nerve roots, and direct electrical stimulation of such misplaced holes and screws activates the adjacent nerve roots, evoking compound muscle action potential (CMAP) responses in muscles from the appropriate myotomes at lower stimulus intensities than those that lie completely contained within the pedicle wall (Figures 9.5A and 9.6A). Stimulus thresholds of less than 4 to 6 mA are suggestive of cortical bony perforation by pedicular instrumentation when the adjacent nerve root is healthy (6,7) (Table 9.5).

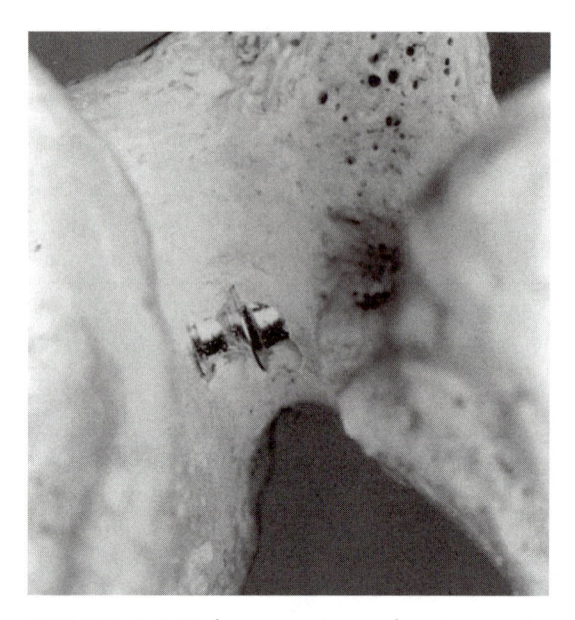

FIGURE 9.4 Cadaver specimen showing a misplaced pedicle screw, a potential source of postoperative irritation or injury to the adjacent nerve root.

Technique

Holes and screws are tested using a monopolar stimulating electrode with a remote anode needle electrode placed in the surgical wound and stimulus-triggered EMG recordings made from appropriate limb muscles. The stimulator is inserted directly into the pedicle hole after drilling. It is preferable to have the stimulator halfway into the hole, so that the uninsulated tip of the electrode is inside the pedicle close to the adjacent nerve root and not deep inside the vertebral body (Figure 9.5A). Screws are tested by touching the stimulator against the exposed shank or port of the screw, taking care to avoid any intervening soft tissue. It is important to test each pedicle hole and screw individually as each is drilled and inserted. A misplaced hole should be redirected and then retested before it is instrumented.

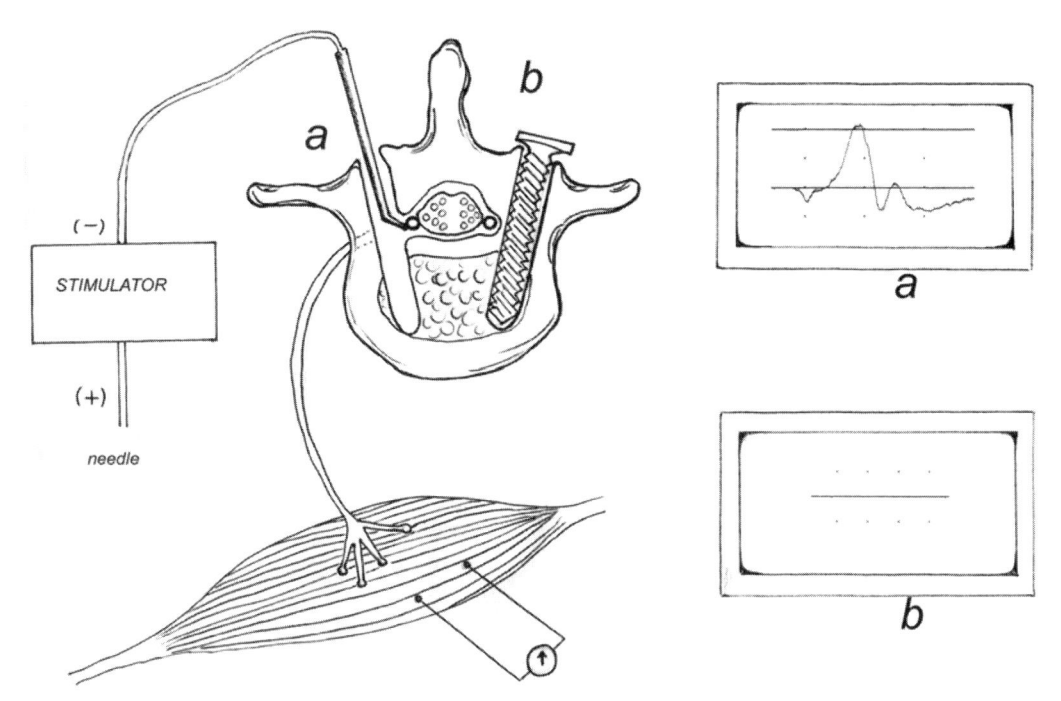

FIGURE 9.5 Stimulus-triggered EMG for detecting pedicular wall breach. A monopolar stimulator is inserted into a pedicle hole or touched against a pedicle screw. A. Holes or screws that have perforated the bony pedicle wall will lie directly against adjacent nerve roots and stimulation activates the adjacent nerve root, evoking a CMAP response. B. Holes or screws that are correctly positioned within the pedicle wall are separated from the adjacent nerve roots by a cortical bony layer, with a high impedance to the passage of electrical current and no evoked CMAP responses.

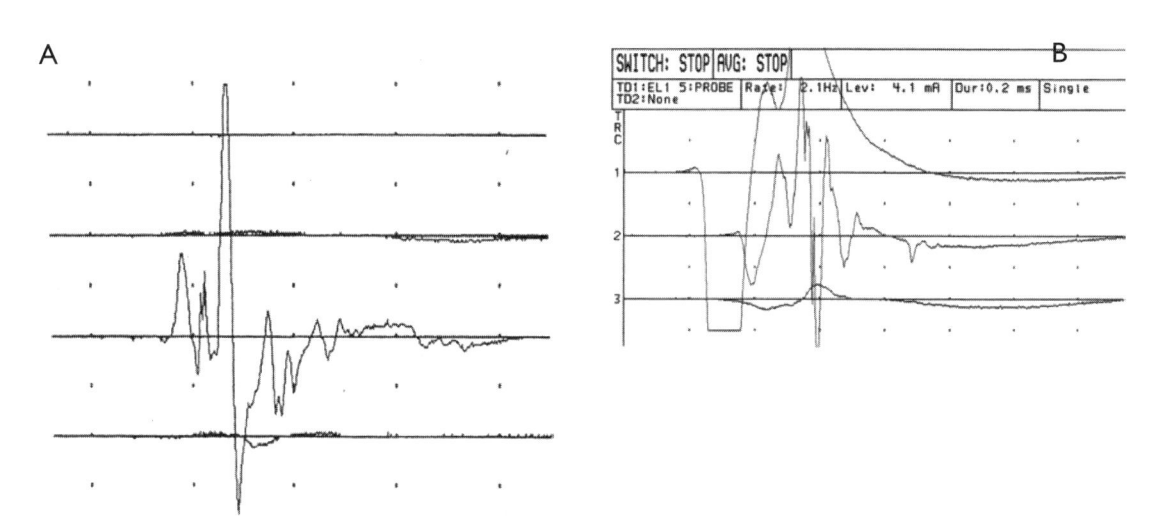

FIGURE 9.6 CMAP responses from intraoperative stimulus-triggered EMG. A. CMAP response in tibialis anterior from stimulation of an L5 pedicle screw at 5.3 mA, suggesting pedicular breach. B. CMAP responses recorded after direct stimulation of exposed cauda equina (as a positive control) at 4 mA. The time base shown is 10 ms/div and the display sensitivity is 50 µV/div.

TABLE 9.5 Stimulus Thresholds for Normal Healthy Nerve Roots, Chronically Compressed Nerve Roots, and Normal and Misplaced Pedicle Holes and Screws*

Structure	Stimulus threshold (mA)
Normal nerve root	(0.2–5.7)
Chronically compressed nerve root	6.3–20
Normal hole	(16.5–44.3)
Normal screw	24 (12.1–35.9)
Misplaced hole	(1–6)
Misplaced screw	(1–6)

*Shown as mean and/or range.
From Maguire et al. (6) and Holland et al. (9).

Redirecting the hole will frequently close off the pedicular perforation with bone fragments pushed outward by the drill bit. Insertion of a pedicle screw may enlarge a previously normal hole causing a wall breach. Finally, some particular brands of pedicle screw have an unusually high electrical resistance based on their metallic composition, so just testing the screw (and not the preceding hole) may give rise to a false-negative result (8).

To save time, each hole and screw can be initially tested at a searching stimulus intensity of 7 to 10 mA. If no CMAP response is identified at this intensity level, then the hole or screw is considered safe. If a CMAP response is identified at the initial searching intensity, the stimulating current is progressively reduced, using recurrent stimulation at 2 Hz, in order to determine the precise stimulus threshold required to evoke the response and hence the probability of pedicular perforation. Pedicle screws or holes with stimulus thresholds of less than 4 mA should be removed and/or redirected. Pedicle screws with stimulus thresholds between 4 and 6 mA are considered borderline and should probably be more closely inspected by the surgeon. The very same technique of stimulus-triggered EMG using a handheld stimulator in the operative field can also be used to identify viable nerve roots during dissection of intraspinal dumbbell and foraminal tumors and spinal surgery for tethered cord release.

Outcome Data

Based on a stimulus threshold of 6 mA or less, the sensitivity of stimulus-triggered EMG for identifying misplaced pedicle screws and hole is more than 90%, significantly exceeding the sensitivity of intraoperative radiography, which is only 63% (6). The probability of a pedicle screw breach increases with decreasing stimulus threshold (7) (Table 9.6).

Precautions

Because the expected result from a correctly placed pedicle screw or hole is negative (i.e., no response at the searching stimulus intensity), it's always a good idea to test a positive control to be sure that the stimulator and amplifier are working properly. This can be accomplished by having the surgeon stimulate an exposed nerve root directly.(Figure 9.6B). It is important to recognize that the stimulus thresholds mentioned above refer to pedicular instrumentation at levels where the bone and adjacent nerve roots are normal and healthy. False-positive stimulus-triggered EMGs can be seen in patients with advanced osteoporosis, presumably because of thin cortical bone

TABLE 9.6 Stimulus Threshold and Pedicle Screw Malposition (Confirmed by Palpation and/or Radiographs) for 4,587 Screws

Stimulus threshold	Probability of screw malposition
>8 mA	0.31%
4–8 mA	17.4%
<4 mA	54.2%
<2.8 mA	100%

From Raynor et al. (7).

with a lower than expected impedance to the passage of the electrical current.

More importantly, false-negative results may be seen in patients with preexisting radiculopathy: the stimulus intensities required to evoke CMAP responses from direct electrical stimulation of nerve roots are higher in the presence of preexisting axonotmetic radiculopathy, sometimes as high as 10 to 20 mA (9) (Table 9.5). Thus the failure to evoke a CMAP response from stimulation of a hole or screw adjacent to a chronically compressed nerve root at the usual searching stimulus intensity of 7 mA will not necessarily exclude a pedicular wall breach at that level, with the potential for further iatrogenic nerve root injury. Clearly, pedicular instrumentation must be tested at higher stimulus intensities when the adjacent nerve root is known to be axonotmetic. Axonotmetic nerve root injury should be suspected in the presence of chronic preoperative radicular motor deficits or abnormal preoperative electromyographic studies.

When possible it is best to first determine the electrical thresholds required to evoke CMAP responses in the appropriate muscles from direct stimulation of the exposed chronically compressed nerve root, and then test the pedicular instrumentation at that level at an appropriately higher intensity (perhaps 5 mA higher) in order to exclude a bony cortical breach. If the nerve root can not be directly tested, for example if there is no laminectomy at that level, then it is probably best to empirically test the holes and screws at a higher searching intensity such as 20 mA.

Once again, EMG cannot be monitored in the presence of total pharmacologic neuromuscular blockade, because nerve activation from electrical stimulation must be transmitted across the neuromuscular junction in order to evoke identifiable CMAP responses.

Finally, one has to be careful using recurrent stimulation to determine a threshold value in the presence of partial neuromuscular blockade, as a physiologically decremental response may suggest a falsely high threshold and lead to a false-negative result. Under these circumstances, it is better to use single shocks at an initial stimulus intensity where a positive response is likely to be significant (e.g., 4 mA).

MONITORING NEUROMUSCULAR BLOCKADE

Background

Nerve activation, whether from mechanical irritation or electrical stimulation, must be transmitted across the neuromuscular junction in order to evoke identifiable myogenic responses. Clearly EMG cannot be monitored in the presence of total pharmacologic neuromuscular blockade. However, muscle relaxation is a critical component of balanced anesthesia. While adequate surgical relaxation may be achieved using inhalation anesthetic agents alone, patients are more likely to move in the absence of specific pharmacologic neuromuscular blockade, and this may compromise patient safety. In addition, many surgeries necessitate simultaneous monitoring of both SEPs and EMG: in the absence of neuromuscular blockers, the higher doses of inhalation anesthetic agents required to maintain adequate muscle relaxation may significantly attenuate cortical SEP responses, and subcortical (cervical) SEP responses may be rendered unreliable by excessive myogenic artifact. Fortunately, EMG can be successfully monitored in the operating room under conditions of partial (as much as 50% to 75%) neuromuscular blockade using carefully titrated doses of short-acting agents such as atracurium or vecuronium.

Neuromuscular blockade has been traditionally monitored by the anesthesiologist during surgery using the number of visible hand twitches after a train-of-four peripheral stimulations to the ulnar nerve at the forearm. However, unfamiliarity with peripheral nerve function and anatomy may result in inaccurate electrode placement and misinterpretation of direct muscle activation as twitches by the anesthesiologist, underestimating the degree of pharmacologic neuromuscular blockade. Muscles from the cranial, cervical, and lumbosacral myotomes have different susceptibilities to the effects of neuromuscular blocking agents. In addition, chronically compressed nerves may have enhanced sensitivity to the effects of neuromuscular blockade. For these reasons, neuromuscular transmission should be monitored using repetitive nerve stimulation from a muscle belonging to the appropriate myotome for the nerves or roots considered at risk from surgery.

Technique

Intraoperative EMG can be monitored in the presence of up to 75% neuromuscular blockade. This is defined as a CMAP response amplitude to a single supramaximal stimulus that is more than 25% of its baseline (preanesthesia) value. In practice, it is rare to set up and test patients prior to induction of anesthesia. It is more usual to monitor neuromuscular transmission in anesthetized patients using repetitive nerve stimulation. Less than 75% neuromuscular blockade corresponds to a decrement of less than 100% over four successive supramaximal repetitive nerve stimulations (10) (Figure 9.7). It is easy to monitor repetitive nerve stimulation from the tibialis anterior muscles during lumbar spine surgery because this muscle is routinely used for EMG monitoring during these cases anyway. The deep peroneal nerve can be stimulated transcutaneously using needle or surface electrodes at the fibula head. Most EMG machines used for intraoperative monitoring will come with repetitive nerve stimulation software. As long as four CMAP responses are identifiable from supramaximal repetitive nerve stimulation at 2 Hz, the degree of neuromuscular blockade is sufficiently low to allow EMG monitoring. (Figure 9.8B and C) Less than four identifiable CMAP responses indicates pharmacologic neuromuscular blockade exceeding 75%, which might lower the sensitivity of EMG monitoring for the detection of intraoperative nerve root injury (Figure 9.8A). The surgeon should be kept apprised of this and may order reversal of neuromuscular blockade if it occurs during a critical phase of surgery.

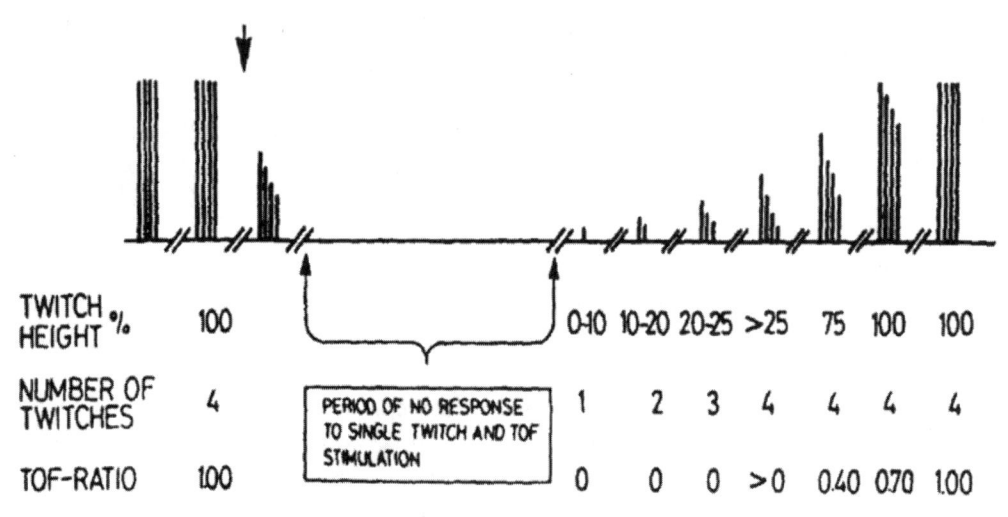

FIGURE 9.7 Relationship between repetitive nerve stimulation (train of four) and degree of neuromuscular blockade. Less than 75% neuromuscular blockade is required for EMG monitoring, which corresponds to less than 25% twitch height and the presence of four twitches on train-of-four repetitive nerve stimulation. [© The Board of Management and Trustees of the British Journal of Anesthesia. Reproduced by permission of Oxford University Press/British Journal of Anesthesia. Viby-Mogensen (10).]

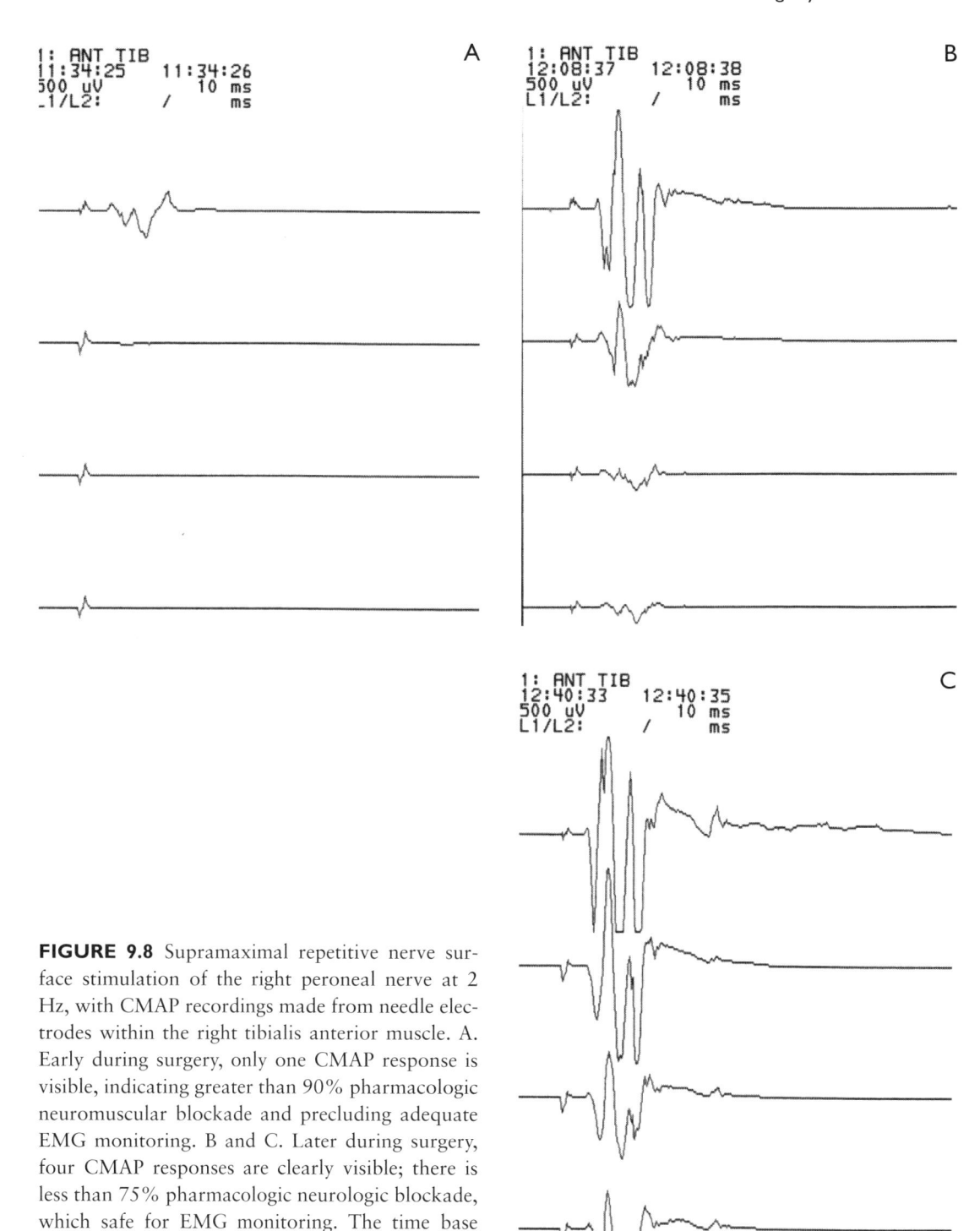

FIGURE 9.8 Supramaximal repetitive nerve surface stimulation of the right peroneal nerve at 2 Hz, with CMAP recordings made from needle electrodes within the right tibialis anterior muscle. A. Early during surgery, only one CMAP response is visible, indicating greater than 90% pharmacologic neuromuscular blockade and precluding adequate EMG monitoring. B and C. Later during surgery, four CMAP responses are clearly visible; there is less than 75% pharmacologic neurologic blockade, which safe for EMG monitoring. The time base shown is 10 ms/div and the display sensitivity is 0.5 mV/div.

TECHNICAL CONSIDERATIONS

Preoperative Studies

It is very helpful to know relevant details of the patient's preoperative neurologic examination and electrodiagnostic testing. It is not always possible to examine every patient personally ahead of surgery. However, it will be possible to review the patient's chart, which should include a neurologic examination and will often include a preoperative EMG report. Many patients undergoing lumbosacral spine surgeries will already have preoperative weakness. Their preoperative EMG reports may show evidence of chronic motor axonal loss from lumbar radiculopathy in the form of low amplitude CMAP responses or denervation on needle EMG examination. These patients have preexisting axonotmetic lumbar nerve root injuries, necessitating special precautions to exclude pedicular breach with stimulus-triggered EMG at those levels.

Recording Electrodes and Parameters

EMG is recorded from limb muscles using paired intramuscular needle or wire electrodes. Subdermal needle electrodes are suitable for most muscles.(Figure 9.9A and B) Monopolar EMG needles (Figure 9.9C) or hooked wire electrodes (Figure 9.9D) can be used for deeper muscles such as iliacus or rectus abdominus. The recording electrodes are placed close together in the muscle belly, and although this arrangement may restrict the area of muscle monitored, it minimizes the risk of detecting volume conducted responses from more distant muscles. Electrodes should be held in place with tape to prevent then from pulling out as the patient is moved and positioned on the table. If necessary, anal sphincter EMG can be recorded using either needle electrodes, or a specialized surface electrode mounted onto a sponge plug.(Figure 9.9E). Urethral sphincter EMG can be recorded using a specialized surface electrode mounted over a Foley catheter (Figure 9.9F).

It is sometimes necessary use to extension cables, depending on where the amplifier box is placed. Paired extension cables can be twisted together to reduce electrical interference (Figure 9.9G). The urethral sphincter electrode should be retrieved at the end of surgery (this will mean the patient's Foley catheter will have to be changed), sterilized, and can be reused. All the other recording electrodes are disposable, but most are sharp and/or potentially contaminated with body fluids, and should be disposed of accordingly. Unless contaminated with body fluids, extension cables are reusable without sterilization.

Typical recording parameters for intraoperative EMG are shown in Table 9.7. One can quickly become very familiar with free-running EMG activity by observing qualitative needle EMG examination in the diagnostic laboratory. However, intraoperative CMAP responses are different from the diagnostic EMG laboratory, and may be less familiar: CMAP from diagnostic motor nerve conduction studies are elicited by supramaximal stimulation with recordings made from carefully placed surface electrodes and are reproducible biphasic responses with amplitudes that correlate with the number of functioning axons present. In contrast, intraoperative CMAP responses are recorded from intramuscular needle electrodes and submaximal stimulation and are highly complicated polyphasic responses with variable onset latencies and response amplitudes.(Figure 9.6A) In effect they are all or nothing responses, although the stimulus threshold can provide some quantitative information regarding nerve function (9).

TABLE 9.7 Typical Recording Parameters for Intraoperative EMG

	Free-running EMG	Stimulus-triggered EMG
Filters	20–10,000 Hz	10–10,000 Hz
Gain	50 µV/div	50 µV/div
Time base	100 ms/div	10 ms/div

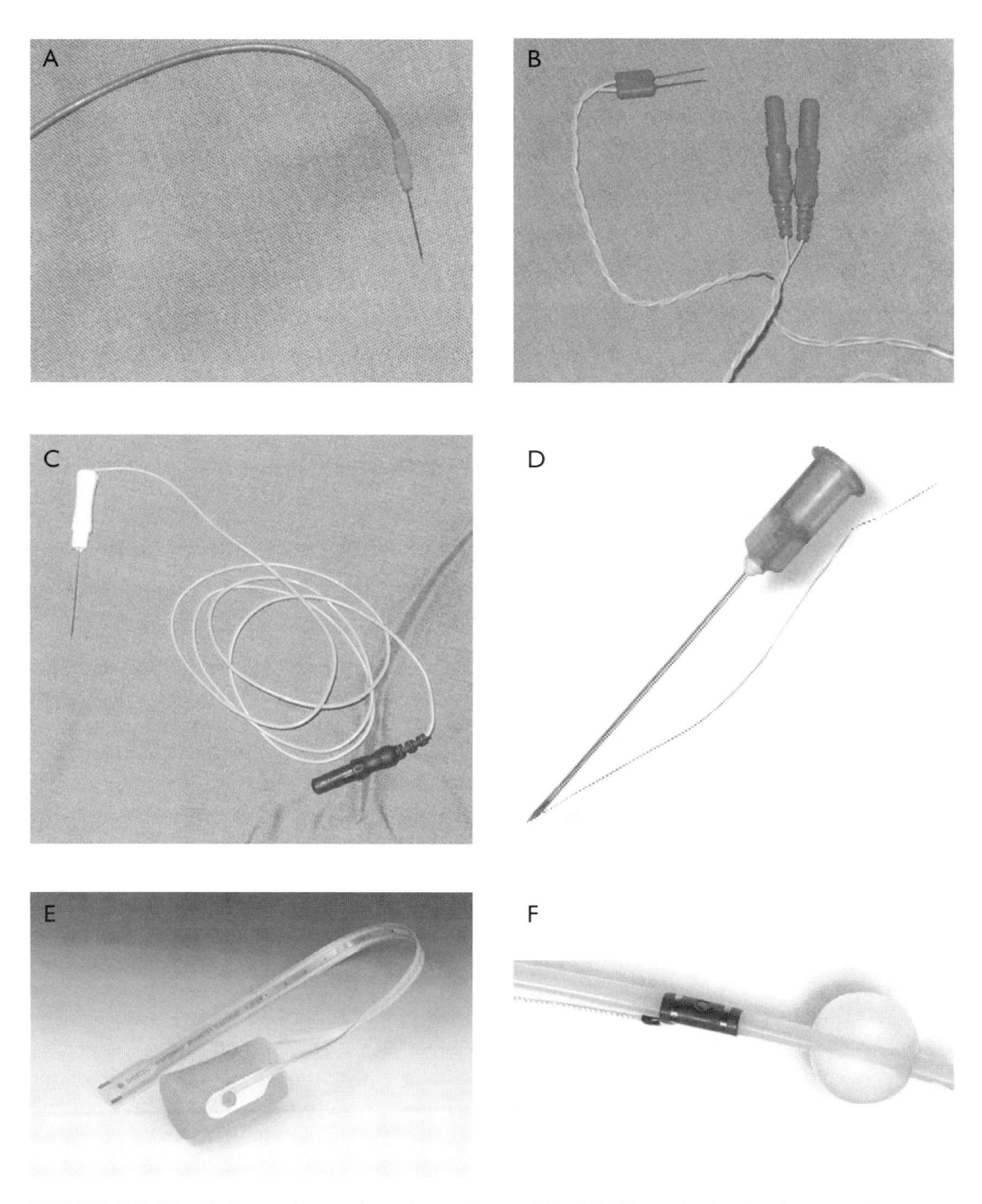

FIGURE 9.9 Stimulating and recording electrodes used for EMG monitoring in the operating room. Subdermal EEG electrodes, either single (A), or arranged in pairs (B), can be used for most muscles. Deeper muscles necessitate either monopolar EMG needles (C) or hooked wire electrodes inserted through a needle (D). E. Anal sphincter EMG can be recorded using surface electrodes mounted on a specialized anal plug sponge. F. Urethral sphincter EMG is recorded from a specialized surface electrode that mounts on to the Foley catheter before it is inserted and lines up with the sphincter muscle. Extension cables can be used if the monitored muscles are not close to the amplifier box.

(contined on next page)

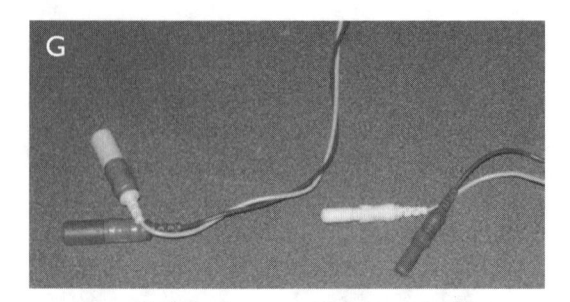

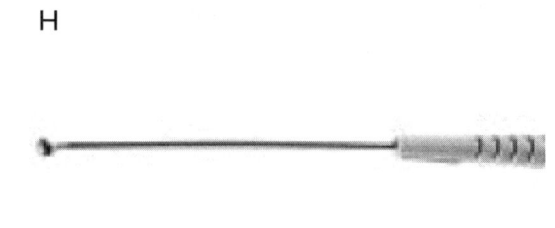

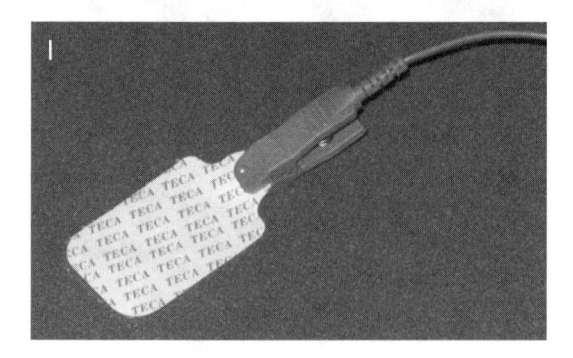

FIGURE 9.9 Paired cables should be twisted together (G) to reduce electrical artifact. A monopolar stimulating electrode (H) is typically used for stimulus-triggered EMG during lumbosacral spine surgery. A large adhesive surface electrode (I) is preferable to a needle for grounding, as it is has a higher contact area which reduces current density in the event of current leakage, thus minimizing the risk of a skin burn.

Stimulating Electrodes and Parameters

A monopolar stimulating electrode is generally preferable during lumbosacral spine surgeries to avoid current shunting from fluid within the operative field. The stimulator is a sterile handheld electrode handed off to the surgeon during the procedure (Figure 9.9H). The anode is a sterile needle electrode usually placed within the wound by the surgeon. The surgeon can insert the stimulator into pedicle holes and touch the stimulator against pedicle screws or any other structure in the operative field.

Although the surgeon holds the stimulating electrode, the technologist controls the electrical stimulator and will need to be sure that it is active when the surgeon wants to stimulate. Stimulation can be with single or recurrent shocks, with a stimulus duration of 0.2 ms and an initial "searching" stimulus intensity of 7 mA. Recurrent shocks are delivered at approximately 2 Hz, usually 2.3 Hz to avoid an exact multiple of 60 and potential artifact, with a stimulus intensity range of 0 to 25 mA. The technologist will need to notify the surgeon if a CMAP response is seen at the searching stimulus intensity and then may be asked to progressively reduce the stimulus intensity and determine the precise stimulus threshold. The stimulating electrode may be reusable, in which case it should be retrieved at the end of surgery and sterilized.

Muscle Selection

Intraoperative EMG monitoring must obviously include muscles appropriate for the nerve roots considered at risk from surgery (Table 9.1). It is important to discuss the case with the surgeon ahead of time to decide which muscles to monitor, as there are a limited number of available recording channels and it may not be possible to relocate recording EMG electrodes after the patent has been prepared and draped for the procedure. Intramuscular EMG electrodes are usually inserted into the anesthetized patient without the assistance of voluntary activation to confirm satisfactory needle placement, and it is important to use muscles that are easily identified using surface landmarks to assure accurate needle placement. It is helpful to have an EMG anatomy atlas readily available in the operating room to check the innervation or location of unfamiliar muscles. Most muscles are innervated by two or more adjacent nerve roots, and accurate localization of nerve root irritation can only be obtained by monitoring multiple muscles simultaneously. For example, abnormal EMG activity recorded from the tibialis anterior muscle is more likely originating from the L4 than the L5 nerve root if abnormal activity is present in the vastus medialis muscle at the same time.

Neuromuscular Blockade

Neuromuscular blockade must be carefully monitored and documented throughout surgery. The expected and preferred result is quiescent EMG monitoring, but quiescent EMG is only meaningful when the technologist is able to demonstrate less than 75% pharmacologic blockade at the same time. Otherwise the false-negative absence of EMG activity may give the surgeon a false sense of security and give rise to a surgical outcome that is worse than it would have been with no monitoring at all. For this reason, the surgeon should be notified right away whenever excessive pharmacologic neuromuscular blockade is detected; he or she will then likely order reversal if approaching a critical phase of the procedure.

Patient Safety

Only one ground electrode should be attached to the patient, preferably a large adhesive surface electrode, which has a higher contact area than a needle and therefore receives a reduced current density in the event of current leakage, thus minimizing the risk of a skin burn (Figure 9.9I). All electrical devices attached to the patient should share the same ground circuit as the EMG machine. The EMG machine should be turned on before any electrodes are attached to the patient and turned off only after all electrodes have been disconnected so as to avoid power surges that could be transmitted to the patient.

There have been skin burns at the site of EMG needle electrode insertion because of current shunting from faulty electrocautery units during surgery; and the following steps should be taken to avoid this: Ground pads from all electrocautery units must be properly positioned to ensure a large area of contact with the patient's skin and placed as close to the surgical site as possible. Each electrocautery unit should contain a built-in ground monitoring system to warn the surgeon in case of circuit discontinuity with a potential for current shunting through other electrodes attached to the patient. Needle electrodes should not be placed in close proximity to electrocautery ground pads and, if possible, should not be placed within the predicted pathway between an active electrocautery electrode and its ground pad. Finally, electrocautery units, EMG monitoring devices, and all operating room electrical circuits should be regularly checked for current leakage.

CONCLUSIONS

NIOM during lumbosacral surgery can be helpful in identifying potential injury to nerve roots. In these types of surgeries, free-running and stimulated EMG are the primary modalities that should be monitored. The NIOM team must also be aware of the presence and extent of neuromuscular blockade. Attention to technique and practice can make this type of NIOM very efficient and efficacious.

REFERENCES

1. Pateder DB, Kostuik JP. Lumbar nerve root palsy after adult spinal deformity surgery. *Spine* 2005;30:1632–1636.
2. Gunnarsson T, Krassioukov AV, Sarjeant R, Fehlings MG. Real-time continuous intraoper-

ative electromyographic and somatosensory evoked potential recordings in spinal surgery: correlation of clinical and electrophysiologic findings in a prospective, consecutive series of 213 cases. *Spine* 2004;29:677–684.
3. Jimenez JC, Sani S, Braverman B, et al. Palsies of the fifth cervical nerve root after cervical decompression: prevention using continuous intraoperative electromyography monitoring. *J Neurosurg Spine* 2005;3:92–97.
4. Fan D, Schwartz DM, Vaccaro AR, et al. Intraoperative neurophysiologic detection of iatrogenic C5 nerve root injury during laminectomy for cervical compression myelopathy. *Spine* 2002;27:2499–2502.
5. Krassioukov AV, Sarjeant R, Arkia H, Fehlings MG. Multimodality intraoperative monitoring during complex lumbosacral procedures: indications, techniques, and long-term follow-up review of 61 consecutive cases. *J Neurosurg Spine* 2004;1:243–253.
6. Maguire J, Wallace S, Madiga R, et al. Evaluation of intrapedicular screw position using intraoperative evoked electromyography. *Spine* 1995;20:1068–1074.
7. Raynor B, Lenke LG, Bridwell K, et al. Correlation between low triggered EMG thresholds and lumbar pedicle screw malposition: analysis of 4587 screws. Presented at the Scoliosis Research Society, 2005.
8. Anderson DG, Wierzbowski LR, Schwartz DM, et al. Pedicle screws with high electrical resistance. A potential source of error with stimulus-evoked EMG. *Spine* 2003;27:1577–1581.
9. Holland NR, Lukaczyk TA, Kostuik JP. A comparison of the stimulus thresholds required to evoke myogenic responses from normal and chronically compressed nerve roots: implications for intraoperative testing during transpedicular instrumentation. *Spine* 1998;23:224–227.
10. Viby-Mogensen J. Clinical assessment of neuromuscular transmission. *Br J Anaesth* 1982;64:209–223.

10 Tethered Cord Surgery

Aatif M. Husain
Kristine H. Ashton

Tethered cord syndrome (TCS) is a congenital condition in which the caudal end of the spinal cord is "tethered" to bone or other inelastic tissue. This tethering produces metabolic changes within the distal spinal cord and nerve roots, causing sensorimotor complications involving the lower extremities as well as anal and urinary sphincter dysfunction. Other cauda equina lesions can produce similar symptoms by affecting the distal spinal cord or nerve roots.

Surgery can prevent progression of symptoms associated with TCS or other cauda equina lesions. This type of surgery involves meticulous dissection of the lumbosacral nerve roots to relieve the tethering or remove the lesion. Injury to nerves supplying the lower extremities or sphincters can occur during the dissection. Neurophysiologic intraoperative monitoring (NIOM) can be used to reduce the possibility of inadvertent injury to neural structures during surgery.

This chapter focuses on NIOM for TCS surgery; however, NIOM for other types of cauda equina surgeries is very similar. Initially relevant anatomy and pathophysiology are discussed, followed by a review of the symptoms and an overview of the surgery for TCS. Finally, the, techniques used for NIOM during TCS surgery and the data supporting their utility are reviewed.

ANATOMY

The anatomy of the conus medularis and cauda equina is important to understand to appreciate the neural elements at risk during TCS surgery and how best to design NIOM paradigms to preserve them. The spinal cord ends between the T12/L1 vertebral level, and L2 and lower nerve roots descend a variable distance prior to exiting the vertebral canal. These descending nerve roots form the cauda equina. Any of them can be affected in TCS.

In addition to motor and sensory innervation to the lower extremities, nerve roots in the cauda equina also contain nerve fibers supplying the urinary bladder and urethral and anal sphincters. The wall of the urinary bladder contains the detrusor muscle, which plays an important role in emptying of the bladder. Contraction of the detrusor muscle is mediated by parasympathetic nerve fibers that arise from the S2, S3, and S4 spinal segments. Preganglionic parasympathetic fibers are initially in the cauda equina and, after exiting the spinal canal, travel in the pelvic splanchnic nerves to synapse in ganglia in the wall of the urinary bladder. Short postganglionic fibers innervate the detrusor muscle and assist with bladder emptying. Sympathetic innervation of the urinary bladder is less important, as it does not aid with emptying. It originates from upper lumbar segments, and preganglionic fibers synapse on the inferior mesenteric ganglion. From there postganglionic fibers travel in the lumbar splanchnic nerves to supply the bladder and assist with relaxation of the detrusor muscle.

Innervation to the anal and external urethral sphincters is under voluntary control from S2, S3, and S4 spinal segments. Nerve roots initially lie in the cauda equina and ultimately form the pudendal nerve. The inferior rectal and perineal branches of the pudendal nerve supply the anal and external urethral sphincters respectively. Damage to the pudendal nerve causes bowel and urinary incontinence. Differential injury to the perineal and inferior rectal nerves is much less likely, but if it were to occur, it would cause problems with one sphincter while sparing the other. These anatomic relations must be considered in designing a NIOM paradigm for TCS surgery.

PATHOPHYSIOLOGY

Spinal cord tethering is frequently associated with various types of neural tube defects, also known as spinal dysraphism. These disorders occur due to abnormal closure of the neural tube, which is responsible for formation of the nervous system during embryonic development. During development, cells of the ectoderm lead to formation of the neural tube, while the mesoderm forms the bony elements, muscles, and meninges. The ectodermal cells proliferate and fold along the margins to make the neural tube, which leads to the formation of the spinal cord up to the level of S2. Meanwhile a group of cells at the caudal end of the neural tube, known as the caudal cell mass, proliferate to make the lower end of the spinal cord, conus medullaris, and filum terminale. After the margins of the neural tube close, the ectoderm separates and forms the overlying skin. The mesoderm (forming the meninges, vertebrae, and muscles) separates the ectoderm from the underlying neural tube. This process is complete by about 6 to 7 weeks of gestation. Thereafter the spinal cord and surrounding tissues continue to grow for the remainder of gestation; however, the elements of the mesoderm grow faster than the spinal cord. Impaired development at any point of this process can lead to spinal dysraphism and tethering to the spinal cord to inelastic tissue.

At the time of birth, the inferior margin of the spinal cord lies at the L1/L2 level; with further growth, the spinal cord moves even higher, to about the T12/L1 level. The upward movement of the spinal cord when the caudal margin in tethered to inelastic tissue results in impaired oxidative metabolism. This leads to the typical symptoms seen with TCS. Surgically releasing the tether results in improved oxidative metabolism and prevents further progression of symptoms.

Although there are many types of spinal dysraphism, they can be separated in to two main kinds, open and occult (Table 10.1). In open spinal dysraphism, an abnormal spinal cord closure is associated with a skin defect overlying the lesion, resulting in a myelomeningocele or myelocele. Myelomeningoceles and myeloceles are associated with other systemic anomalies, such as Arnold-Chiari malformation, scoliosis, congenital heart disease, and tethering of the spinal cord to low-lying structures. These anomalies are readily diagnosed at birth or in utero with ultrasound and surgically corrected early in life. The tethering of the spinal cord is also released at the time of surgery.

Occult spinal dysraphism refers to a series of abnormalities in which the spinal cord malformation is covered by skin (see Table 10.1). A lipomyelomeningocele, also called a spinal lipoma, consists of adipose tissue extending from subcutaneous tissues to the dorsal aspect of the spinal cord, tethering it inferiorly. This is one of the commonest causes of TCS. A dermal sinus consists of an epithelium-lined tract extending from the skin surface to the spinal cord. There is often an epidermoid tumor asso-

TABLE 10.1 Classification of Spinal Dysraphism*

Open spinal dysraphism	Occult spinal dysraphism
Myelomeningocele	Lipomyelomeningocele
Myelocele	Dermal sinus
	Diastematomyelia
	Terminal myelocystocele
	Thickened filum terminale

*There are other rare types of spinal dysraphism; these are not discussed here.

ciated with a dermal sinus. Diastematomyelia, or split-cord malformation, occurs when bony or cartilaginous tissue divides the spinal cord into two halves. Often, an overlying skin abnormality is associated with diastematomyelia. A terminal myelocystocele involves dilation of the central canal at its terminus to form a balloon-like structure. This defect is associated with heterotropia in the brain and vertebral anomalies as well. In filum terminale syndrome, a thickened filum terminale is attached to the dura mater or extradural tissue and tethers the spinal cord. Upon release, the spinal cord usually retracts upward a few centimeters. There are several other rarer types of spinal dysraphism that can also cause TCS; the reader is referred to more comprehensive texts on the subject for details (1).

SYMPTOMS

It is important to recognize symptoms and signs of TCS, as early surgery may not only prevent progression but also lead to improvement. When TCS is associated with open spinal dysraphism, diagnosis is easy and early treatment almost universal. Although occult spinal dysraphism and associated TCS may be harder to diagnose, it is no less important to treat.

The clinical presentation of TCS can be protean. Neurologic features can involve the motor and sensory systems and anal and urinary sphincters. Motor manifestations include weakness and asymmetric length of the lower extremities, reflex asymmetry, and atrophy. Involvement of the lower spinal cord may cause spasticity and hyperreflexia. Sensory involvement leads to patchy areas of numbness, a saddle area of diminished sensation, and paresthesias in the legs. Urogenital involvement leads to incontinence, recurrent urinary tract infections, and sexual dysfunction. Fecal incontinence can also occur owing to involvement of the anal sphincter. Abnormalities of the musculoskeletal system may occur and include scoliosis, hip subluxation, and club feet. Various skin manifestations of occult spinal dysraphism may also be present, such as subcutaneous lipomas, tufts of hair in the lower back, dermal sinus, or a caudal appendage.

The diagnostic modality of choice for TCS and spinal dysraphism is magnetic resonance imaging (MRI). MRI can often show the source of the tethering of the spinal cord and associated spinal cord and vertebral anomalies (Figure 10.1). In young children and in utero, ultrasound can be used to make the diagnosis of spinal dysraphism, but its

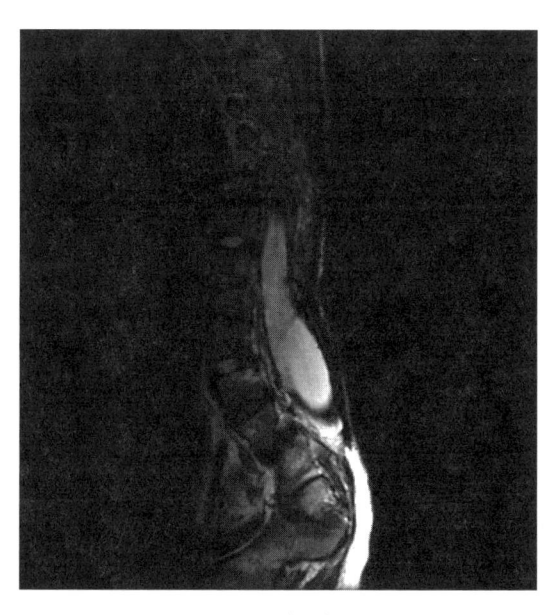

FIGURE 10.1 A T2-weighted MRI showing a terminal myelocystocele and tethered spinal cord.

sensitivity is not as great as that of MRI. When an MRI cannot be obtained, a computed tomography (CT) myelogram can be considered, but that too does not resolve the anatomy as well as an MRI.

SURGICAL CONSIDERATIONS

The surgical procedure used for TCS will depend on the underlying etiology. An overview of the surgical procedure used for TCS is presented here; for details of operative technique, standard neurosurgical texts should be consulted (1). The patient is positioned prone and a skin incision is made over the pathologic spinal segments. After dissection of skin and subcutaneous tissue, a laminectomy is performed to expose the dura mater. The dura mater is cut to reach the lesion and the nerve roots of the cauda equina. The nerve roots are identified and freed of adhesions. The filum terminale or other tether is identified and cut if possible. The underlying spinal dysraphism is corrected. Once the dissection is complete, the dura mater is closed with a dural graft. The soft tissues are then opposed in layers.

During dissection of the cauda equina, injury to neural elements can occur. To reduce the chance of this, a surgical microscope is used. Although meticulous dissection can reduce complications, neural tissue often cannot be identified even with the use of a microscope. This may lead to inadvertent injury. NIOM provides a physiologic method of assessing tissue within the surgical field and thus to isolate nerves from other nonneural tissues. Additionally, NIOM can help localize nerve roots to particular levels. Finally, NIOM can help determine if neural tissue is present within the tether.

NIOM PARADIGM

NIOM has been used in various forms during TCS surgery. Motor, sensory, and sphincter function has been monitored, and often more than one modality is performed. A review of the modalities that can be used is presented below.

Motor System Monitoring

During TCS surgery, the motor system is monitored with electromyography (EMG) of lower extremity muscles. The muscles monitored depend on the level at which surgery is being performed and the number of channels available. Common muscles that should be considered for any TCS surgery include the following: quadriceps femoris (rectus femoris or vastus lateralis) (L2, L3, L4), tibialis anterior (L4, L5), extensor hallucis longus (L5, S1), one of the hamstrings (L5, S1, S2), gluteus maximus (L5, S1, S2), and medial gastrocnemius (S1, S2).

Several types of electrodes can be used to record EMGs; however, subdermal needle electrodes are used most often. A pair of electrodes is inserted near the motor point of each muscle to provide a bipolar recording. These electrodes can be applied quickly after the patient has been anesthetized and can be secured easily. Both normal and abnormal activity can be detected by these electrodes. In obese patients, subdermal needle electrodes may not reach muscle; even in this situation, however, they can detect activity of interest reliably. As an alternative, wire electrodes can be used in these patients so that intramuscular recordings can be more reliably obtained. Surface electroencephalography (EEG) cup electrodes have also been used. They cannot reliably detect neurotonic discharges (see below), take longer to apply, and are less sensitive than subdermal needle electrodes.

Two types of EMG are monitored in TCS surgeries: spontaneous and stimulated. Monitoring for spontaneous EMG activity is performed throughout the surgical procedure. Irritation of a nerve in the surgical field will produce compound muscle action potentials

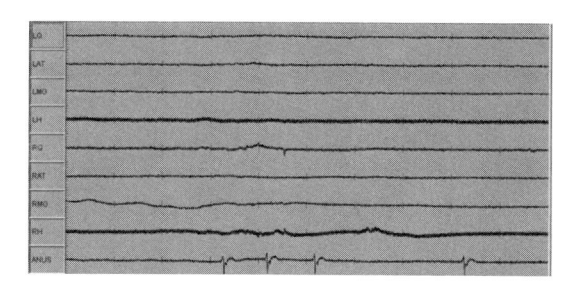

FIGURE 10.2 Isolated spontaneous CMAP that occurred due to irrigation of the surgical field. Because the response is seen mostly in the anal sphincter muscle, the lower sacral nerve roots were most likely irritated. Time base is 100 ms per division (1 second full screen) and amplitude is 100 µV per division. LQ = left quadriceps femoris (vastus lateralis); LAT = left anterior tibialis; LMG = left medial gastrocnemius; LH = left hamstring (semitendinosus); RQ = right quadriceps femoris (vastus lateralis); RAT = right anterior tibialis; RMG = right medial gastrocnemius; RH = right hamstring (semitendinosus).

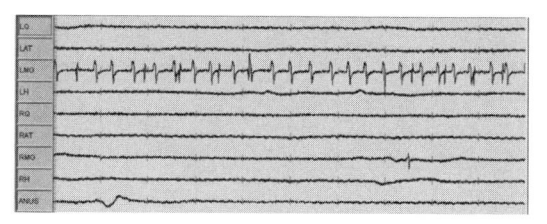

FIGURE 10.3 A run of neurotonic discharges from the anal sphincter that occurred during dissection of the cauda equina. Time base is 100 ms per division (1 second full screen) and amplitude is 100 µV per division. LQ = left quadriceps femoris (vastus lateralis); LAT = left anterior tibialis; LMG = left medial gastrocnemius; LH = left hamstring (semitendinosus); RQ = right quadriceps femoris (vastus lateralis); RAT = right anterior tibialis; RMG = right medial gastrocnemius; RH = right hamstring (semitendinosus).

(CMAPs) in muscles innervated by that nerve (Figure 10.2). Isolated CMAPs can occur with irrigation or manipulation of nerves or during dissection. When CMAPs occur in longer trains, called neurotonic discharges, they imply nerve injury (Figure 10.3). The surgeon should be alerted when neurotonic discharges are noted so that further and permanent nerve injury can be prevented. With modern NIOM equipment, EMG bursts can be interfaced with a loudspeaker so that all personnel, including the surgeon, can hear the CMAP and neurotonic discharges. It should be remembered that needle electrodes will record other types of spontaneous activity, such as fibrillations, positive sharp waves, and fasciculations, which are not related to the surgery but are rather due to the preexisting illness. These discharges should not be misinterpreted as neurotonic discharges.

Stimulated EMG is used when structures within the surgical field need to be stimulated to determine if they contain neural elements (Figure 10.4). A bipolar stimulating electrode is usually used for this purpose, and an electrocautry forceps can be used as such an electrode. Bipolar stimulating electrodes are advantageous over monopolar electrodes since they allow more focal current delivery. Sometimes, however, a monopolar electrode is used to stimulate parts of a large lesion (such as a tumor) to determine which parts contain neural elements.

A wide range of stimulation intensities have been suggested for screening for neural elements in the surgical field. Using a constant-voltage stimulator with a duration of 200 µs, an intensity of 0.05 to 1.0 V is needed to stimulate nerve roots in children and 0.1 to 7 V adults (approximately 0.1 to 10 mA for a constant-current stimulator). The filum terminale is stimulated prior to transection. Some investigators recommend increasing the stimulation intensity to 100 V to stimulate the filum terminale (2). These investigators advocate that greater than a 100-fold difference must exist between the intensity needed to activate motor roots and nonneural tissues such as the filum terminale. Commonly, however, such high stimulation intensities are not used, and if a response is not noted with a 10-V (or 20-mA) stimulation, the structure is

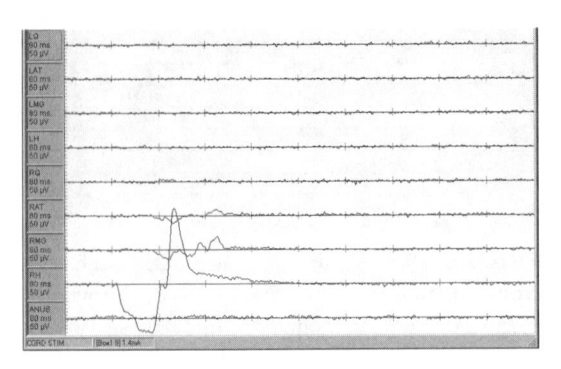

FIGURE 10.4 Evoked response from stimulation of the right S1 nerve root (stimulated EMG). Notice the response in the right hamstring (semitendinosus) muscle, the main muscle of those being monitored, innervated by the S1 nerve root. Time base is 80 ms per division (800 ms full screen) and amplitude is 50 µV per division. LQ = left quadriceps femoris (vastus lateralis); LAT = left anterior tibialis; LMG = left medial gastrocnemius; LH = left hamstring (semitendinosus); RQ = right quadriceps femoris (vastus lateralis); RAT = right anterior tibialis; RMG = right medial gastrocnemius; RH = right hamstring (semitendinosus).

assumed to not contain neural elements. Lower stimulation intensities limit current spread.

Sensory System Monitoring

Sensory pathways can be monitored during TCS surgery by performing tibial somatosensory evoked potentials (SEPs). Techniques used for monitoring SEPs are described in Chapter 2. During TCS surgery, the tibial nerve is stimulated near the medial malleolus and subcortical or cortical waveforms are recorded from scalp and nonscalp electrodes. A 50% drop in amplitude of the response or a 10% prolongation in latency is considered significant and should prompt a surgical alarm that neural elements may be compromised.

Tibial SEPs can also be recorded from an epidural electrode inserted by the surgeon rostral to the site of surgery. This electrode records the SEPs directly from the dorsal surface of the spinal cord and has a much better signal-to-noise ratio than scalp-recorded potentials. Averaging only a few repetitions results in a reproducible response. The disadvantages of epidural electrodes include that they must be placed by the surgeon. Slight movement of the electrode can result in a change in morphology of the response and may prompt a false-positive interpretation. There are no amplitude and latency change criteria that are considered significant in epidural recordings. Rather, if there is a substantial simplification of the epidural response, neural compromise should be suspected. Loss of cortical, subcortical, or epidural SEP responses is concerning for damage to the cauda equina.

SEPs can also be used to identify neural elements in the surgical field. Structures resembling dorsal roots can be stimulated by the surgeon using a handheld bipolar stimulating electrode. Cortical and subcortical responses are recorded from scalp and nonscalp electrodes, as is done with tibial SEPs. If stimulation of the structure results in a reproducible response, it is a dorsal root. This method is seldom used, as it is time-consuming and requires the surgeon to hold the stimulating electrode while the average is completed. If the stimulating electrode moves during the averaging, a new trial should be started.

SEPs from branches of the perineal nerve (branch of the pudendal nerve) have also been used during TCS surgery to minimize the risk of urinary or sexual dysfunction. The dorsal penile nerve is stimulated with the cathode and anode applied to the dorsal surface of the penis; for stimulation of the clitoral nerve, the cathode is placed on the clitoris and the anode in the adjacent labium. Surface electrodes can be used to stimulate the dorsal penile nerve, but needle electrodes are needed to stimulate the clitoral nerve. Cortical and subcortical responses are recorded from the same electrodes as used for recording tibial SEPs. This technique is also seldom used, as both the dorsal penile and clitoral nerves are small and difficult to stimulate, and many repetitions are needed to obtain reproducible responses, thus increasing feedback time to the surgeon.

Sphincter Function Monitoring

Anal or urinary sphincter dysfunction is a devastating complication of cauda equina surgery. By monitoring sphincter function, the risk of this complication can be reduced. The anal and external urethral sphincters and detrusor muscle can be monitored.

Anal sphincter monitoring is the easiest and is performed most commonly. Monopolar subdermal needle electrodes (similar to those used to perform EMG monitoring) are inserted percutaneously in the anal sphincter muscle after the patient haa been anesthetized. At least two needles are inserted on opposite sides of the sphincter and referenced to each other. Two additional needles can be placed in the two remaining quadrants of the sphincter (Figure 10.5). The latter needles can serve as backup electrodes in case the primary ones become unusable. The needles must be secured well so that they will not be dislodged during positioning and surgery (Figure 10.6).

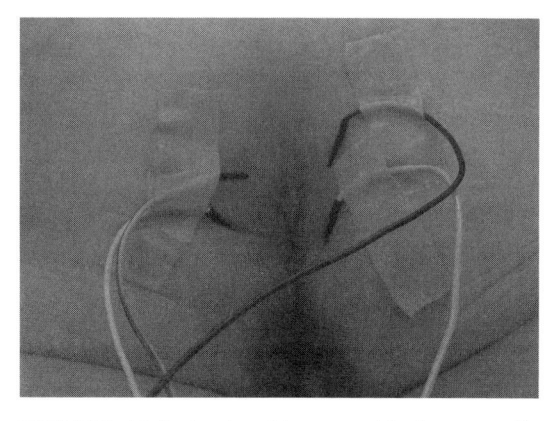

FIGURE 10.5 Anal sphincter with four needle electrodes, one in each quadrant. Two needles are used for a bipolar recording, with the other two needles providing redundancy.

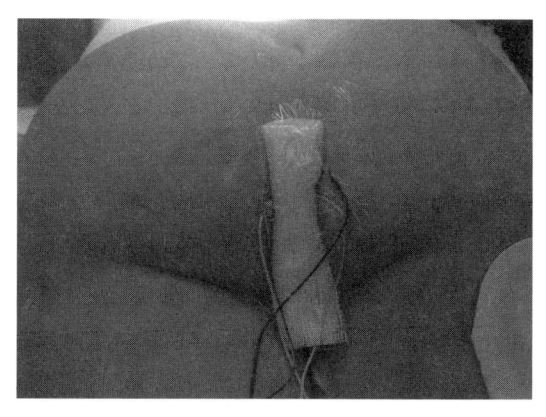

FIGURE 10.6 Anal sphincter needle electrodes secured in place to prevent dislodgement during positioning and surgery.

These electrodes can record free-running EMG activity, including neurotonic discharges and stimulated EMGs.

Another method for recording anal sphincter activity is with surface electrodes. Anal plug electrodes are available, which contain two or four imbedded platinum electrodes. The plug is inserted into the rectum after induction of anesthesia. This electrode must be secured, as it is also susceptible to dislodgement. The platinum electrodes serve as surface EMG electrodes and record stimulated EMGs. Free-running EMG and neurotonic discharges can also be detected with these electrodes, but they are less reliable than needle electrodes for this purpose.

The external urethral sphincter surrounds the proximal part of the urethra and is not accessible percutaneously. Consequently needle electrodes cannot be inserted into this sphincter. To monitor the external urethral sphincter, a specially made ring electrode is attached to a Foley catheter 1 to 2 cm distal to the bulb. This ring electrode serves as a bipolar surface electrode that records stimulated and free-running EMGs. This electrode must be positioned carefully; its slippage will result in it being too distal in the urethra and unable to record sphincter activity. Sometimes a urologist is needed to position this electrode correctly.

The detrusor muscle can be monitored during TCS as well. This muscle is responsible for contraction of the urinary bladder. Since the detrusor muscle cannot be monitored with needle electrodes inserted directly into it or with surface EMG electrodes, changes in bladder pressure are used as surrogate markers for muscle integrity. Prior to surgery, a cystometrogram is performed to determine the capacity of the bladder. At the time of surgery, a Foley catheter is inserted and attached to a three-way flow adapter, which is attached to a manometer. The bladder is filled with fluid to capacity (determined by the cystometrogram). Contraction of the detrusor muscle causes an increase in bladder pressure, which is measured by the manometer. This type of monitoring is cumbersome to set up and requires urologic evaluation prior to surgery. Additionally, during surgery, sustained high-frequency stimulation in the operative field is needed to induce detrusor muscle contraction. When the contraction occurs, it is delayed for several seconds. This results in a delay in providing feedback to the surgeon.

UTILITY OF NIOM IN TCS SURGERY

It is very difficult to establish conclusively that NIOM improves outcomes in patients undergoing surgery for TCS; data on other cauda equina lesions are even sparser. There is no study comparing outcomes in patients who underwent TCS surgery with and without NIOM with other variables being kept constant. Changes in surgical technique, the introduction of new surgical technology, the skill of the surgeon, and lack of surgical outcomes data make comparisons very difficult.

Despite these difficulties, several studies provide insights on the utility of NIOM in TCS surgeries. A retrospective review from one center compared outcomes of three surgeons who performed TCS surgeries (3). Two of the surgeons had no adverse outcomes and the third had neurologic complications in 12% of patients. SEP NIOM was used in 7% and 17% of patients, and EMG NIOM was used in 11% and 63% of cases by the first two surgeons. The third surgeon used only EMG NIOM in only 8% of patients. Whereas this seems to suggest that the use of NIOM led to fewer complications, that may not necessarily be the case. In this series, the third surgeon used the operating microscope much less often and had a higher percentage of re-do operations, which carry a higher morbidity.

In 72 children undergoing TCS surgery without NIOM, improvement in sensorimotor and sphincter function was noted in 43% and 42%; deterioration in the same functions occurred in 9%, and 12% (4). In series where NIOM was used, outcomes have ranged from no complications to results similar to those seen when NIOM was not used. Studies using only EMG NIOM have reported new motor weakness in 0% to 6% of patients (5,6). Additionally, in one study, the surgical procedure was altered in 50% of patients as a result of NIOM findings (a decision having been made not to resect tissue owing to the presence of neural elements) (7).

As discussed previously, monitoring of motor, sensory, and sphincter function can be done in patients undergoing TCS surgery. However, is monitoring all of these modalities necessary? Motor system monitoring with free-running EMG is of benefit, since neurotonic discharges can warn the surgeon when nerves are compromised. Stimulated EMG is useful in identifying neural elements, especially prior to resection. Studies cited above demonstrate the utility of these techniques.

The utility of tibial and other SEP NIOM is less clear. It has been noted that tibial SEP monitoring does not protect sensory nerve roots (8). This is probably because SEPs are mediated through several nerve roots. Injury to a single root is unlikely to alter the response enough to raise an alarm (6). SEP monitoring is useful when injury to neural structures is gradual, as occurs with spinal cord injury due to scoliosis. This allows reproducible responses to be obtained, the surgeon to be notified, and corrective action taken before permanent damage occurs. In TCS surgery, there is potential for injury to peripheral nerves (roots). By the time a reproducible SEP response is obtained and the surgeon alerted, the nerve damage has often already occurred. These factors reduce the utility of SEP monitoring during TCS surgery.

Preserving sphincter function is an important part of TCS surgery. Consequently, monitoring sphincter function is routinely recommended. However, there is less agreement on which sphincter(s) to monitor. Since the anal and external urethral sphincters are supplied by branches of the pudendal nerve, it has been suggested that monitoring of the anal sphincter is sufficient (5). However, others have noted that since different branches of the pudendal nerve supply these two sphincters, differential damage to one branch may result in selective injury (8). The detrusor muscle is supplied by the S2, S3, and S4 spinal segments, which are the same segments providing innervation to the pudendal nerve and anal sphincter. Thus monitoring the anal sphincter may serve as a surrogate monitor for the detrusor muscle as well. Critics of this approach have argued that the detrusor muscle is innervated by the pelvic splanchnic nerves, which can be selectively damaged (9).

PROPOSED PARADIGM FOR NIOM IN TCS SURGERY

In developing a paradigm to provide NIOM for TCS surgery, the neurophysiologist must ensure that all modalities providing useful information are monitored. The paradigm discussed below is one that is used in the authors' practice.

Needle electrodes are placed in the following muscles bilaterally: vastus lateralis, tibialis anterior, medial gastrocnemius, and semitendinosus. Each muscle is displayed in a separate channel. Additionally, two to four needles are placed in the anal sphincter; anal sphincter EMG is displayed in a single channel. If the NIOM machine being used has only eight channels, some of the lower extremity muscle groups are not recorded; which ones are left off depends on the spinal level of the surgery.

During dissection, free-running EMG is monitored from the muscle groups noted above. The time window is set at 0.5 to 1 second full screen, as this allows better recognition of neurotonic discharges. When these discharges are noted, the surgeon must be alerted, as they signify nerve injury. Depending on the muscle group from which neurotonic discharges are recorded, the neurophysiologist can determine which nerve roots were most likely irritated. When stimulated EMG is used, a time window of 100 to 500 ms full screen should be used. This allows separation of the stimulus artifact from the response. The stimulation intensity at which the response occurs should be noted.

TECHNICAL CONSIDERATIONS

As noted above, the modalities that are most consistently monitored during TCS surgery are free-running and stimulated EMG. Technical issues relevant to NIOM for these types of surgeries involve preparing for and monitoring EMG. In some centers tibial nerve SEP monitoring may also be performed.

Preparation

Although occasionally performed in adults, surgery for TCS is most commonly performed in children. The NIOM technologist must be comfortable with setup and monitoring in children. Unlike other types of monitoring, all patients are able to undergo EMG monitoring. However, some conditions may make the monitoring more difficult. Obesity may make the EMG signals more difficult to obtain, since the recording needles may not reach the muscles. Despite this, EMG signals are usually quite large and still recordable. Severely atrophied muscles are sometimes difficult to monitor. In such patients, isolating the muscles of interest may be difficult, and the needle electrode may mistakenly be placed in an adjacent muscle.

Standard NIOM equipment can be used to monitor TCS surgeries. Most modern NIOM machines have 16 channels, which can be arranged to accommodate stimulated and free-running EMGs in any variety of views. Needle electrodes are used most often to monitor EMG discharges from muscles. When these electrodes are used, two needles are adjacent near the motor point of the muscle and bipolar recording montages used. The needle electrodes are available in twisted pairs, color coded for ease of placement and setup. They are disposable and usually come presterilized. Surface electrodes can also be used; however, they are less sensitive in evaluating spontaneous EMG activity. If these electrodes are used, the active electrode must be placed on the belly of the muscle and reference near a bony point (belly-tendon method). Two surface electrode placed close together near the motor point of a muscle will result in excessive cancellation. Regardless of which type of electrode is used, the NIOM technologist must make certain that enough electrodes are available for all muscle groups to be monitored. Additionally, the technologist must have various types of stimulating electrodes with which the surgeon can stimulate structures within the surgical field (described below).

Preoperative studies are typically not needed for TCS patients who will be undergoing only EMG monitoring. However, if tibial nerve SEPs are to be used, preoperative tibial SEPs should be obtained. If the surgeon has particular concerns about the patient's clinical status, a diagnostic EMG can be helpful in identifying abnormal muscles.

Since the NIOM technologist needs to apply only needle electrode in TCS patients, he or she may not meet the patient until after induction, as only then can the needle electrodes be applied. However, the technologist should make an effort to meet the patient (and if this is a child, the parents) in the preoperative holding area. During this time the procedure and the role of the NIOM team should be explained to the patient and family members. At this time the technologist may use a skin marking pen to mark the site where needle electrodes will be inserted. This is particularly useful, since during this time the patient can participate in the examination, which makes it easier to identify muscles. After induction, the muscles become harder to identify.

Procedure

Needle electrodes are applied after the patient has been induced. As noted previously, a selection of muscles innervated by the entire lumbosacral region is necessary for thorough monitoring. Monitoring is usually done bilaterally. A typical set of muscle to be monitored would include the vastus lateralis, tibialis anterior, medial gastrocnemius, semitendinosus, and gluteus maximus and the anal sphincter. Electrode placement should be done by the NIOM technologist after his or her hands have been washed and gloved. Needle electrodes can be inserted into the leg muscles after the skin has been cleaned with alcohol. The electrodes are kept in place with tape of the technologist's choice. The patient's leg may be wrapped with an Ace bandage for extra security, or the surgeon may have ordered sequential compression devices (SCDs), which also help to keep the electrodes secure.

Once the patient has been turned prone, the anal sphincter electrodes must be placed. This is a more challenging set of electrodes, both to place and to keep secure. The anus is visualized by separating the buttocks, and a needle electrode is placed on each side (or in each quadrant for added redundancy) (Figure 10.5). A rolle of gauze covered by Tegaderm helps secure these electrodes (Figure 10.6). It is especially important to check the impedances of these electrodes before the surgery begins to be sure they are properly inserted and secure. Anal plug electrodes especially designed for surface EMG monitoring of the anal sphincter are also available, but they are harder to secure in place and do not provide as good a signal. The needle electrodes work very well once the application technique has been mastered.

There are very few restrictions for anesthetic regimen in patients undergoing TCS. Paralytics may not be used for most cases in which EMG monitoring is necessary. A single dose of a short-acting neuromuscular blocking agent can be used during induction, as it will have worn off by the time the dura mater is opened. These drugs should not be used once EMG monitoring becomes necessary.

After the patient has been positioned, the NIOM technologist should once again check impedances of all the electrodes to make sure that none have been inadvertently pulled out. The electrodes are then connected to the preamplifier. A comment should be made on the record at the start of the procedure documenting the anesthetics being used and other physiologic parameters. It is advisable for the technologist to shake the electrode wires or touch the electrodes if they are accessible to be sure the entire system is working. As only EMG is monitored in most cases, a baseline is not obtained. However, the free-running EMG should be evaluated to see if spontaneous activity such as fibrillations and positive sharp waves are present. By noting their presence at this time, their presence during critical points in the surgery can be appropriately interpreted. Unlike many of the types of cases, the technologist is not needed during exposure but should inform the surgeon or the circulating nurse of his or her whereabouts. The technologist should return to the operating room before the dura mater is opened.

Free-running EMG is monitored the entire time the dura mater is open. A time window of 1 second full screen is useful in reviewing free-running EMG. Sensitivity settings range from 50 µV to 2 mV per division.

Nerve roots may be irritated, and the surgeon should be informed when spontaneous activity is seen. Some surgeons may prefer to hear the EMG activity themselves, in which case the sound on the monitoring equipment should be turned up to a volume that the surgeon can hear. The NIOM team will still need to tell the surgeon which nerve roots are being irritated by noting which muscles generate the spontaneous activity.

Stimulated EMG is also frequently used in TCS. An appropriate triggered EMG program should be used. The time window for stimulated EMG should be 100 ms full screen. This will allow the responses, which occur around 20 to 30 ms after stimulation, to be in the middle of the screen. The sensitivity is usually set between 100 µV and 5 mV per division. The surgeon will stimulate different structures within the field to map nerve roots and nonneural structures. A stimulating forceps (bipolar stimulator) that plugs into the EP machine works particularly well. Alternatively, a stimulating probe (monopolar stimulator) with a needle electrode inserted into the wound serving as a reference can also be used. The monopolar stimulating electrode produces more current spread and therefore is less specific. After the type of stimulating electrode to be used is chosen, there are two ways to stimulate. One is to keep the current on a preset intensity (for example, 3.0 mA) and move the electrode to search for responses. The other method is to keep the probe in the same location and increase the current until a response is seen. The method used is the surgeon's choice. The filum is stimulated prior to cutting to make certain that it does not contain nerve roots. In stimulating the filum, the current intensity should be increased to about 10 V (or 20 mA) to make certain that there is no neural element within it. Some authors have recommended using an intensity as high as 100 V (2). Upon stimulation of the filum, no response should be seen.

During removal of lipomas during TCS, a carbon dioxide (CO_2) laser may be used. If that is the case, protective CO_2 laser goggles should be worn by all personnel in the operating room while the laser is in use. The laser is a heat-producing device; while it is in use, thermal injury or irritation to nerve roots may occur. Consequently, when the laser is being used, the NIOM team should be alert to neurotonic discharges.

The NIOM team must be in direct communication with the surgeon during TCS. If the neurophysiologist is in the operating room, he or she should communicate directly with the surgeon regarding any significant findings. If the neurophysiologist is monitoring the case remotely, any nerve root irritation is communicated to the surgeon by the technologist. The technologist and the neurophysiologist should be in communication via whatever method is set up at the operating institution. Today this is often via a chat function on a computer; however, telephone communications are also used. The immediacy of an EMG case requires that the technologist communicate with the surgeon directly in the operating room. The neurophysiologist may also communicate with the surgeon via speakerphone. Whichever communication method is used, the technologist should keep notes about stimulation levels, responses, what the surgeon is stimulating, any alarms given to the surgeon, and other relevant notes.

Postprocedure

After termination of the surgery, the needle electrodes should be removed before the patient awakens from anesthesia. This applies particularly to the anal sphincter electrodes. The needle electrode sites should be checked for bleeding. If bleeding is present, pressure should be applied to those areas and they should be cleaned with an alcohol pad. Additionally, the technologist should ensure that no needle tip has broken and lodged in soft tissue. If this has occurred, the surgeon should be informed immediately so that the tip can be surgically removed. Needle electrodes are disposable and should be discarded in an appropriate container.

The NIOM team should try to examine the patient after surgery. Particularly important is motor examination of the lower extremities. Bowel and bladder function is harder to assess and cannot be done immediately after surgery. It is important to ultimately obtain this information so that changes in monitoring and examination can be correlated.

A summary report of the monitoring should be written following the procedure. This report should include the patient's name, medical record number, age, gender, date, names of the surgeon, neurophysiologist, and technologist, surgical procedure, modalities monitored, NIOM machine used (if there more than one is available), summary of events including changes in NIOM, warnings given to the surgeon, and responses to them. Postoperative follow-up should be documented if available. This report should be kept on file in the department and a copy should be sent to the neurophysiologist. A system of keeping the digital files for each case should be determined at each institution based on the NIOM equipment's capabilities and the volume of monitoring data generated. Snapshots of the EMG responses may be kept as part of the patient's record if desired.

The NIOM machine should be maintained by the hospital's biomedical engineering department. It is inspected on an annual basis. Any problems or suspected problems should be reported immediately, and the equipment should be sequestered. All maintenance stickers should be up to date. It is the responsibility of the NIOM technologist to inspect the sticker upon use of the equipment to be sure it is not outdated.

FUTURE DIRECTIONS

Future research will likely lead to better monitoring techniques for patients undergoing TCS surgery. Electrodes for monitoring the external urethral sphincter and the detrusor muscle are likely to become easier to use and more reliable. Studies evaluating the stimulus thresholds for various structures before and after untethering may help guide surgery. New stimulating probes will be able to switch between monopolar and bipolar stimulation, allowing easier and more precise delivery of stimuli.

Ultimately more studies will be needed that compare outcomes of patients undergoing TCS surgery with and without NIOM. By keeping other variables stable, this would provide conclusive evidence not only of the utility of NIOM but also of the types of NIOM to use.

CONCLUSIONS

TCS can be associated with many different types of spinal dysraphism. Surgery for TCS is often necessary to prevent progression of symptoms. Sensorimotor worsening and sphincter dysfunction are common complications of surgery. NIOM with free-running and stimulated EMGs from the muscles of the lower extremities and anal sphincter may reduce the morbidity of the surgery.

REFERENCES

1. Muraszko KM. Spinal dysraphism in the adult and pediatric populations. In: Grossman RG, Loftus CM, eds. *Principles of Neurosurgery*, 2nd ed. Philadelphia: Lippincott-Raven, 1999: 59–75.
2. Quinones-Hinojosa A, Gadkary CA, Gulati M, et al. Neurophysiological monitoring for safe surgical tethered cord syndrome release in adults. *Surg Neurol* 2004;62:127–133; discussion 133–135.
3. Albright AL, Pollack IF, Adelson PD, Solot JJ. Outcome data and analysis in pediatric neurosurgery. *Neurosurgery* 1999;45:101–106.
4. Anderson FM. Occult spinal dysraphism: a series of 73 cases. *Pediatrics* 1975;55: 826–835.
5. Kothbauer K, Schmid UD, Seiler RW, Eisner W. Intraoperative motor and sensory monitoring of the cauda equina. *Neurosurgery* 1994;34:702–707; discussion 707.
6. von Koch CS, Quinones-Hinojosa A, Gulati M, et al. Clinical outcome in children undergoing tethered cord release utilizing intraoperative neurophysiological monitoring. *Pediatr Neurosurg* 2002;37:81–86.
7. Phillips LH II, Jane JA. Electrophysiologic monitoring during tethered spinal cord release. *Clin Neurosurg* 1996;43:163–174.
8. Krassioukov AV, Sarjeant R, Arkia H, Fehlings MG. Multimodality intraoperative monitoring during complex lumbosacral procedures: indications, techniques, and long-term follow-up review of 61 consecutive cases. *J Neurosurg Spine* 2004;1:243–253.
9. Shinomiya K, Fuchioka M, Matsuoka T, et al. Intraoperative monitoring for tethered spinal cord syndrome. *Spine* 1991;16:1290–1294.

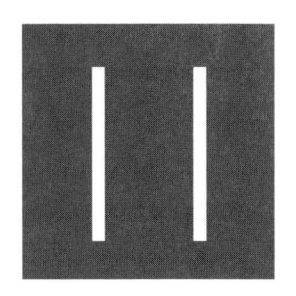

11 Selective Dorsal Rhizotomy

Daniel L. Menkes
Chi-Keung Kong
D. Benjamin Kabakoff

The first report on the effectiveness of dorsal rhizotomy as a treatment for spasticity was published in 1913 (1). However, it was not until late in the last century that a systematic approach using selective dorsal rhizotomy (SDR) techniques came into widespread use. Electrophysiological methods for selectively ablating abnormal sensory nerve rootlets, thus sparing normal sensory rootlets, were proposed by Fasano et al. and later by Peacock et al. (2–4). These methodologies came into more widespread use after standardized neurophysiologic intraoperative monitoring (NIOM) techniques were reported by Staudt et al. (5). This chapter discusses the background, indications, and NIOM SDR procedural techniques performed for treatment of spasticity. It should be stated that there are numerous variations on this technique, which are employed at the various hospitals that utilize NIOM. Nonetheless, this chapter is based on those techniques that have been previously cited and those based on a meta-analysis of SDR techniques (6). Those centers with extensive experience often modify these procedures based upon their own experience. However, those who perform these studies on an infrequent basis or who do not have extensive experience with this technique ought to use the standards published in the literature, which are summarized in this chapter.

BACKGROUND

SDR was introduced primarily as a treatment for children with cerebral palsy (CP). The etiology of CP is idiopathic in most instances, although perinatal injury to the pyramidal and/or extrapyramidal motor systems is thought to be responsible. Irrespective of the cause, the net effect, in cases of the more common spastic types of CP, is to reduce upper motor neuron inhibitory influences on the spinal cord. This relative reduction of descending inhibitory influences in the corticospinal pathways results in relative overactivity of the affected muscles, leading increased tone (i.e., spasticity). Spasticity is thought to be enhanced by sensory input onto the anterior horn cells that is unopposed by the descending inhibitory influences of the corticospinal tract. SDR is based on the hypothesis that reducing the degree of abnormal sensory input into the spinal reflex arc will result in diminished spasticity.

More than 70% of patients diagnosed with CP have the spastic type, which results from corticospinal or "pyramidal" tract dysfunction. These are the patients who are most likely to respond to SDR. However, there are other subtypes of CP that manifest with extrapyramidal dysfunction, such as dyskinetic, ataxic, and choreoathetotic movements. There are also "mixed types" of CP that manifest pyramidal and extrapyramidal dysfunction. However, it is only the patients with pure spastic CP who demonstrate a benefit from SDR.

The spastic forms of CP may be subdivided based on the distribution of limb involvement. In spastic diplegia, four limbs are affected, but the lower extremities are more severely affected than the upper extremities.. SDR tends to be most effective for this group of patients. "Spastic quadriplegia" refers to equal degrees of weakness and spasticity in all four limbs. This type is less amenable to SDR. The spastic hemiplegia subtype, in which half of the body is affected, is most commonly observed after full-term births (7). Although some of these patients may benefit from SDR, it is recommended only after other treatments have proven ineffective. Thus, SDR tends to be considered for patients with the spastic diplegia subtype of the spastic cerebral palsies.

The goal of SDR is to reduce spasticity so that the patient regains a greater degree of mobility. The initial reports of dorsal rhizotomies did not discriminate between normal and abnormal sensory nerve input, as it was assumed that removing all sensory input would provide the best result. However, complete dorsal rhizotomy with its resulting hypotonia may complicate rather than benefit the patient's course of postoperative rehabilitation. This is particularly true for those whose legs are weak and who require some degree of leg spasticity for weight bearing while walking. Nonetheless, some authors have questioned the benefit of SDR, stating that nonselective rhizotomy may provide similar results (8). Despite publications that question the utility of SDR, a recent meta-analysis demonstrated that SDR plus physical therapy was effective in reducing spasticity in children with spastic diplegia and that this benefit directly correlated with the amount of sensory nerve afferent tissue resected (6). Given this report, SDR should be considered as part of a comprehensive approach for the treatment of patients with spasticity due to increased abnormal sensory afferent input.

INDICATIONS

As previously discussed, SDR is generally recommended for those people with spastic forms of CP who do not rely on their spasticity to ambulate. Patient selection is very important for the success of SDR. Since SDR is primarily an operation for spasticity reduction, it should be considered for children who have normal intelligence, well-preserved muscle strength, and good selective motor control. Patients with dystonia, ataxia, or other involuntary movements usually do not benefit from SDR. It must be emphasized that SDR represents only the initial phase of spasticity treatment. With few exceptions, an intensive course of postoperative rehabilitation lasting several months to 1 year is required in order to achieve the maximum possible benefit from SDR. It is also worth noting that the number of patients referred for SDR by pediatric neurologists is diminishing over time in favor of intrathecal pumps (Leshner RT, personal communication). Intrathecal pumps using diazepam or lorazepam deliver more of the therapeutic agent to the target site while minimizing systemic side effects. Thus, it is likely that SDR will come to be viewed as a second-line procedure for those persons who do not obtain adequate relief of their symptoms from intrathecal pumps. While intrathecal pumps have the advantage of being reversible, they have their own inherent complications, including infection, bleeding, misdirection of the catheter, and meningitis. Therefore those patients who experience these adverse effects ought to be considered for SDR as well.

NIOM TECHNIQUES

The basics of NIOM including patient positioning, proper use of anesthetics, and the importance of proper clinical neurophysiologic techniques are reviewed in earlier chapters. SDR requires monitoring of electromyographic (EMG) activity generated by motor unit action potentials (MUAPs). Therefore the use of muscle paralytic agents should be minimized in order to perform this procedure properly. Since some institutions use pudendal somatosensory evoked potentials (SSEPs) during this procedure, it is imperative that the anesthetic agents chosen for this surgery permit the optimal recording of SSEP waveforms as well.

Preoperative Preparation

The technologist applies recording electrodes, surface or needle, to muscles innervated by the L2 to S2 nerve roots bilaterally. The muscles usually recorded are the thigh adductors, quadriceps femoris (e.g., rectus femoris or vastus lateralis), biceps femoris, tibialis anterior, gastrocnemius, and external anal sphincter (5). Because surface recordings do not discriminate between individual muscles, it is more meaningful to discuss the SDR NIOM procedure on the basis of muscle groups. Even if subdermal needles are used, the needles may not be of sufficient length or placed with enough accuracy such that one can be certain that all myogenic activity is generated only by one named muscle. For simplicity, the muscles are discussed as though the MUAPs recorded were generated primarily by the muscle named in Table 11.1. Of all these muscle groups, the thigh adductors and the knee extensors (e.g., quadriceps femoris) deserve additional attention. Although both the thigh adductors and quadriceps femoris are innervated by the L2 to L4 motor nerve roots, abnormal responses from the thigh adductors should favor resection of the nerve rootlet, as described in the next section. The purpose is to improve scissoring due to thigh adductor spasticity, which is common in children with CP, yet preserve adequate knee extensor tone, which may be required for weight bearing. Institutions can use additional or other recording muscles depending on the preferences of the clinical neurophysiologist, the operating surgeon, or both. Irrespective of the target muscles examined, it is important to ensure that there is adequate representation of the L2-S2 nerve roots bilaterally as part of the intraoperative monitoring procedure.

Recording parameters should be set for optimal EMG recording. Common settings are a bandpass of 10 Hz to 5 kHz, a sweep of 200 ms, and a gain of 100 to 200 μV per division. However, others have used a bandpass of 30 to 3000 Hz with a 60-Hz notch filter (5). As discussed in the technical section, 60-Hz notch filters should be avoided whenever possible. Although variations of this bandpass are used elsewhere, in no instance should a bandpass narrower than 30 to 3,000 Hz be

TABLE 11.1 NIOM Muscle Monitoring

Muscle	Nerve innervation	Root innervation
Thigh adductors	Obturator*	L2-L4
Quadriceps femoris	Femoral	L2-L4
Tibialis anterior	Deep peroneal	L4-L5
Short head of biceps femoris	Sciatic†	L5-S1
Gastrocnemius	Tibial	S1-S2
External anal sphincter	Pudendal	S2-S4

*The adductor magnus has dual innervation from the obturator and sciatic nerves.
†The peroneal division of the sciatic nerve innervates the lateral hamstrings (short head of the biceps femoris), whereas the tibial division of the sciatic nerve innervates the medial hamstrings (long head of the biceps femoris).

used, as this will eliminate some of the signal under consideration.

Although the original studies were often performed with paper recordings, digital recordings may be used instead. One of the authors (CK) prefers paper recordings, as this expedites EMG comparisons during the operation. Unlike electroencephalography (EEG), postrecording reformatting and reanalysis is hardly ever required. Therefore there is no significant advantage to digital recordings other than facilitating data storage. Irrespective of the recording method used, the gain should be adjusted depending on the amplitude of the EMG response. Additional details regarding the technical aspects of this monitoring procedure will also be presented. The remainder of this chapter discusses the procedure regarding gross anatomic identification of the nerve roots, verification of optimal anesthetic levels, and dorsal rootlet selection for ablation.

Anesthetic Induction

Although previously discussed, it must be reiterated that cooperation between the surgeon, the anesthesiologist, and the NIOM team is of paramount importance. The anesthesiologist should use short-acting neuromuscular blocking agents so that EMG recordings can proceed soon after intubation. The optimal use of anesthetic agents is discussed elsewhere, but it is worth mentioning that isoflurane levels should be maintained between 1.0% and 1.4%, as it has been noted that changes of as little as 0.1% to 0.2% can adversely affect the NIOM procedures (5). Therefore it is imperative that optimal anesthesia with minimal variability be used throughout the NIOM procedure.

Exposure/Anatomic Identification

The surgeon exposes the conus medullaris and the cauda equina through a midline incision with the patient lying prone. The sensory nerve roots from L1 to S2 are identified in the operative field. The surgeon usually accomplishes this by identifying the conus medullaris where the spinal cord ends and the cauda equina begins. Although variant anatomy exists, the S1 nerve root tends to be the largest nerve root in the lumbosacral region. The S2 nerve root should be smaller than the more rostral S1 nerve root. Once the nerve roots have been identified bilaterally, anesthetic verification can proceed.

Stimulation and Recording Parameters

Stimulation is performed using a constant-voltage stimulator, as opposed to a constant-current stimulator. The stimulation is performed with a square-wave pulse 0.1 ms in duration at 50 Hz for 1 second. Restated, a 1 second train of 50 Hertz square wave pulses, each of 0.1 ms duration, is given for the specific voltage selected. The surgeon holds the nerve root or rootlet with a pair of blunt-tipped nerve hook electrodes of opposing polarity that are insulated except at the tip, where the stimulation will occur (Figure 11.1). The surgeon must ensure that the neural structure is not held under tension, is clear of the cerebrospinal fluid, and that the tip separation is between 5 and 10 mm. The voltage is gradually increased until a response is noted either clinically or electromyographically. Two distinct portions of the procedure require

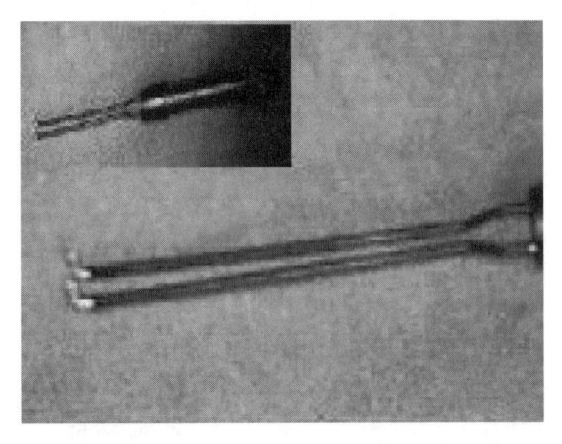

FIGURE 11.1 Stimulating hook electrode.

this type of stimulation—anesthetic verification and dorsal rootlet selection—discussed later in this section.

A minimum of 11 pairs of electrodes should be used for recording; 5 pairs for each lower extremity and one pair devoted to the anal sphincter. The recording sites should include the thigh adductors, quadriceps femoris, short head of the biceps femoris, tibialis anterior, gastrocnemius, and the anal sphincter muscles bilaterally (Table 11.2, Figure 11.2). It is important to monitor the anal sphincter in order to preserve sphincter function. Therefore nerve rootlets with triggered EMG activity from the anal sphincter should be divided with caution. If excessive ablations are performed, the patient may develop urinary and/or bowel incontinence due to reduction of sphincter tone.

Surface or subdermal needle electrodes are used for limb muscle recordings, as discussed later. Figure 11.3 depicts the use of subdermal recording electrodes. Irrespective of the method used for recording limb EMG activity, needle electrodes are preferred for anal sphincter monitoring.

Anesthetic/Nerve Root Verification

There are two phases involved in this portion of the procedure. The first is to confirm that the levels of anesthesia are appropriate for nerve root testing. Lightly anesthetized patients have continuous background muscle artifact, whereas too deeply anesthetized patients demonstrate no reflex movement with stimulation of the posterior rootlets (5). Therefore the ratio between anterior and posterior nerve root threshold may be used to assess the anesthetic level. The threshold to stimulation is determined as the minimum voltage required to elicit a visible twitch or EMG response in the target muscle(s). At least two trials at this intensity should be conducted in order to ensure reproducibility. For example, stimulation of the left L3 nerve root should result in a response in the left thigh adductors and quadriceps femoris muscles. The anterior or ventral roots, which contain the motor efferent fibers, require much less stimulation than do the dorsal roots, which contain the sensory afferent fibers (5). The ventral roots usually require 1% to 2% of the stimulus needed to evoke a response in the same target muscle as did the dorsal root. This may be expressed as threshold ratio (TR), which is defined as follows:

Threshold ratio (TR) = (dorsal root threshold) / (ventral root threshold)

The optimal threshold ratio should be between 50 and 100. A ratio greater than 100 is usually considered to indicate too deep a

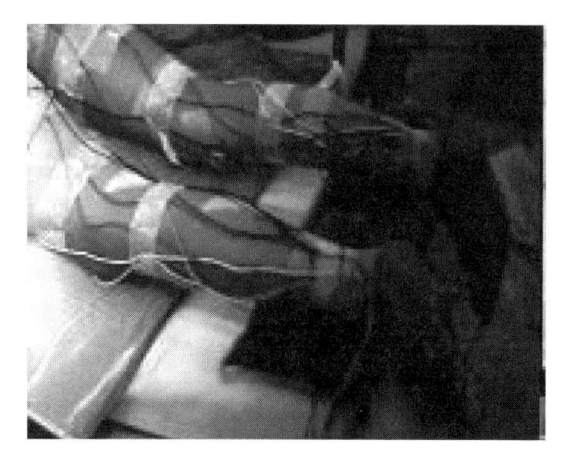

FIGURE 11.2 Patient preparing to undergo SDR surgery.

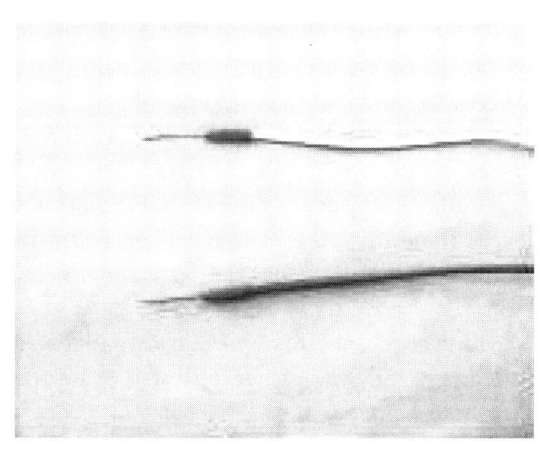

FIGURE 11.3 Subdermal needle electrodes.

TABLE 11.2 Standard Montage for SDR Monitoring

G1 electrode	G2 electrode	Innervation	LFF	HFF	Time/horizontal division (ms)	Voltage/vertical division (μV)
LAL	LAL	L2–L4	10 Hz	5 KHz	200	100
LVL	LVL	L2–L4	10 Hz	5 KHz	200	100
LBF	LBF	L4–S1	10 Hz	5 KHz	200	100
LAT	LAT	L4–L5	10 Hz	5 KHz	200	100
LG	LG	S1–S2	10 Hz	5 KHz	200	100
RAL	RAL	L2–L4	10 Hz	5 KHz	200	100
RVL	RVL	L2–L4	10 Hz	5 KHz	200	100
RBF	RBF	L4–S1	10 Hz	5 KHz	200	100
RAT	RAT	L4–L5	10 Hz	5 KHz	200	100
RG	RG	S1–S2	10 Hz	5 KHz	200	100
LAS	RAS	S3–S4	10 Hz	5 KHz	200	100

L = left; R = right; AL = adductor longus; VL = vastus lateralis; BF = biceps femoris; AT = anterior tibialis; G = gastrocnemius; AS = anal sphincter; G1 = grid 1 electrode; G2 = grid 2 electrode; LFF = low-frequency filter setting; HFF = high-frequency filter setting; ms = milliseconds; μV = microvolts.

level of anesthetic agent. A dorsal nerve root threshold greater than 30 V is indicative of excessive anesthesia (5). Tables 11.3 and 11.4 summarize the threshold and threshold ratio criteria for identification of an optimum anesthetic level and for proper separation of the mixed nerve root into its dorsal and ventral subcomponents. If a TR greater than 100 is identified, the amount of administered anesthetic agent should be reduced and testing repeated after an appropriate time interval. By contrast, TR less than 10 usually indicates incorrect identification of the nerve rootlets. In such instances it is important to ensure that the ventral and dorsal roots have been properly identified and separated. All ventral and dorsal nerve roots from L2 to S2 are tested individually in order to ensure that the proper level of anesthetic agent is being used and to confirm definitive separation of the dorsal from the ventral nerve roots.

In practice, the first nerve root pair to be tested is usually the S1 nerve roots. When the threshold voltage of the S1 ventral root is achieved, approximately 200 mV, should result in knee flexion and ankle plantar flexion without any associated toe flexion or anal sphincter contraction. The threshold voltage should result in either a visible twitch and/or definite EMG activity in the target muscle(s). By contrast, the dorsal root threshold should then be on the order of 10 to 20 V or 50 to 100 times the motor threshold. The S2 nerve root is then tested in a similar manner except that stimulation of the S2 ventral root should cause ankle plantar flexion and toe flexion in the absence of knee flexion. This confirmation of the S1 and S2 nerve roots is important, since the anatomic identification of S1 is not always easy. Because stimulation of an L5 nerve root may give a response similar to that of S1, it is always necessary to test the next caudal root in order to confirm that the first tested root is S1. After these levels have been determined to have optimal recording parameters, the process of identifying abnormal sensory nerve roots begins.

Dorsal Nerve Rootlet Selection

Most surgeons divide the dorsal roots to be tested into three to five subcomponent

TABLE 11.3 Threshold Ratios and Interpretation

Threshold ratio	Interpretation	Corrective action
100	Excess anesthesia	Reduce anesthetic
50–100	Optimal level	None
10–50	Borderline	Reassess anatomy/anesthetic levels
10	Low dorsal root threshold	Reassess anatomy

TABLE 11.4 Nerve Root Thresholds and Interpretation

Dorsal root threshold (V)	Interpretation	Corrective action
> 30	Excess anesthesia	Reduce anesthetic
10–30	Optimal level	None
≤ 10	Low dorsal root threshold	Ensure absence of ventral roots

rootlets (Figure 11.4). Some surgeons routinely section half of the L1 nerve rootlets without EMG testing in order to reduce hip flexor spasticity (9). The L1 nerve root should be identified by counting upward from the previously identified S1 and S2 nerve roots (5). The L1 nerve root is then identified and separated into dorsal and ventral components. These roots are then examined in order to determine the ventral threshold, the dorsal threshold, and the threshold ratio. If the dorsal root threshold is between 10 and 30 V with a TR between 50 and 100, the dorsal root is subdivided into three to five subsections. Each of these subsections is individually tested in order to determine whether that subcomponent sensory rootlet is normal or abnormal. This decision is based upon the distribution and pattern of the response to dorsal rootlet stimulation. This decision process is repeated at all levels caudal to the first level tested, L1 or L2, and then contralaterally.

Testing of the subcomponent rootlets begins with reducing the voltage to 30% of the threshold voltage for the entire dorsal root. The voltage is gradually increased until EMG activity and/or a visible twitch is noted in the appropriate ipsilateral target muscle. Figure 11.5 lists the various types of EMG responses that may result from stimulation. Decremental, squared, or decremental-squared responses are considered normal. By contrast, incremental, multiphasic, clonic, and sustained EMG responses are considered abnormal. Other abnormalities include the activation of muscles outside of the nerve root territory, which is considered to be the equivalent of hyperreflexia. Depending on the degree of spasticity, between 30% and 60% of all rootlets are resected.

"Secondary" criteria for abnormalities include low-threshold criteria, abrupt responses, and irregular responses (5). Low threshold is as an "unexpected" decrease in threshold of more than 50% from the previous rootlets tested. For example, if all previous rootlets had thresholds between 50 and 150 V, then a threshold less than or equal to 25 V would be considered abnormal. An abrupt response is a "vigorous, strong" myo-

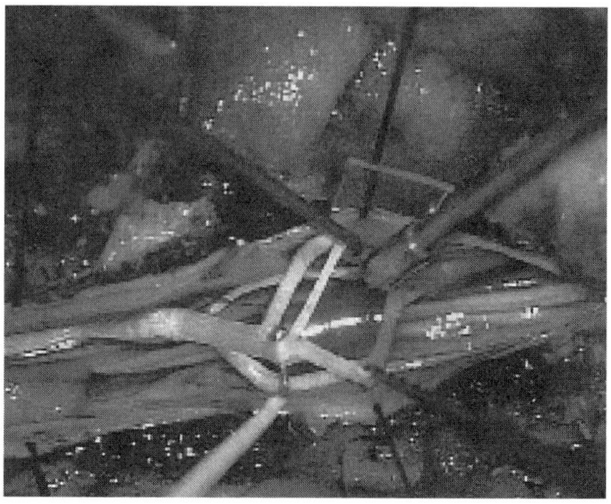

FIGURE 11.4 Sensory root division into subcomponent rootlets. Courtesy of Dr. KY Yam, Consultant Neurosurgeon, Tuen Mun Hospital, Hong Kong, China.

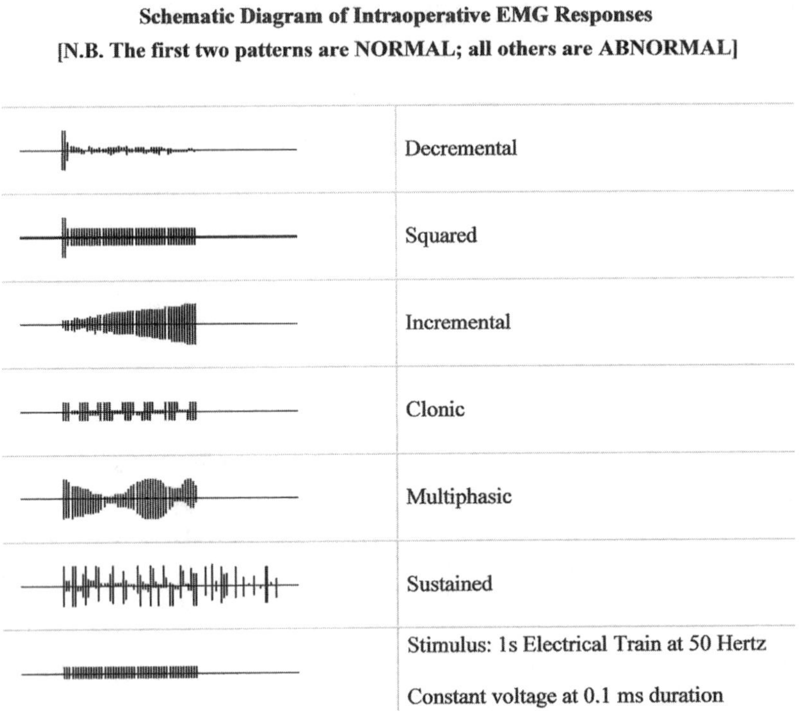

Schematic Diagram of Intraoperative EMG Responses
[N.B. The first two patterns are NORMAL; all others are ABNORMAL]

Waveform	Pattern
	Decremental
	Squared
	Incremental
	Clonic
	Multiphasic
	Sustained

Stimulus: 1s Electrical Train at 50 Hertz

Constant voltage at 0.1 ms duration

FIGURE 11.5 Patterns of EMG discharges from nerve rootlets. The first two patterns are normal; all others are abnormal.

genic response after a small incremental increase in voltage from stimulus intensities that previously evoked no responses. An irregular response is a fluctuation in EMG amplitude throughout the 1-second stimulus interval where the amplitude ratio of the highest to lowest amplitude was greater than or equal to 2. Of all these "secondary abnormalities," an abrupt response is considered to be most indicative of pathology, whereas a low threshold is the least. Some laboratories do not consider these secondary findings to represent definite abnormalities.

Dorsal Nerve Rootlet Sparing

Rootlets associated with anal sphincter responses at any of the sacral levels should be spared in order to reduce the probability of urinary or anal sphincter dysfunction. Some investigators do not spare an S1 level rootlet if a "small response" over the anal sphincter is noted and the response is otherwise abnormal (5). However, one should err on the side of caution in sectioning S1 rootlets. By contrast, anal sphincter responses resulting from lumbar rootlet stimulation are considered to be a manifestation of pathological reflex activity such that these rootlets need not be spared. Stimulation of sensory nerve rootlets that result in no response with 30-V stimulation, assuming that all other optimal recording parameters are present, are considered to be normal and should not be resected.

It is good practice to reassess all of the nerve roots that were not resected on the first round of testing. The remaining rootlets should be retested in order to ensure that no abnormal roots were overlooked in the first instance. If a nerve rootlet is abnormal on the second pass, a third test is indicated in order to ensure that a "borderline rootlet" is not sectioned. Many patients with CP already have reduced bowel and bladder capacity on the basis of reduced descending inhibition, similar to the spasticity mechanism noted in limb musculature. Therefore it is highly recommended not to section additional dorsal nerve rootlets in the sacral region, as this may lead to sphincter dysfunction.

TECHNICAL CONSIDERATIONS

Unlike most NIOM techniques, clinical neurophysiologic methods used in SDR identify abnormal neural structures for ablation rather than monitoring normal structures to ensure their protection. NIOM for SDR identifies the overactive sensory rootlets contained within the dorsal root so that these rootlets can be severed, whereas the normally functioning rootlets are spared. Given the relative preservation of normal sensory afferent input as well as the redundancy and overlap of the sensory coverage of the dorsal roots, resulting sensory deficits are minimized.

Preparation

Evoked (triggered) and spontaneous EMG are the techniques for displaying and recording the electrophysiological activity of the nerve rootlets. While evoked EMG is the primary modality for identifying the more problematic nerve rootlets, spontaneous EMG is useful for ensuring that high-quality information is available when needed. If a problem occurs, as with an electrode interface or lead, it can be noted and corrected quickly rather than being discovered when vital information is required. The evoked EMG is triggered by the technologist at the direction of the surgeon, who holds the bipolar stimulating probe on the rootlet to be tested.

Any NIOM device that is FDA-approved for use in the surgical suite and can simultaneously display a minimum of 11 channels of EMG activity may be used for an SDR procedure. However, it should be recalled that a total of 22 EMG recording leads will be required, as there are 5 pairs (10 leads) for the lower extremities and 1 pair for the anal sphincter. The display of 11 channels of spontaneous EMG and the display of 11 channels of evoked EMG do not have to be present at the same time. To help speed electrode preparation and aid in troubleshooting, a handheld impedance meter (Z-meter) with digital display is extremely helpful. If waveforms are to be printed in the operating room, a rapid laser printer should be used.

The bipolar stimulator for the surgeon, an extender lead, and at least one spare set should be sterilized in accordance with the hospital's infection-control policy. The patient should be instructed to take a bath or shower the night prior to surgery. No lotion or oil, such as bubble bath with skin emollients, should be used anywhere on the body in the perioperative period, so that tape will adhere well to the skin. A minimum of 22 disposable surface electrodes and 4 subdermal electrodes, or 26 subdermal electrodes (these numbers include some spares) should be available. Labels for each pair of electrodes are recommended. Twisted pairs of subdermal electrodes are quicker and easier to apply. Such electrodes are also preferred because they reduce the degree of electromagnetic interference (EMI).

The following pairs of limb leads should be placed bilaterally: thigh adductors, quadriceps femoris, biceps femoris, tibialis anterior, and gastrocnemius muscles. A ground should be placed on either leg just below the buttocks. These leads may be either subdermal leads or surface electrodes. The advantage of surface electrodes is that of saving time in the surgical suite, since these electrodes can be applied prior to the surgery. However, the patient must be able to tolerate the skin preparation. The patient should be informed what to expect regarding skin preparation for surface electrode application. In contrast, subdermal leads should be inserted after the patient is anesthetized. Subdermal leads are applied to the right and left sides of the anal sphincter muscles after cleaning the area with alcohol wipes. The surgeon should insert the subdermal needles tangentially below the right and left side of anal skin parallel to the sagittal plane of the patient. Because the needle track is quite visible, the risk of creating a fistula is low. However, the risk may be lessened by having the surgeon place a gloved, lubricated finger into the anus while slowly advancing the needle into the muscle. This will allow the surgeon to detect any approach of the subdermal needle into the anal canal. The needle need not be perfectly placed within the muscle, as the EMG activity recorded from the sphincter is readily obtained even with an approximate placement. Irrespective of the methodology used, the anal sphincter leads forms its own pair. The left anal sphincter lead is referenced to the right, as noted in Table 11.2. Therefore a total of 11 pairs or 22 EMG leads are used for monitoring; five for each lower extremity and a pair for the anal sphincter.

For disposable surface electrodes, each electrode site should be prepared with a FDA-approved skin preparation using a 6 inch (about 15 cm) Q-tip. It may be helpful to stretch the skin between two fingers of the free hand to make lower impedance contact easier to achieve. Excess skin preparation should be wiped off with a washcloth prior to placing the electrode on the skin. It is useful to squirt a small amount of EEG electrode gel underneath each pad in order to reduce impedance. The electrodes in each pair should be approximately 3 to 6 cm apart. These should not be shorted together with electrolyte or other conductive material. In verifying interelectrode impedances, it is best to have as many electrodes plugged into the Z-meter as possible, as the displayed reading is the sum of the impedance of the electrode being tested plus the impedance of the remainder of the electrodes in parallel. The addition of more electrodes into this reference should result in a low impedance value, which should approximate zero impedance in the ideal situation. The optimum range of interelectrode impedance is less than 5,000 ohms. However, in some cases it may not be possible to achieve this range. In such situations, it is best to prepare the pair such that they are both as low and as balanced or equivalent as possible. To ensure that the electrodes are properly connected to the recording machine, the electrodes may be touched one by one to check if movement artifacts appear on the corresponding trace.

It is recommended that a twitch-level monitor, as used by anesthesia personnel, be used to verify and document the twitch level on one of the lower extremities. Only two additional stimulating electrodes are required, as the recording leads are already present on the anterior tibialis and gastrocnemius muscles. The cathode is placed approximately 2 to 3 cm medial to the fibular head on soft tissue, medial to the bone. The anode is placed approximately 5 cm rostral to the cathode in the lateral part of the popliteal fossa. These leads stimulate the peroneal nerve.

The recording leads for each leg (if not already twisted and paired) should be bundled together (tape works well) and braided to increase the artifact rejection of EMI, which is almost invariably present in the surgical environment. A 60-Hz notch filter should not be used unless absolutely necessary. Many sources of EMI in the operating room environment generate frequencies at 60 Hz or at one of its harmonic frequencies. Therefore omitting the 60-Hz notch filter increases the probability of detecting faulty recording leads.

The twitch-level channel consists of either the right or left leg (anterior tibialis to gastrocnemius muscles) filtered as above and set to approximately 2 mV per division and with a time base of 3 ms per division. The stimulation is applied four consecutive times at a 2-Hz rate. A pulse width of 0.2 ms is usually satisfactory.

The nerve stimulator, which is usually built into the NIOM device, is set up with a maximum intensity limit of 100 V, a pulse width of 0.1 ms, recurrent stimulus rate of 50 Hz, and a train length of 1 second. If the stimulator is not built into the NIOM device, connect its **trigger out** to the **external trigger input** of the NIOM device. It is important to discuss the anesthesia protocol with anesthesia personnel in order to ensure that any muscle relaxants will have been metabolized by the time that the surgeon is ready to proceed with nerve stimulation. The twitch-level monitor will confirm that the muscles can respond appropriately.

All stimulating leads, extenders, and recording leads are plugged in and their satisfactory functioning is verified. This should be documented by storing a sample waveform. All leads should be continually observed to ensure that no new sources of EMI, such as cautery, drills, intravenous pumps, etc., have been introduced that will significantly interfere with monitoring. Any faulty leads are corrected, and electrical interference is reduced. Once the nerve stimulator is needed, it will be connected to the sterile stimulating extender leads by the surgeon or the surgeon's assistants.

Procedure

The NIOM technologist should be skilled and experienced in all aspects of NIOM, as the information provided will be utilized to cut nerve roots permanently. It is also imperative that a clinical neurophysiologist who is experienced with this procedure be present throughout the operation.. Excellent communication between technologist, neurophysiologist, surgeon, and anesthesia personnel is essential. If the technologist notes a technical problem or anything else that is vital to the procedure, it should be communicated without delay to enable rapid correction. The thresholds determined by the technologist may be utilized by anesthesia personnel to alter the administration of anesthesia.

Before and during the exposure, as cautery permits, the recording leads should be checked continuously with spontaneous EMG recordings in order to verify that all leads are working. The spontaneous EMG waveforms should be stored periodically. If the NIOM device has a built-in impedance meter, the impedance of the recording leads should be checked and stored. Any faulty recording leads should be corrected as soon as possible. By careful preparation and setup, the need for troubleshooting will be minimized. The twitch level should be monitored periodically and waveforms stored.

After the exposure is complete, the surgeon will request stimulation of the nerve roots and rootlets. Numerous individual nerves, which can be posterior nerve roots, anterior nerve roots, or the individual rootlets, will be stimulated. The surgeon should state which nerve root (anterior or posterior and level) or nerve rootlet is to be tested. For each root, a threshold is determined by slowly increasing the stimulating intensity and applying the stimulation singly or automatically at relatively lengthy intervals (e.g., 0.5-Hz rate) until an EMG response is detected. For anterior nerve roots, the threshold should be very low (likely less than 5 V), whereas for posterior nerve roots, it will be much higher (likely 20 to 100 V). As the stimulation is applied directly to a nerve, there is a possibility of damaging the nerve and of movement by the patient. Therefore, the threshold should be determined by starting at a very low intensity and increasing in small increments. For each threshold, the stimulation intensity, the level of the root (and whether anterior or posterior), and which muscles responded should be noted. Also, whether single stimulations or a train of stimuli was necessary to elicit a response should be recorded. This documentation should be readily available for reference if required.

When directed by the surgeon, a train of stimuli is applied to a root whose threshold for stimulation has been pre-determined. The initial stimulation intensity should be approximately one third of the pre-determined threshold. The intensity should be increased if needed to get a response. The neurophysiologist must assess the elicited waveform(s) and determine if it is a normal or abnormal response and provide an explanation if needed. The above procedure is repeated numerous times. Occasionally the same nerve will be tested more than once. The threshold ratios and the absolute nerve root threshold may be used to determine if the anesthetic level is optimal, as noted in the previous section.

Postprocedure

All leads should be removed at the end of the surgical procedure, preferably while the patient is still anesthetized, then discarded. Infection-control procedures established by the hospital where the procedure is performed should be followed at all times. Any NIOM equipment that is to be reused, such as stimulators, recording electrodes, and other hardware, should be sterilized in accordance with established standards. A report documenting the significant findings should be created.

CONCLUSIONS

SDR is a surgical procedure that can permanently reduce the effect of spasticity in persons affected with spastic forms of CP, so that greater degrees of movement are possible. The patients must be carefully selected, as this procedure is most beneficial to persons with certain subtypes of CP. SDR is performed by identifying the anatomic level of the dorsal roots, carefully separating them into four to five subcomponent rootlets, testing the rootlets with NIOM procedures, and ablating the abnormal sensory rootlets that are contributing to the patient's spasticity. Close cooperation between the surgeon, the anesthesiologist, and the NIOM team is required to ensure that only the abnormal rootlets are sectioned and that every attempt is made to spare sphincter function. This requires careful attention to detail regarding the muscles monitored, the type and level of anesthesia used, NIOM recording techniques, and the proper interpretation of the resulting EMG discharges when a dorsal rootlet is stimulated.

REFERENCES

1. Foerster O. On the indications and results of the excision of posterior spinal roots in men. *Surg Gynecol Obstet* 1913;16:463–474.
2. Fasano VA, Barolat-Romana G, Zeeme S, Sguazzi A. Electrophysiologic assessment of spinal circuits in spasticity by direct dorsal root stimulation. *Neurosurgery* 1979;4: 146–151.
3. Peacock WJ, Arens LJ, Berman B. Cerebral palsy spasticity, selective posterior rhizotomy. *Pediat Neurosci*. 1987;13:61–66.
4. Peacock WJ, Staudt LA, Nuwer MR. A neurological approach to spasticity: selective posterior rhizotomy. In: R. Wilkins R, Rengachary S, eds. *Neurosurgery Update II*. New York: McGraw Hill, 1990:403–407.
5. Staudt LA, Nuwer MR, Peacock WJ. Intraoperative monitoring during selective posterior rhizotomy: technique and patient outcome. *Electroencephalogr Clin Neurophysiol* 1995;97:296–309.
6. McLaughlin J, Bjornson K, Temkin N, et al. Selective dorsal rhizotomy: meta-analysis of three randomized controlled trials. *Dev Med Child Neurol* 2002;44:17–25.
7. Pharoah PO, Platt MJ, Cooke T. The changing epidemiology of cerebral palsy. *Arch Dis Child Fetal Neonatal Ed* 1996;75:F169–F173.
8. Logigian EL, Wolinsky JS, Soriano SG, et al. H reflex studies in cerebral palsy patients undergoing selective posterior rhizotomy. *Muscle Nerve* 1994;17:539–549.
9. About selective dorsal rhizotomy. Saint Louis Children's Hospital, accessed on November 10, 2006, at http://www.stlouischildrens.org/tabid/96/itemid/1540/About-Selective-Dorsal-Rhizotomy.aspx.

12 Peripheral Nerve Surgery*

Brian A. Crum
Jeffrey A. Strommen
James A. Abbott

Neurophysiologic monitoring of peripheral nerves during surgery is an extremely valuable procedure that provides vital, real-time information to the surgical team. Preoperative neurophysiologic testing provides the surgeon with valuable data to assist with decision making; however, there is information that simply cannot be garnered from these studies, and intraoperative studies help bridge this gap. Monitoring of peripheral nerves has been described and studied for nearly 40 years and been the subject of several reviews (1–7). Neurophysiologic intraoperative monitoring (NIOM) requires a skilled and knowledgeable team (neurophysiologists and technologists) who ensure rapid and accurate acquisition and interpretation of neurophysiologic data. It also requires a good working relationship with the entire surgical team. Communication with the surgeon(s) is vital in assisting with surgical decision making between sometimes quite divergent surgical plans. Accurate and timely communication with the anesthesiologist is also important, as certain anesthetic agents can have detrimental affects on neurophysiologic studies. Having a peripheral nerve NIOM plan prior to surgery is ideal to maximize the efficiency and utility of the studies.

The goal of this chapter is to provide a background in the equipment, techniques, and interpretation of intraoperative peripheral nerve stimulation and recording. Additionally, the NIOM approach to several specific peripheral nerve disorders is addressed.

UTILITY OF NIOM IN PERIPHERAL NERVE SURGERY

There are many uses for peripheral nerve NIOM. It can be used to identify peripheral nerves in the surgical field. Localizing preexisting disease processes along the course of a nerve is also possible. Functional continuity across a preexisting lesion can also be determined. Monitoring can prevent damage to intact nerves during surgery. Finally, NIOM is useful in selecting fascicles of nerves for resection or biopsy.

Surgery on peripheral nerves is most often performed for focal trauma or compression. The preoperative clinical examination is critical in evaluation of these patients to answer the four questions below.

Is this a neurologic problem? The neurologic examination should answer this ques-

---

*Portions of this chapter are reproduced with permission from the AANEM Minimonograph "Peripheral Nerve Stimulation and Monitoring During Operative Procedures" in *Muscle Nerve*, 2007;35:159-170.

tion, though in some patients the motor examination can be clouded by pain or poor effort. The sensory examination is notoriously subjective and occasionally difficult to rely on for that reason.

To which nerve(s) does the problem localize? This relies on the clinician's knowledge of peripheral nerve anatomy and innervation patterns. A full discussion of this is best reserved for general or peripheral neurology textbooks.

Where along the course of the nerve is the damage? Again, this relies on the clinician's knowledge of innervation patterns to muscles and to skin. One must also take into account the typical sites of compression and the mechanism of injury.

Is the lesion complete? A complete lesion is a clinical judgment based on the findings of no motor or sensory function distal to a point of nerve injury. It is important to realize that after injury, there may be axonal regrowth, which can be occurring but not detectable by the clinical examination as the axons may not yet have reached their targets. This is one of the main reasons to employ peripheral nerve NIOM, as the finding of continuity of axons across a lesion may be detectable in a timely fashion only in this way.

Preoperative neurophysiologic studies help to compliment the clinical evaluation to answer all of the above questions. Again, given the time it takes for reinnervation to occur after injury, even preoperative neurophysiologic studies may not be able to determine whether a lesion is complete or not or, stated in another way, whether or not there is functional continuity across a lesion.

As mentioned, peripheral nerve NIOM is used to determine continuity across an injured segment of nerve or for precise localization of a lesion. Following an axonal injury, Wallerian degeneration will occur back to the level of the nerve injury. Axonal regeneration may then proceed from the lesion, moving distally at a rate of about 1 mm per day. Following this, reinnervation of the end organ must occur for functional recovery. After axons reach a muscle, there may be a several weeks to months of delay before this reinnervation can be detected, initially by neurophysiologic means (nascent motor unit action potentials) and then by visible voluntary contraction (8). Depending on the distance from lesion to end organ, therefore, a variable period of time must then pass to see clinical and neurophysiologic signs of reinnervation. By the time one concludes there is no reinnervation by using these means, the opportunity for a surgical approach to reinnervation (i.e., nerve grafting) may be lost, as the best results are obtained if surgery is performed in the first 6 to 12 months. In a proximal sciatic lesion, for example, that much time or more would be required to conclude from a clinical or standard neurophysiologic measurement that there is no reinnervation to the anterior compartment of the leg.

In this setting only intraoperative assessment can make an early determination of whether there is functional continuity of axons across a lesion at a time when surgical intervention is most likely to be successful. Visual inspection is of great importance in an anatomically continuous lesion as nerve thickening and neuroma formation may indicate a lesion without functional continuity. There is, though, no visual way to reliably determine functional continuity of axons, especially regenerating ones. Eliciting a muscle twitch [or a compound muscle action potential (CMAP)] downstream from a site of peripheral nerve stimulation indicates functional continuity of that section of nerve. A response from direct muscle stimulation or from stimulation of an adjacent nerve must be excluded. Additionally, only a few functioning axons are needed to elicit a CMAP, which may not turn out to be functionally useful. An absent response, though, could mean either a lesion in continuity (without muscle reinnervation yet) or a complete lesion. The presence of a nerve action potential (NAP) across a lesion, therefore, remains the "gold standard" to determine functional nerve continuity and therefore the type of surgical approach. A NAP can be obtained in the setting of a lesion that appears complete clinically and by routine preoperative neurophysiologic testing (2). Lesions in continuity are treated with neurolysis and are not grafted, as they have a high likelihood of a good outcome. About 90% of those patients experience a good outcome (2). Lesions with no NAP transmitted are thought to have no chance of spontaneous reinnervation and are thus treated by grafting or nerve transfer (2,6).

If there is no NAP across a lesion, a second possibility is that there may be continuity and the potential for axonal regeneration that is being stunted by compression of fascicles by scarring within the nerve itself. An internal neurolysis can then be performed, allowing outgrowth of these regenerating axons. This carries with it some risk for neural damage and disruption of regenerating axons and is generally not performed. Unfortunately, the distinction between the above two possibilities is impossible neurophysiologically and must be made by the surgeon, taking into consideration the appearance of the nerve (2,9). In some settings, although a NAP is recorded across the lesion, part of the nerve appears significantly injured and fascicular NAP recordings are helpful. Single fascicles are stimulated; those that demonstrate continuity are left alone and those that do not are treated with primary repair or fascicular grafting (3).

Peripheral nerve NIOM can be called upon to assist with localization of a lesion along a nerve. When a response is present on stimulating at one point on a nerve and then not present on stimulating at another point, the localization of the lesion between these two points is clear. A neurapraxic lesion that does not completely block all conduction through it, though, will lead to responses being recorded with both proximal and distal stimulation (across a lesion). The response with proximal stimulation may be longer in duration (temporal dispersion), lower in amplitude (partial conduction block), and arrive at the recording electrodes with a longer latency than would be expected (focal slowing). Inching is a technique of stimulating at short, incremental steps across a lesion, making assessments of the change in morphology and latency of the evoked waveforms recorded distally (10). If one inches at 1-cm increments, assuming a conduction velocity of 50 m/s, the onset of each successive waveform should be separated by 0.2 ms. A longer latency difference between two sites of stimulation may indicate a focal lesion. Also, the stimulus threshold may increase just as one enters a diseased segment of nerve, again helping to precisely localize an area of abnormality. As the main goal of inching is to localize focal lesions more precisely, it is useful in the intraoperative setting when this localization has not been provided by preoperative neurophysiologic studies.

PERIPHERAL NERVE NIOM TECHNIQUES

Nerve Conduction Studies

Nerve conduction studies are performed with stimulation and recording of motor, sensory, or mixed nerves, yielding a NAP. Potentials can also be recorded over muscle (CMAP) or centrally over spine or scalp [evoked potentials (EPs)]. Many factors will dictate which of these (or which combinations) is used, which will then dictate the type of equipment necessary and the regimen of anesthesia that should be utilized.

Intraoperative peripheral nerve stimulation is given directly to the surgically exposed nerve (Figure 12.1). A bipolar stimulator is held in place by the surgeon with cathode directed toward the recording electrodes. The interelectrode distance is usually 3 mm, although this distance is dictated by the size of the nerve. A larger nerve, such as the sciatic, demands a larger interelectrode distance, such as 7 mm. The proper orientation of the stim-

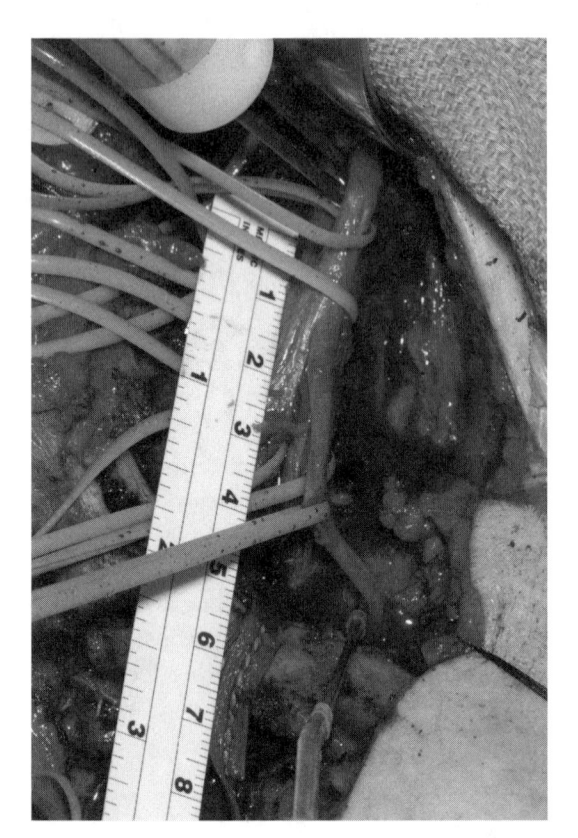

FIGURE 12.1 Intraoperative peripheral nerve bipolar stimulation electrodes (bottom) and recording electrodes (top).

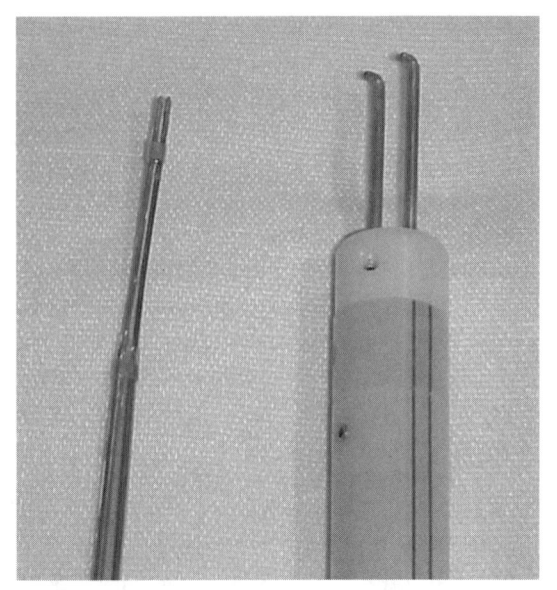

FIGURE 12.2 Bipolar electrodes. Left: pointed-tip electrodes often used for stimulation. Right: hook electrodes often used for recording.

ulating electrodes is important, and visual confirmation of correct placement by the neurophysiologist or technologist in the operating room is useful. Monopolar stimulation with the cathode on the nerve and the anode some distance away can be done when the proper bipolar orientation is impossible. This should generally be avoided, however, as stimulation cannot be more precisely focused, leading to current spread to adjacent nerves and muscles and potentially farther down the nerve than desired. Bipolar stimulation affords less current spread. A tripolar stimulating electrode can also be used (2,11). In this arrangement, a single cathode is between two anodes, further focusing the site of stimulation while minimizing stimulus artifact. Special stimulating electrodes, some with hooks or very small pointed tips, often need to be used (Figure 12.2).

Hook electrodes allow the nerve to be elevated out of the surgical field to avoid contact with excessive fluid thus reducing current spread. The authors use stimulating electrodes made of a silver solder alloy; these are gas-sterilized or autoclaved after surgical procedures.

The amount of stimulation required to depolarize the underlying axon is much less than that needed for percutaneous stimulation. Excessive stimulation must be avoided to limit current spread down the stimulated nerve and to other nearby nerves and muscles and to decrease the stimulus artifact, which is amplified with a shorter distance between the stimulating and recording electrodes. A square-wave pulsed stimulus with duration of 0.05 ms and intensity of only a few milliamperes (1 – 5 mA) is usually sufficient for depolarization of the axonal membrane in a supramaximal fashion. Of note, short-duration stimulation of this type is more likely to preferentially activate motor axons (12). For constant-voltage stimulation, intensities of 25 to 50 V are used (13). It is important to remember that, in diseased nerves, higher stimulus intensity may be needed to reach threshold. It is the authors' practice to increase the stimulus intensity up to 20 to 25 mA if no response is initially obtained. These higher intensities, however, result in more stimulus artifact and more likely evoke volume-conducted responses than true NAPs (see below). As the size of the NAP is small (microvolts), averaging of one to five responses is often helpful; although when a response is present, it is usually visible after the first stimulus (Figure 12.3).

NAP recordings take place along the course of the stimulated nerve. The distance between the cathode and the active, recording electrode should be at least 4 cm to minimize stimulus artifact. Recording is with a bipolar arrangement, with an interelectrode distance of 3 to 5 mm. A wider separation is used when there is a longer distance between the cathode and recording electrode, allowing the longer traveling wave to completely pass under the active electrode before passing under the referential electrode. The farther the separation, however, the more likely extraneous noise and stimulus artifact will be seen as different by the two recording electrodes and, thus, not rejected or cancelled out in common mode. The nerve may need to be lifted out of the surgical field, similar to the site of stimulation. The recording electrodes are held in place by the surgeon, and again visual confirmation of the correct orientation (active electrode toward the cathode) is important. The size of the recording electrodes should match the size of the recording nerve. A three-pronged electrode with ground-active-referential arrangement has also been used. The same electrodes can be used for either stimulating or recording, depending on whether they are connected to the amplifier or stimulator. Bipolar point electrodes are generally used for stimulation and the curved hook electrodes for recording (Figure 12.1). The ground electrode is a flat metal plate that is placed under the patient and separate from the ground used for cautery.

As the NAP waveforms contain frequencies in the 1-kHz range, using filter settings of 5 to 10 Hz for the low-frequency (high-pass) filter and 2 to 3 kHz for the high-frequency (low-pass) filter are appropriate. Occasionally it is helpful to increase the high-frequency filter to better separate the NAP waveform from the stimulus artifact (11). The NAP amplitude is usually less than 100 µV, so a gain of 20 to 50 µV per division is utilized. The latency depends on the length between stimulating and recording electrodes. A simple guide is 1 ms per 5-cm distance (assuming 50 m/second conduction velocity). A time base of 0.5 ms per division is reasonable, increasing this for longer distances.

When the goal of intraoperative peripheral nerve studies is to determine the degree of continuity or the exact location of a peripheral nerve lesion, stimulation and recording will need to be done on both sides of the lesion. The orientation will vary depending on the accessibility to the nerve. In assessing for continuity, it is important to realize that the presence of only few large myelinated axons can produce a response with relatively normal conduction velocity, latency, and threshold; therefore it is most useful to assess the amplitude or, at minimum, the presence of the NAP to determine the number of functioning axons across a lesion. A NAP proves the existence of a large number (over 4,000) of functioning, medium-sized, myelinated axons (1). Stimulation is usually performed proximal to the lesion with recording distal. In localizing

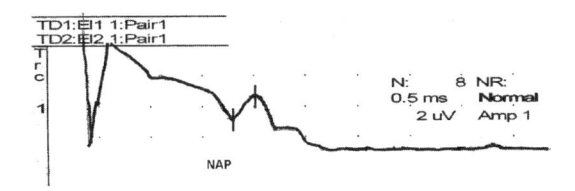

FIGURE 12.3 Nerve action potential with a peak latency of about 2 ms. Horizontal gain 0.5 ms per division; vertical gain 2 microvolts per division.

lesions, recording electrodes are placed proximally and the stimulating electrodes are moved proximal to, then into, then distal to the suspected lesion, assessing for a change in morphology of the waveform.

As mentioned above, CMAP recordings are of limited utility in determining functional continuity, although they can be used in localizing lesions. Recording CMAP has the advantage of amplification of responses as each axon innervates and activates hundreds to thousands of muscle fibers. Amplitudes are measured in millivolts, as opposed to microvolts in NAP recordings. CMAP recording is performed with surface (as in routine nerve conduction studies), subcutaneous, or intramuscular electrodes (Figure 12.4). Subcutaneous recordings are done with needle electrodes placed above or into the muscle of interest. Fine, longer intramuscular wires placed with the use of a hollow needle can also be utilized. Both intramuscular and subcutaneous recordings limit the size of the recording area, thereby reducing extraneous noise in the recording. Intramuscular recordings, though, do this to a much greater degree, recording from only a small part of a muscle and therefore reflecting activity in only a fraction of the axons that might be stimulated intraoperatively. They also tend to introduce more noise than subcutaneous EEG electrodes. They are not suitable for NIOM when one is interested in the amount of innervation to a muscle. Wire electrodes are used most often for deep muscles or those that are small or from which recording is difficult (i.e., rhomboids, laryngeal muscles). Subcutaneous recordings are favored at the authors' institution, given the ease of placement and quiet recordings.

Needle Electromyography

Monitoring needle electromyography (EMG) activity during surgery can give relatively noninvasive, real-time information regarding the status of motor axons. This is most often used in NIOM when a surgical procedure places motor axons at risk of injury. This includes spinal roots during spine surgery or peripheral or cranial nerves during limb or skull base surgery. A recording electrode placed in a muscle can be used to identify abnormal activity, namely neurotonic discharges. Neurotonic discharges are high-frequency bursts of motor unit action potentials (MUAPs) either firing briefly or in more prolonged trains (14). These bursts or trains are made up of MUAPs firing at 30 to 100 Hz. Neurotonic discharges are caused by mechanical irritation to axons, including traction, stretch, manipulation, or saline irrigation. They must be distinguished from irregular voluntary MUAPs occurring under light anesthesia or from other electrode or surgical (i.e., electrocautery) artifacts. Although neurotonic discharges are sensitive indicators of nerve irritation, their presence

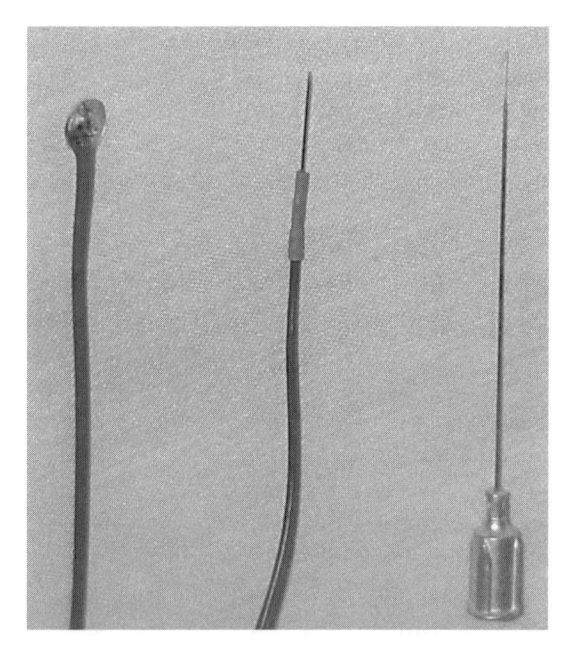

FIGURE 12.4 Electrodes used for compound muscle action potential recording. Left: surface electrode. Middle: needle electrode for subcutaneous recording. Right: fine intramuscular wire electrode introduced in hollow needle which is then removed with fine wire "hooked" into place in muscle.

does not always indicate damage to axons and their absence does not guarantee lack of damage. Neurotonic discharges are, for example, common in some spine surgeries, although postoperative radiculopathy is rare (15). It is important to note that sharp transection of a nerve may produce no neurotonic discharges. These discharges are less likely to be produced after mechanical stimulation in previously damaged nerves. They can still be recorded with neuromuscular blocking agents producing up to 75% block as measured by CMAP amplitude (16).

Free-running recording can be achieved with subcutaneous needle electrodes, often referencing a nearby muscle to limit the number of channels required. One channel could have the medial gastrocnemius muscle referenced to the anterior tibialis, the next vastus medialis muscle referenced to the rectus femoris, and so on. Abnormal activity may not, therefore, be localized precisely to one muscle. If such localization is vital, then each channel should be made to represent separate muscles, with two electrodes placed in each muscle. Fine-wire electrodes can also be used, with the active recording surface being a small bared tip. This is most useful for deep or small muscles (i.e., rhomboid and laryngeal muscles), especially when a more selective recording from a single muscle is vital. As the fine-wire electrodes record from a smaller area of muscle, subcutaneous needle electrodes are preferred to maximize the chance of detecting neurotonic discharges.

TECHNICAL PROBLEMS

Given the importance of acquiring accurate information quickly, as it may guide surgical decision making, several potential technical problems must be understood. Low temperature of nerves is inevitable in NIOM, leading to slowed conduction velocities and higher amplitudes. Since temperature cannot be increased during NIOM, the effect of low temperature must simply be kept in mind. Most analysis is done looking at a presence or absence of a potential or a change in a potential at nearby recording sites. These parameters are unlikely to be significantly affected by the cool temperatures during NIOM. Peripheral ischemia from a blood pressure cuff can impair nerve conduction studies, and it is recommended that if a tourniquet is in place for 60 minutes on the limb of study, it should be let down for at least 20 minutes before beginning NIOM studies. The operating room is an electrically hostile environment. Surgical instruments, beds, machines, and lights all can contribute, especially in the form of 60-Hz interference. Limiting fluorescent lights and any electrical motors or electrocautery devices during recording is helpful.

Stimulus artifact can be a challenge. Making sure that the electrodes are lifted out of a wet field is important. The lowest stimulation intensity at the least duration possible should be used to achieve supramaximal stimulation. The distance between stimulation and recording electrodes can be increased if exposure in the surgical field permits. Recording electrodes can be arranged in a monopolar fashion, with the referential or inactive electrode in adjacent tissue perpendicular to the active electrode.

Muscle artifact caused by volume conduction from nearby sources can also distort the NAP. Proper orientation of the electrodes and grounding must be assured. The placement of the stimulating and recording electrodes can be reversed, stimulating distally. This can help to reduce the amount of activation of nearby muscles innervated by more proximal branches from the nerve being studied. Neuromuscular blocking agents can be utilized to eliminate this artifact as well.

When a NAP is not obtained or there is trouble getting the response, it is useful to record a NAP over a normal portion of nerve. This acts as a control to ensure functioning of the whole NIOM system. If there is no visible twitch in a downstream muscle and no elicited electrical response, one must also ensure that the stimulation is indeed occurring. The stimulating electrodes then are placed on a nearby known functioning nerve or muscle to assess for twitch. Even in the setting of neuromuscular blocking agents, direct stimulation of muscle should result in a twitch.

NAP and CMAP recordings are minimally affected by anesthesia. If CMAPs are being recorded, neuromuscular blocking agents should be minimized or not used at all. If, however, a neuromuscular blocking agent is used, a peripheral stimulator with a train-of-four recording is done to monitor the degree of block (amplitude change from the first to the fourth stimulus). CMAP responses can still be obtained if there is a less than 100% decrement over the four successive supramaximal repetitive nerve stimulations (16). As mentioned above, neuromuscular blocking agents may be desirable for NAP studies in which muscle artifact must be eliminated.

NIOM FOR SPECIFIC DISORDERS

Ulnar Neuropathy at the Elbow

Ulnar neuropathy at the elbow (UNE) is the second most common entrapment mononeuropathy, trailing only median neuropathy at the wrist (carpal tunnel syndrome). While NIOM is not often used for UNE surgery, it can be useful in certain instances. The two main anatomic sites of compression at the elbow are the cubital tunnel, formed by the two heads of the flexor carpi ulnaris, and the retroepicondylar groove between the medial epicondyle and the olecranon. The surgical approach to compression at these two levels is different: simple decompression with entrapment at the cubital tunnel, and ulnar nerve transposition or epicondylectomy if entrapment is more proximal in the retroepicondylar groove.

Preoperative neurophysiologic studies may confirm UNE but not localize the lesion to one of these sites (8,17). Factors that contribute to this include variability in anatomic location of these two potential entrapment sites, selective involvement of fascicles in the ulnar nerve, technical difficulties with overstimulation (especially at the below-elbow site), and anastomotic nerve connections. Last, as is often the case, the lesion may be predominately axonal and not easily localized by inching. The degree of intraoperative neurophysiologic abnormality is often more severe than expected based on routine preoperative studies (2). Intraoperative studies may even show abnormalities when routine nerve conduction studies across the elbow are normal (18). Additionally, compression may be at a more distal site than expected (19,20). Intraoperative ulnar nerve studies are therefore useful when localization is needed to guide the type and site of surgical intervention.

The ulnar nerve is usually easily exposed surgically. If possible, stimulation and recording should be performed on a normal portion of the nerve to ensure a working system. Then, recording proximally, the stimulating electrodes are placed at intervals closer, into, and distal to the area in question. An assessment is made for changes in stimulus threshold and NAP amplitude, latency, and morphology as stimulation moves into the abnormal segment of nerve. Based on intraoperative ulnar nerve studies, the site of compression is most commonly at or just proximal to the retroepicondylar groove/ medial epicondyle (2,18,21). In fact, a 30-year study at Louisiana State University demonstrated compressive ulnar neuropathies localized to the epicondyle level in over 97% of cases (18). Cubital tunnel localization was seen more frequently in other studies (20,22). Based on these findings, the NIOM team should begin stimulating across the epicondylar region. If no clear abnormalities are seen, the segment of nerve across the cubital tunnel should be assessed. If these sites are normal, it is important to realize that rarely the ulnar nerve can be compressed at sites distal to the cubital tunnel, within or as it exits the flexor carpi ulnaris (20,23).

Median Neuropathy at the Wrist

Median neuropathy at the wrist is the most common upper extremity entrapment neuropathy. Routine neurophysiologic studies are excellent at confirming the clinical diagnosis of carpal tunnel syndrome (24). As in UNE, intraoperative studies are rarely performed, given the relative ease of the decompressive procedure and the lack of uncertainty in localization.

In one approach to intraoperative median nerve studies, stimulation of the nerve was performed in 5-mm increments proximal to, through, and distal to the carpal tunnel, with surface recording over the thenar eminence (21). The most abnormal segment with respect to focal slowing or conduction block corresponded to the segment of most abnormal-appearing nerve. In the remainder of cases, the slowing involved two or more 5-mm segments. The site of the most abnormal conduction was within the first 10 to 20 mm just distal to the proximal border of the flexor retinaculum. Immediately upon release of the median nerve in the carpal tunnel, latencies have been noted to improve or remain the same (25,26).

Another technique has been described in which the median nerve is stimulated in the region of the carpal tunnel with recording of the sensory digital branches on the third digit (27). This technique demonstrated that the most abnormal segment (most conduction slowing and amplitude reduction) was the distal part of the carpal tunnel. This also correlated with the area of highest intracarpal tunnel pressure measurements.

Common Peroneal Neuropathy at the Knee

The common peroneal nerve can be compressed or damaged as it traverses the fibular head at the knee. As in median neuropathy at the wrist and UNE, localization with routine neurophysiologic studies is usually possible. Intraoperative peroneal nerve studies can be performed for localization and to determine nerve continuity (21). A large series of surgically treated common peroneal neuropathies revealed that often there was no transmission of a NAP across the lesion, which led to nerve graft repairs. Most patients in this series of 318 cases had suffered traumatic peroneal neuropathies. Nontraumatic cases with compression or entrapment at the knee (51 of 318) were more likely to have recordable NAPs (42 of 51) and thus undergo neurolysis as opposed to nerve grafting (28).

Use in Operating on Nerve Tumors

Peripheral nerve tumors are rare. They are broadly separated into neural sheath tumors and non–neural sheath tumors. Examples of the former include benign entities such as neurofibromas (with or without neurofibromatosis type I) and schwannomas. Sarcomas (neurogenic, fibrosarcoma, spindle cell, synovial, or perineurial) are malignant neural sheath tumors. Non–neural sheath tumors include ganglion cysts, lipomas, hypertrophic neuropathy (although some of these may be inflammatory), vascular tumors, and desmoid tumors. Metastatic carcinoma can affect nerves; most commonly this is from a lung or breast primary. The location for these peripheral nerve tumors varies, with the brachial plexus and upper extremity being most common, followed by the lower extremity and rarely the lumbosacral plexus (29,30).

The use of NAP recordings can be helpful intraoperatively. A stimulator can be used to localize peripheral nerve if the architecture or anatomy is confusing. Functioning fascicles are identified in order to protect them if at all possible and thereby limit postoperative neurologic deficit. In most cases, complete tumor removal takes precedence and fascicles may need to be sacrificed. Typically, fascicles involved by tumor are usually nonfunctioning (6).

Use in Selecting Fascicles for Nerve Biopsy

Rarely, given a focal or multifocal process, a nerve biopsy will be required of a proximal or nontraditional nerve (i.e., not the sural or superficial peroneal). Targets include nerve root, brachial plexus, or fascicles of proximal or distal nerves. These biopsies are useful, leading to diagnoses such as lymphoma, focal inflammatory neuropathy, or sarcoidosis, which all have varying treatments and prognoses. Clinical examination, preoperative neurophysiologic testing, and imaging studies with three-tesla magnetic resonance imaging (MRI) can all localize pathology to certain nerves or parts of nerves (i.e., the peroneal division of the sciatic nerve). During the procedure, however, when the surgeon is faced with actually removing sections of these nerves, it is crucial to remove that part of the nerve with the highest chance of a pathologic diagnosis and the lowest chance of causing a new postoperative deficit. Visual assessment made by the surgeon upon exposure of the nerve at the time of biopsy is helpful. Neurophysiologic testing can further add to this important assessment.

Just prior to biopsy, direct stimulation is applied to the individual fascicles in question. An assessment is made by the presence or absence of a downstream twitch in muscles innervated by the nerve, or by recording from muscle (with surface or needle electrodes) or nerve (as a NAP) as described earlier. This allows for the identification of functioning and nonfunctioning fascicles. In this manner, a biopsy can be performed with the highest diagnostic yield and lowest risk.

TECHNICAL CONSIDERATIONS

Preparation

In preparation for peripheral nerve NIOM, it is important to realize that the neural structures that will be monitored are actually generally already damaged. This damage can usually be estimated by preoperative examination and neurophysiologic studies. If there has been complete damage to the nerve, there is no risk of further damage to that nerve, although surrounding nerves and portions of nerves that are not completely damaged are at risk. This is especially important for surgery on tumors of peripheral nerve. The modalities that are monitored are NAPs and CMAPs.

There are no specific contraindications for peripheral nerve monitoring given the very low stimulus intensities used with direct nerve stimulation. If the patient has abnormal nerves—for example, underlying peripheral neuropathy—this may affect the stimulus threshold. As the presence or absence of the response (not the latency, amplitude, or conduction velocity) is the main parameter being assessed, usually this is not significantly altered in a generalized neuropathic process. The interpretation of NIOM data when using higher stimulus intensities, though, introduces more troubles with stimulus artifact and volume conduction.

The equipment includes an eight-channel EMG machine with bipolar stimulating and recording electrodes. A square metal ground is used separate from the electrocautery ground. Needle electrodes or tin-disk, reusable surface electrodes are used for recording CMAPs. Occasionally, a fine wire intramuscular electrode is used for deeper muscles. Needle electrodes come sterile and are opened at the time of use. The stimulators are gas-sterilized and opened in sterile field. Preoperative NCS and EMG studies are done to determine the damage to individual peripheral nerves and the type of surgical approach.

Before surgery, the patient is told that he or she will have electrical monitoring of the nerves and muscles during the surgical procedure. As the intensities of stimulus are very low, there is no risk of permanent damage or postoperative complication related to the NIOM. There may be mild bruising if needle electrodes are used for recording, but this is very minimal. If the patient is on anticoagulation, usually this is stopped for the surgical procedure.

Procedure

Prior to monitoring, the NIOM team reviews the patient's history and examination as well as the preoperative electrophysiologic studies. They also confer with the surgical team to determine a consensus on the type of monitoring to be done and the type of information to be obtained. Recording electrodes are held in place on the nerve or a needle electrode is used in the subcutaneous tissue for recording CMAPs. Taping or pasting of electrodes onto the skin is usually not necessary. An electrode cream is used for the metal ground. Inhalation anesthesia does not affect peripheral nerve monitoring. Neuromuscular blockade is avoided except at times when one is attempting to distinguish a NAP from volume-conducted motor responses. For baseline studies, a normal portion of nerve is tested if possible. A small bipolar electrode is used for stimulating and a larger hooked bipolar electrode for recording (Figure 12.1).

After surgical exposure, NAP studies are attempted across the lesion to assess for continuity. One complication that can occur is volume conduction from nearby activated muscles, which can be misinterpreted as a NAPs or CMAPs. Careful attention to technical detail as well as using neuromuscular blockade can be helpful. As the surgeons are holding the stimulating electrodes, they should be alerted when stimulation begins. Visual confirmation of correct electrode placement and nerve-to-electrode contact is important. The red electrodes are designated "active" (active recording electrode and cathode for nerve stimulation), so the instructions are "red to red" for NAP studies. The nerves often need to be held up out of a wet surgical field. Constant communication with the surgical and anesthesia team is vital prior to and during NNIOM.

Postprocedure

Postsurgical monitoring is not necessary in most cases. All needle electrodes are removed and counted. The skin is assessed at the site of the needle puncture, and if there is any excessive bruising, the operating room nurse or surgical team is alerted and the patient is seen in follow-up postoperatively by the technologist until any complication, such as bruising, resolves. At the end of the procedure, the final NIOM results are discussed with the surgical team to ensure acquisition of proper information to assist with surgical decision making. A final report is written by the neurophysiologist in charge of the NIOM and entered into the patient's records. The highlights of the NIOM are also typically included in the surgeon's operative note. The reusable surface electrodes are cleaned with alcohol, the needle electrodes are discarded, and the stimulators are gas-sterilized. Updates of the software for the monitoring system are performed periodically.

SUMMARY

Performing high-quality intraoperative monitoring of peripheral nerves is a challenging endeavor. With the proper equipment, training, and techniques, vital neurophysiologic information can be obtained quickly, interpreted, and input given to the surgical team. Specifically, this includes identification of peripheral nerves, determination of continuity of peripheral axons, and localization of peripheral nerve lesions. This information can then be utilized to maximize the effectiveness and safety of surgical intervention.

REFERENCES

1. Kline DG, Hackett ER, May PR. Evaluation of nerve injuries by evoked potentials and electromyography. *J Neurosurg* 1969;31:128–136.

2. Kline DG, Happel LT. A quarter century's experience with intraoperative nerve action potential recording. *Can J Neurol Sci* 1993; 20:3–10.
3. Terzis JK, Dykes RW, Hakstian RW. Neurophysiologic recordings in peripheral nerve surgery: a review. *J Hand Surg* 1976;1:52–66.
4. Brown WF, Veitch J. AAEM minimonograph #42: intraoperative monitoring of peripheral and cranial nerves. *Muscle Nerve* 1994;17: 371–377.
5. Slimp JC. Intraoperative monitoring of nerve repairs. *Hand Clin* 2000;16:25–36.
6. Spinner RJ, Kline DG. Surgery for peripheral nerve and brachial plexus injuries or other nerve lesions. *Muscle Nerve* 2000;23:680–695.
7. Harper CM. Preoperative and intraoperative electrophysiologic assessment of brachial plexus injuries. *Hand Clin* 2005;21:39–46.
8. Kline DG, Hudson AR, Zager E. Selection and preoperative work-up for peripheral nerve surgery. *Clin Neurosurg* 1992;39:8–35.
9. Oberle J, Antoniadis G, Rath SA, Richter HP. Value of nerve action potentials in the surgical management of traumatic nerve lesions. *Neurosurgery* 1997;41:1337–1344.
10. Campbell WW. The value of inching techniques in the diagnosis of focal nerve lesions. *Muscle Nerve* 1998;21:1554–1556.
11. Tiel RL, Happel LT, Kline DG. Nerve action potential recording method and equipment. *Neurosurgery* 1996;39:103–109.
12. Veale JL, Mark FR, Rees S. Differential sensitivity of motor and sensory fibres in human ulnar nerve. *J Neurol Neurosurg Psychiatry* 1973;36:75–86.
13. Nelson KR. Use of peripheral nerve action potentials for intraoperative monitoring. *Neurol Clin* 1988;6:917–933.
14. Daube JR. Assessing the motor unit with needle electromyography. In: Daube J, ed. *Clinical Neurophysiology*. Philadelphia: Davis, 1996:271.
15. Gunnarsson T, Krassioukov AV, Sarjeant R, Fehlings MG. Real-time continuous intraoperative electromyographic and somatosensory evoked potential recordings in spinal surgery: Correlation of clinical and electrophysiologic findings in a prospective, consecutive series of 213 cases. *Spine* 2004;29:677–684.
16. Holland NR. Intraoperative electromyography. *J Clin Neurophysiol* 2002;19:444–453.
17. Harper CM. Peripheral nervous system monitoring. In: Daube J, ed. *Clinical Neurophysiology*. Philadelphia: Davis, 1996: 465–466.
18. Kim DH, Han K, Tiel RL, et al. Surgical outcomes of 654 ulnar nerve lesions. *J Neurosurg* 2003;98:993–1004.
19. Campbell WW, Pridgeon RM, Sahni SK. Entrapment neuropathy of the ulnar nerve at its point of exit from the flexor carpi ulnaris muscle. *Muscle Nerve* 1988;11: 467–470.
20. Campbell WW, Pridgeon RM, Sahni SK. Short segment incremental studies in the evaluation of ulnar neuropathy at the elbow. *Muscle Nerve* 1992;15:1050–1054.
21. Brown WF, Veitch J. AAEM minimonograph #42: intraoperative monitoring of peripheral and cranial nerves. *Muscle Nerve* 1994;17: 371–377.
22. Campbell WW. The value of inching techniques in the diagnosis of focal nerve lesions. Inching is a useful technique. *Muscle Nerve* 1998;21:1554–1556.
23. Campbell WW. AAEE case report #18: ulnar neuropathy in the distal forearm. *Muscle Nerve* 1989;12:347–352.
24. American Association of Electrodiagnostic Medicine, American Academy of Neurology, American Academy of Physical Medicine and Rehabilitation. Practice parameter for electrodiagnostic studies in carpal tunnel syndrome: summary statement. *Muscle Nerve* 2002;25: 918–922.
25. Eversmann WW, Ritsick JA. Intraoperative changes in motor nerve conduction latency in carpal tunnel syndrome. *J Hand Surg Am* 1978;3:77–81.
26. Yates SK, Hurst LN, Brown WF. Physiological observations in the median nerve during carpal tunnel surgery. *Ann Neurol* 1981;10: 227–229.
27. Luchetti R, Schoenhuber R, Alfarano M, et al. Carpal tunnel syndrome: correlations between pressure measurement and intraoperative neurophysiologic nerve study. *Muscle Nerve* 1990;13:1164–1168.
28. Kim DH, Murovic JA, Tiel RL, Kline DG. Management and outcomes in 318 operative common peroneal nerve lesions at the Louisiana State University Health Sciences Center. *J Neurosurg* 2004;54:1421–1429.

29. Kim DH, Murovic JA, Tiel RL, et al. A series of 397 peripheral neural sheath tumors: 30-year experience at Louisiana State University Health Sciences Center. *J Neurosurg* 2005;102:246–255.

30. Kim DH, Murovic JA, Tiel RL, et al. A series of 146 peripheral non-neural sheath nerve tumors: 30-year experience at Louisiana State University Health Sciences Center. *J Neurosurg* 2005;102:256–266.

13 Cerebellopontine Angle Surgery: Microvascular Decompression

Cormac A. O' Donovan
Scott Kuhn

Microvascular decompression (MVD) surgery is frequently performed for cranial neuralgias that are refractory to medical treatment. These include trigeminal neuralgia (TN), hemifacial spasm (HFS), and glossopharyngeal neuralgia (GPN). The basis for the surgery is that arterial compression of the nerves at the root entry/exit zone gives rise to the symptoms of pain and hyperactivity of muscles seen in these conditions. Hearing loss due to injury of the vestibulocochlear nerve was a common complication of these procedures; but with advances in neurophysiologic intraoperative monitoring (NIOM), this complication has been greatly reduced. In some types of MVD surgery, NIOM can assist in determining when adequate decompression of the nerve has been achieved.

In this chapter a brief discussion of the basic anatomy, pathology, clinical features and surgical techniques of MVD surgery is presented. This is followed by a detailed review of NIOM modalities used to reduce the morbidity of these surgeries. NIOM modalities used in other types of brainstem pathology, such as tumors, are discussed elsewhere.

CLINICAL SYNDROMES

Trigeminal Neuralgia

Anatomy and Pathology

The trigeminal nucleus consists of a collection of nuclei centered in the pons but extending from the midbrain to the medulla. Sensory fibers from the face enter the trigeminal ganglion and then enter the brainstem before going to the mesencephalic, main sensory, or spinal nucleus of the trigeminal nerve. Three types of sensory fibers are contained within the trigeminal nerve. Large A beta fibers subserve discriminative touch. These large-diameter fibers enter the main sensory nucleus before joining the medial lemniscus to ascend and enter the thalamus. Small A delta and C fibers subserve pain and temperature. These fibers travel caudally before entering the subnucleus caudalis of the spinal nucleus before entering the spinothalamic tract which ascends to enter the thalamus. A alpha fibers serve as stretch and tendon receptors and synapse directly in the mesencephalic nucleus which serves as a dorsal root ganglion for these fibers. They then synapse on the motor nucleus of trigeminal nerve, which innervates the muscles of mastication.

In patients with TN, the lateral mesencephalic segment of the superior cerebellar artery (SCA) lies medial to the trigeminal nerve and compresses it from the rostromedial direction. The superior petrosal vein (SPV) may be an additional cause of compression in approximately 50% of cases and may be the sole cause in a minority. Occasionally ectatic vertebral or basilar arteries are the responsible vessels in older patients. This may be in part related to atherosclerosis of the arteries, causing tortuosity and propensity to compress the trigeminal nerve.

Clinical Features

TN usually occurs after the age of 50 years with severe unilateral lancinating facial pain that occurs episodically and frequently clusters. The pain is most commonly described as stabbing and electric shock–like, but in atypical cases it can be associated with constant, dull, burning, aching pain. Stimuli such as touching the face, chewing, other facial motions, and cold breezes can induce an attack of TN. The patient is usually pain-free between attacks and may avoid triggers such as talking or eating in fear of inducing an attack. The actual attacks may last only a few seconds. Bilateral cases are rare; however, at times TN may occur as part of a syndrome of multiple cranial neuropathies.

The majority of cases of TN are idiopathic, with a secondary cause, such as multiple sclerosis, being found in about 15%. Magnetic resonance imaging (MRI) sequences with 3D volume acquisition and 0.8-mm thin cuts can detect vascular loops causing trigeminal nerve compression in up to 80% of cases. Initial treatment is usually with antiepileptic drugs (AEDs), tricyclic antidepressants, and baclofen, but randomized controlled trials demonstrating definite efficacy of these medications are lacking.

Hemifacial Spasm

Anatomy and Pathology

The facial nerve has sensory, motor, and autonomic components and is susceptible to vascular compression owing to its long intracranial course. The motor fibers arise in the pons and travel around the abducens nucleus to emerge from the caudal pons. The facial nerve travels with the vestibulocochlear nerve in the internal auditory canal before passing into the facial canal and uniting with the geniculate ganglion. It supplies innervation to the stapedius, chorda tympani, and posterior belly of digastric muscles before entering the stylomastoid foramen and passing into the parotid gland. In the parotid gland it divides into five branches, temporal, zygomatic, buccal, mandibular, and cervical, innervating muscles of facial expression. The temporal nerve is an important branch that innervates the mentalis muscle. This branch is often stimulated in HFS MVD surgeries, as discussed later.

In patients with HFS, electrical stimulation of one branch of the facial nerve causes spasms of muscles supplied by other branches. This has been called the anomalous or lateral response. This phenomenon is due to abnormal activity at the facial nerve root entry zone secondary to vascular compression, which induces hyperexcitability of the facial nerve nucleus. This anomalous response can be confirmed by electromyography (EMG).

HFS is caused by a blood vessel, usually a branch of the posterior inferior cerebellar artery (PICA), pulsating against the facial nerve root as it leaves the brainstem. Rarely HFS can be caused by a vein causing compression in the same location. This irritation causes abnormal signals to travel back to the facial nerve nucleus, which becomes hyperactive, producing the anomalous response and HFS.

Clinical Features

HFS is defined as unintended twitching of one side of the face. It typically begins in the upper face or lower eyelid and spreads over years to involve other areas of the face. Involvement of eye and mouth musculature interferes with vision, talking, eating, and playing wind instruments. On occasion branches to middle ear muscles may be involved, causing clicking, and a loud noise may trigger the spasm. It usually presents in middle age and both sexes are equally affected, as are all races. The maximum extent of symptoms usually occurs within 2 years, and they rarely improve spontaneously. HFS very infrequently involves other cranial nerves ipsilaterally or bilaterally. Sensation is normal over the face. Precipitants for attacks include fatigue, anxiety, and reading.

The abnormal vascular loop causing compression of the facial nerve is difficult to visualize on MRI, but MRI is recommended to rule out the rare possibility of HFS being caused by a tumor. Needle EMG shows irregular, brief, high-frequency bursts (150 to 400 Hz) of motor unit potentials, which are synchronized. Oral medications, including benzodiazepines and AEDs, are generally ineffective. Botulinum toxin has been used with some success. If medications do not control symptoms, MVD surgery is considered.

Glossopharyngeal Neuralgia

Anatomy and Pathology

The glossopharyngeal nerve arises from many different nuclear complexes in the medulla. These include the tractus solitarius, nucleus ambiguus, and inferior salivatory nucleus. Fibers leave the medulla between the inferior olive and cerebellar peduncle and exit the skull through the jugular foramen. The glossopharyngeal nerve is in close proximity to the vagus and accessory nerves in the jugular foramen and then lies between internal jugular vein and internal carotid artery. It travels beneath the styloid process and then lies along the lateral wall of the pharynx near the inferior border of the stylopharyngeus muscle. The principal function of the glossopharyngeal nerve is sensory, and it forms the afferent arm of the gag reflex.

Clinical Features

Glossopharyngeal neuralgia (GPN) is characterized by paroxysmal attacks of pain in the posterior pharynx, tonsils, back of tongue, and middle ear. The pain attacks are brief and occur spontaneously or can be precipitated by movement such as chewing, swallowing, talking or sneezing. Syncope may occur infrequently due to vagus nerve involvement. Whereas GPN can be due to lesions such as a cerebellopontine angle (CPA) tumor, the majority are idiopathic. The occurrence rates are rare with a frequency one hundred times less than TN. GPN usually occurs in men after the age of 40 years. MRI often does not localize the abnormal blood vessel causing compression of the glossopharyngeal nerve. Oral medications are generally ineffective; however, some patients respond to carbamazepine; atropine may be used if syncope coexists. Applying anesthetic solution to affected area of mouth and throat provides temporary relief and is often used as a diagnostic test for the disorder. When medications are ineffective in controlling the pain, MVD is considered.

SURGICAL TECHNIQUE

Surgical techniques for MVD of the different cranial neuralgias involve variations on the lateral suboccipital approach to the CPA. The CPA can be divided into superior, middle, and inferior regions in considering the goals for each approach. Each approach is considered on its merits for providing access to and visualizing the various foramina, cranial nerves, arteries, and veins. Three of the commonest approaches are (a) the infratentorial lateral supracerebellar approach (ILSA), which is used for decompression of the trigeminal nerve; (b) the lateral suboccipital infrafloccular approach (LSIA), which is used for access to the facial nerve; and (c) the transcondylar fossa approach (TFA), which is used for access to the glossopharyngeal nerve. The skin incisions for the ILSA and LSIA are placed medial to the hairline, and may extend from just above the asterion (a surface landmark at the level of the upper third of the pinna) down to the level of the digastric groove. The incision for TFA is more extensive in the shape of a horseshoe.

Surgery for Trigeminal Neuralgia

The ILSA is used for trigeminal neuralgia decompression. It allows the nerve to be approached from the tentorial surface, which reduces the likelihood that a retractor will be placed injuriously on the facial and vestibulocochlear complex. During dissection, excessive use of electrocautery near the vestibulocochlear nerve can result in thermal injury to that nerve, which may cause postoperative hearing loss. The SCA is usually the source of compression of the trigeminal nerve and can be visualized easily in its medial and anterior relationship to the root entry zone of the nerve into the brainstem. Less commonly, the anterior inferior cerebellar artery (AICA) is the source of the compression with a redundant loop of artery lying in the same anatomic relationship to the root entry zone.

After draining cerebrospinal fluid (CSF) along the trajectory of the approach or from the ambient cistern, initial caudal and medial retraction of the cerebellar hemisphere usually reveals the trigeminal nerve lying deep to the superior petrosal venous complex. This complex is usually coagulated and sectioned to facilitate additional cerebellar retraction. Overly vigorous retraction can result in tension on the vestibulocochlear nerve, leading to hearing loss. The trigeminal nerve is usually found to be compressed by the SCA at the point where it is bifurcates into rostral and caudal trunks. Venous compression alone, or in combination with arterial compression, of the trigeminal nerve can be seen and may predispose to recurrence of the facial pain as tiny veins not seen at operation may enlarge postoperatively.

Once the nerve and vessel are identified, attention is directed at mobilizing the blood vessel away from the root entry zone of the nerve. This usually requires releasing arachnoid bands with sharp dissection. The artery is frequently quite muscular and may resist initial attempts to displace it from the position it has occupied for decades. Once the vessel is mobilized, kinking or vasospasm of branches to the vestibulocochlear nerve may produce ischemia and postoperative hearing loss. The vasospasm can be reversed by positioning the vessel in a different location or with papaverine soaked gel foam. A Teflon pad is placed in such a way as to buffer the nerve from continued pulsations and to prevent the nerve from returning to its original, offending location. The retractor is then removed, and the dura mater and the suboccipital musculature are closed.

Complications directly related to nerve injury include ipsilateral hearing loss most commonly, followed by facial paresis, trochlear nerve palsy, and facial numbness. Excessive manipulation of the brainstem can cause a brainstem infarct, cerebellar hematoma, and supratentorial hematoma.

Surgery for Hemifacial Spasm

The LSIA is typically used for MVD of the facial nerve. The decompression involves freeing the nerve from a loop of the PICA in the majority of patients; the AICA and vertebrobasilar artery can also be the offending blood vessels in some patients. The craniotomy is similar in size to that performed for patients with TN, although the epicenter is lower at the mid portion of the sigmoid sinus to allow better visualization of the facial and vestibulocochlear nerve complexes. This lower orientation of the approach facilitates placement of the retractor on the inferolateral surface of the cerebellum, avoiding possibly injurious placement on or near the facial and vestibulocochlear nerves. Identifying lower cranial nerves before they enter their respective foramina and opening the arachnoid mater to identify the choroid plexus are key aspects of the approach. A dural incision is made from the upper border of the sigmoid sinus to the inferior margin. A Teflon sponge is placed between the brainstem and the offending vessel, with care not to compress the facial or vestibulocochlear nerve more than necessary to achieve a durable result.

Surgery for Glossopharyngeal Neuralgia

MVD surgery of the glossopharyngeal nerve can be an alternative or sequel to rhizotomy or sectioning of its branches. Different approaches are used and include the TFA. Retraction of the cerebellum superiorly and medially allows the surgeon to locate the jugular foramen and expose the glossopharyngeal and vagus nerves. Care is taken to avoid the occurrence of hypotension and tachycardia through stimulation of the glossopharyngeal and vagus nerves. Much like MVD surgery for TN, in these surgeries the vestibulocochlear nerve is at risk from excessive traction when the cerebellum is being retracted, thermal injury from electrocoagulation, and ischemia due to interruption of vascular supply to the nerve.

MONITORING TECHNIQUES

Among the most frequent complications of MVD surgery for cranial neuralgias is ipsilateral hearing loss from injury to the vestibulocochlear nerve. This injury may be due to traction, ischemia, or electrocoagulation, as described above. Brainstem auditory evoked potentials (BAEPs) have been used to prevent this complication. Excessive manipulation of the brainstem can cause injury to the pons or midbrain. Since BAEP monitoring will be unable to detect injury to the upper brainstem, median nerve somatosensory evoked potentials (SEPs) have occasionally been used to monitor for this rare complication. Facial nerve electromyography (EMG) has been used to confirm adequacy of decompression (explained below). Sensory and motor trigeminal nerve monitoring is not usually performed during MVD surgery, rather can be of utility in rhizotomy and tumor surgery of involving the brainstem.

Details of BAEP, median nerve SEP, and facial nerve EMG monitoring have been discussed elsewhere in this book, but specifics related to MVD surgery are presented here. Because of similarities in surgical approaches and potential complications, NIOM for all three types of cranial neuralgias are discussed together.

Brainstem Auditory Evoked Potentials

BAEP monitoring is the most commonly used NIOM modality for MVD surgeries. It provides early warning of injury to the vestibulocochlear nerve, which can lead to postoperative hearing loss. This allows the surgeon to modify the procedure prior to permanent damage. It is important to realize that BAEPs are not an absolute measure of hearing. Despite complete loss of BAEPs, hearing may still be preserved, and when BAEPs are present, hearing may occasionally still be impaired. Despite these limitations, BAEP are among the most sensitive tests for hearing assessment in an anesthetized patient.

Technique

Details of the methodology of BAEP acquisition have been discussed previously in this book. Issues particularly relevant to MVD surgery are discussed here. Recording electrodes, either electroencephalographic (EEG) cup or subdermal needle, are placed at Cz and bilateral mastoid processes or medial surface of the earlobes. Most often a Cz-Ai and Cz-Ac montage is used, with positivity displayed upward (Figure 13.1). Often BAEP responses from both ears are obtained.

In the outpatient laboratory, BAEPs are obtained with broadband clicks delivered through earphones. These are large and cover most of the pinna. Earphones are impractical for use in the operating room as they invade the surgical field and cannot be secured. Consequently, in the operating room, the

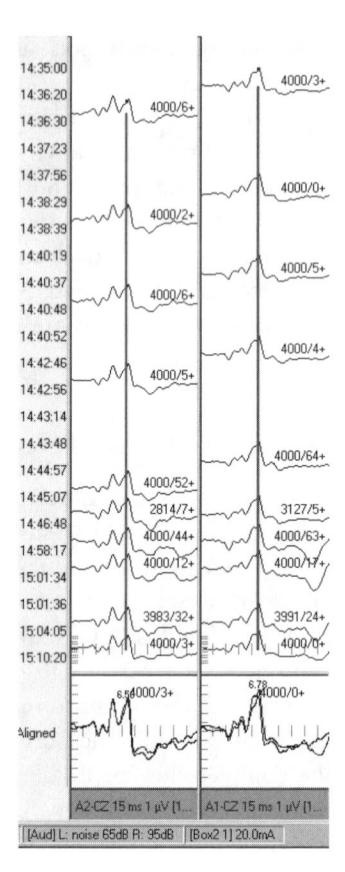

FIGURE 13.1 BAEP waveforms obtained with stimulation of the right ear during MVD surgery for TN. Notice that there is no significant change in wave V latency. No alerts were raised for the surgeon during this procedure. [Reproduced with permission from reference (1).]

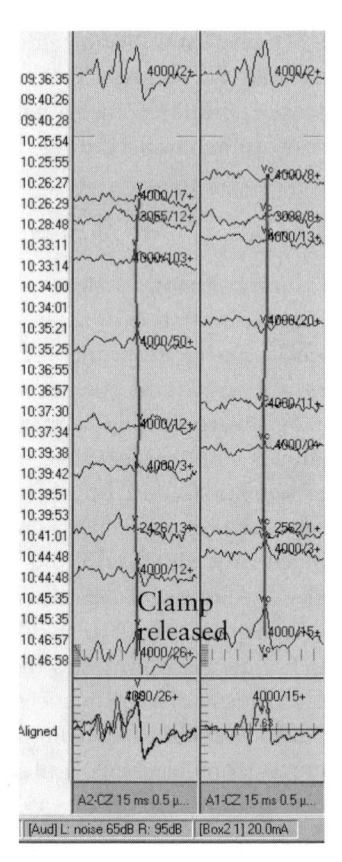

FIGURE 13.2 BAEP waveforms obtained with stimulation of the right ear during MVD surgery for TN. Robust responses are obtained at baseline prior to draping the patient. After draping and positioning, there is loss of the BAEPs. When clamps retracting the pinna are released, the BAEPs return. The transducer tubing was kinked with the clamps. [Reproduced with permission from Husain (1).]

BAEP stimulus is delivered through transducers that connect to plastic tubing with a sponge collar at the end. The sponge collar is secured in the external auditory canal. The plastic tubing adds about 1 ms to the absolute latencies of the waveforms. This is irrelevant in NIOM, as the patient serves as his or her own control, and it is the change from baseline that is most important. When the patient is being draped for surgery, the pinna is often clamped away from the surgical field. This may cause kinking of the plastic tubing, resulting in loss of BAEP waveforms (1). Releasing and repositioning the clamps corrects this problem (Figure 13.2).

It is important to optimize the stimulation characteristics of the broadband clicks to minimize the amount of time it takes to obtain a reproducible average. The recommended stimulation rate is about 30 per second. In the outpatient laboratory, slower stimulation rates are often used, as faster rates result in prolongation of the interpeak latencies (IPL). Again, this is irrelevant in NIOM, as the patient serves as his or her own control. Rates of about 50 per second do not result in quicker acquisition of a reproducible response, as at this rate the amplitude of the waveforms is smaller. Thus more repetitions are needed before a reproducible response is seen. Alternating clicks are used as the intensity of stimulation is high, resulting in a significant stimulation artifact. Because the polarity of the clicks alternates between condensation and rarefaction, the stimulus artifact is minimized.

Effects of Anesthetics

BAEPs have the advantage of being relatively insensitive to anesthetics. Regardless of the type of inhalation or intravenous anesthetic agent used, there is little effect on BAEP waveforms. These agents can cause up to a 0.1- to 0.2-ms prolongation of absolute latency, but it occurs at the start of the case and does not confound interpretation. Temperature and blood pressure have a more significant effect. Wave V latency increases by 0.2 ms per degree (centigrade) drop in temperature (2). Similarly, if anesthetics result in a drop in blood pressure, wave V amplitude drops and latency increases. Neuromuscular blocking agents do not have a significant impact on BAEPs.

Interpretation

Wave V of the BAEP is followed closely in MVD surgeries. Somewhat empirically, a latency prolongation of 1 ms or an amplitude decrement of at least 50% has historically been considered significant and indicative of traction or heat related injury to the vestibu-

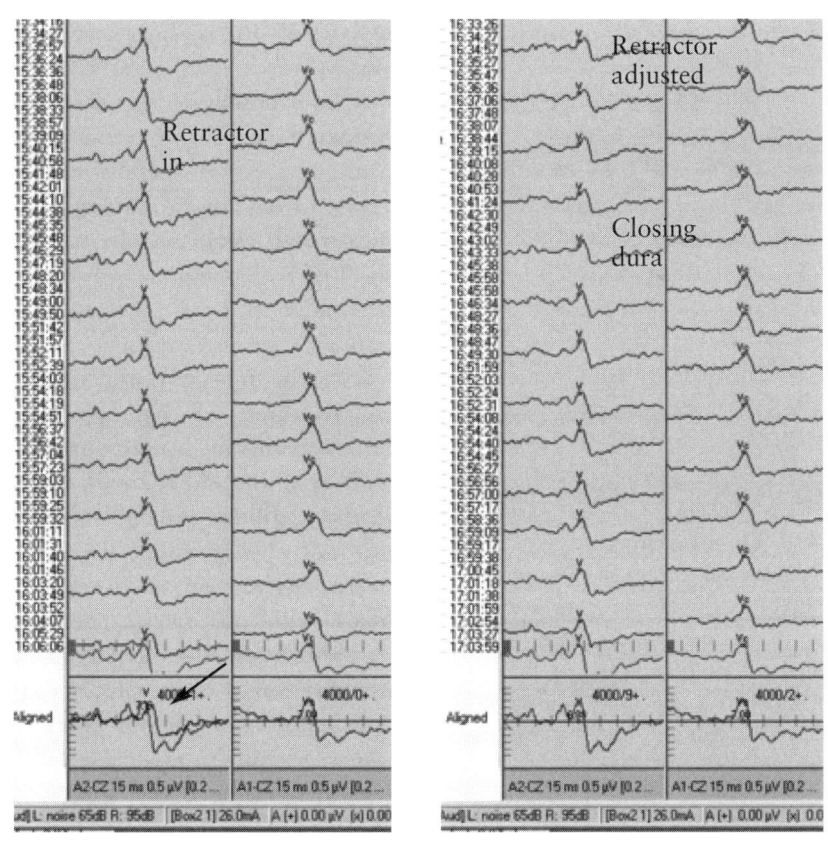

FIGURE 13.3 BAEP waveforms obtained with stimulation of the right ear during MVD surgery for TN. There is a 0.6-ms prolongation of wave V latency and greater than 50% drop in amplitude (arrow). Because of the amplitude drop, an alert is raised and the surgeon adjusts the retractor. Wave V gradually returns to baseline. [Reproduced with permission from Husain (1).]

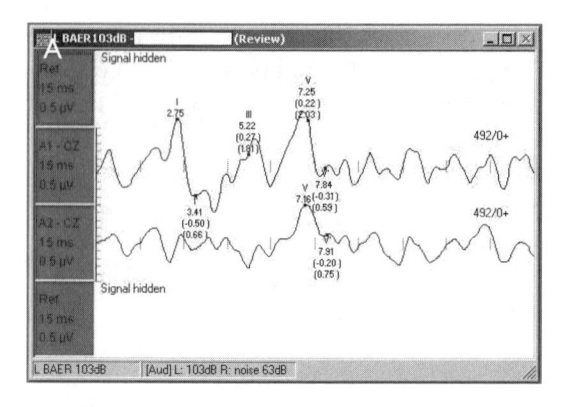

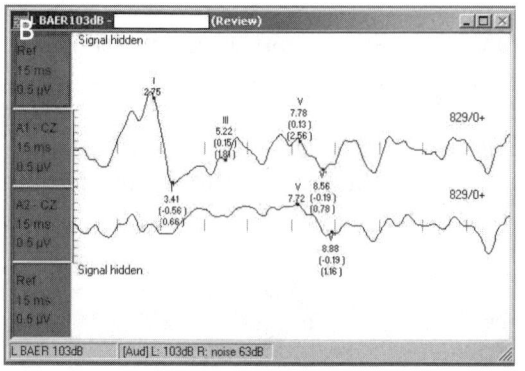

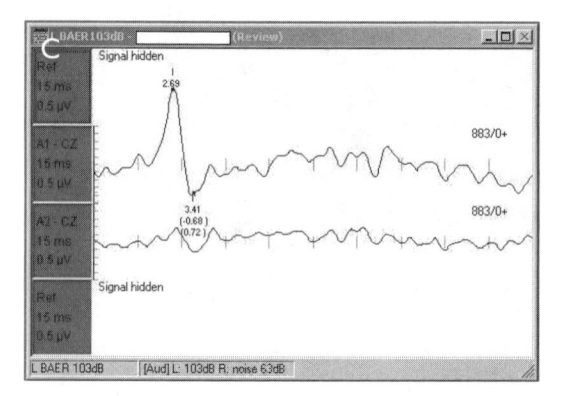

FIGURE 13.4 BAEP waveforms obtained with stimulation of the left ear during MVD surgery for TN. A robust BAEP is seen at the start of the surgery (A). After the retractor is in place, there is gradual loss of wave V amplitude and prolongation of latency (B). Eventually the wave V disappears completely (C). This patient had postoperative hearing loss.

locochlear nerve. When this degree of change is noted, a warning is typically given to the surgeon (Figure 13.3). Recently it was suggested that, in patients undergoing MVD surgery, it is only when there is a complete loss of wave V that there is a higher chance of hearing loss (3) (Figure 13.4A, B, and C). This is in distinction to BAEP changes observed during CPA tumor surgery. In the latter scenario, much smaller latency changes have been found to be associated with hearing loss.

The wave I–V IPL has also been used as a marker for vestibulocochlear nerve injury. A prolongation of 1 ms is considered significant. The wave I–V IPL is not affected by changes in absolute latency of the wave I, as may occur with temperature or anesthetic changes. This may theoretically make this a more sensitive marker for vestibulocochlear nerve injury; however, in practice these changes are usually not clinically significant.

A significant change in wave V latency or wave I–V IPL is suggestive of injury to the vestibulocochlear nerve. This injury is often due to traction if the cerebellum is being retracted. In this situation, the surgeon will often remove the retractor and pause the surgery for a few minutes until the BAEPs improve. If electrocautery is being used when the BAEP change is noted, the injury may be thermally induced. The surgeon may again pause the surgery and suspend use of the electrocautery. It is important to use a bipolar electrocautery in these procedures, as that limits spread of heat to surrounding tissues. Both traction and thermally mediated injury to the vestibulocochlear nerve is manifest by gradually increasing wave-V latency or decreasing amplitude. If wave V is suddenly lost (within one or two averages), the injury is most likely due to ischemia, suggesting interruption of blood supply to the vestibulocochlear nerve. Whereas traction and thermal injury are often reversible, ischemic injury typically is permanent. Some patients appear to be more sensitive to changes in BAEP. Patients with preexisting brainstem lesions, such as multiple sclerosis plaques, may loose BAEPs much more quickly yet have no hearing loss postoperatively.

Before warning the surgeon of a significant change in BAEP, the NIOM team must ensure that the change is not due to artifact or nonsurgical factors. If the BAEP responses are poorly reproducible, a change in wave-V latency or amplitude may occur with successive averages. The surgeon should be informed of the lack of reliability of the data. Loss of the wave I along with loss of the wave V often implies failure of the stimulating system. This may occur if fluid seeps into the external auditory canal; because of this, the technologist should ensure that an adequate seal is obtained around the ear insert. Also, as noted above, kinking of the stimulator tubing when the pinna is clamped forward may result in the loss of BAEPs. Dislodging or malfunction of the transducer can produce similar changes (Figure 13.5). Blood pressure and anesthesia rarely cause significant changes. All these changes should be recognized as not due to surgery and the surgeon informed accordingly.

Although loss of wave I is often due to technical factors, it rarely can occur due to ischemia of the cochlea. During surgery, excessive manipulation of the AICA or labyrinthine artery can cause vasospasm and ischemia of the cochlea, leading to loss of wave I. Injury to these vessels would have the same outcome. This results in postoperative hearing loss.

A wave-V latency shift of 1 ms and amplitude reduction of 50% are accepted as warning criteria for alerting the surgeon. Many neurophysiologists will alert the surgeon to smaller shifts in latency and decrements in amplitude. This allows the surgeon to know which surgical manipulations are causing the changes. When a significant change is noted, the surgeon will have a better understanding of which process must be halted or undone.

Rarely cases are described in which BAEP monitoring shows no significant change, yet the patient has a postoperative deficit. One such case involved a patient undergoing MVD surgery for TN. Bleeding was encountered during the surgery and there was transient loss of wave V. However, by the end of surgery, the BAEPs were close to baseline values. The patient has a postoperative hemiplegia due to a midbrain stroke (2). It should be remembered that BAEPs assess auditory pathways only up to the rostral pons; consequently lesions occurring higher in the neuroaxis will not be detected. Because of this some laboratories routinely perform median nerve SEP in patients undergoing MVD surgeries.

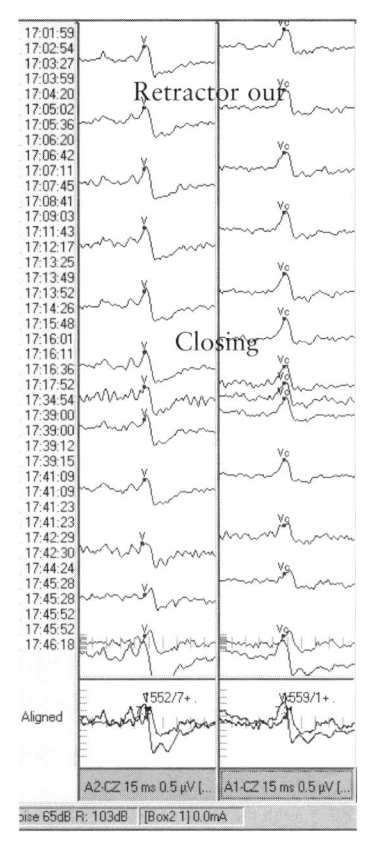

FIGURE 13.5 BAEP waveforms obtained with stimulation of the right ear during MVD surgery for TN. The retractor is removed near the top of the data stack shown. Near the end of the surgery (bottom of the data stack), there is gradual loss of amplitude and prolongation of latency of wave V. Notice also that wave I is no longer clearly seen. In this case the stimulator had been dislodged toward the end of surgery, preventing effective stimulation. [Reproduced with permission from Husain (1).]

Vestibulocochlear Nerve Action Potential

Vestibulocochlear nerve action potentials (NAPs) have been used to monitor auditory function intraoperatively and might offer some advantages over BAEPs (4). Practical experience with this shows that inadvertent changes in electrode position and need for surgical placement of electrodes that interferes with the surgery limits their implementation on a more widespread basis.

Technique

Vestibulocochlear NAPs, as their name implies, are recorded directly over the proximal part of the vestibulocochlear nerve. A cotton wick electrode attached to a malleable wire is placed on the nerve by the surgeon proximal to the site at which traction injury typically occurs. The weight of the electrode may keep it in place; alternatively, it can be sutured. The cotton wick electrode is a monopolar electrode with the reference usually at a distance. Specially made bipolar electrodes have also been used to record NAPs.

The stimulation setup for NAPs is the same as that for BAEPs. The rate of stimulation can be slower, however, since the NAP is a high-amplitude triphasic response. At times the response is evident even without averaging. Thus even with a stimulation rate of 1 per second, very rapid feedback can be given to the surgeon about the integrity of the nerve. However, often the NAPs will be obtained in conjunction with the BAEPs, in which case the high stimulation rates will be used. Because these responses are of high amplitude, a display sensitivity of 1 to 10 µV per division can be used. Filter settings are the same as for other NAPs.

Effects of Anesthetics

Like BAEPs and other NAPs, these responses are little affected by anesthetics. Inhalation and intravenous anesthetics have little effect on vestibulocochlear NAPs. Similarly, neuromuscular blocking agents do not alter these responses. As with other NAPs, a drop of temperature can increase the amplitude of these responses. This may occur frequently, as exposure of the nerve during MVD surgery results in a drop in local temperature. Only extremes of blood pressure change affect the vestibulocochlear NAPs.

Interpretation

The vestibulocochlear NAPs obtained with a monopolar electrode is a triphasic response. The initial wave is a positive and represents the nerve depolarization volley approaching the electrode. The second, large peak is negative and represents the depolarization of the nerve under the electrode. The final wave is positive and represents the depolarization volley moving away from the electrode. Injury to the nerve is manifest by loss of the large negative and second positive waveform. Persistence of the initial positive component implies that the volley comes toward the electrode but is interrupted by a lesion prior to reaching it.

Traction and thermal damage to the vestibulocochlear nerve produces a prolongation of latency and drop in amplitude of the NAP. Exactly how much of a decrement in amplitude or prolongation in latency is significant has not been established; most authors raise an alert when at least 50% of the amplitude is lost. Prior to alerting the surgeon of the loss of the NAPs, nonsurgical causes must be excluded. Many of the same reasons for stimulation failure listed above for BAEPs apply to NAPs as well. A unique reason for changes in NAP is movement of the cotton wick recording electrode. If the electrode moves off the nerve during surgery, the amplitude of the NAPs that it records will change dramatically. Consequently, whenever a significant change in NAPs is seen, the surgical team must be asked to confirm that the recording electrode is still in position.

The vestibulocochlear NAP has enabled surgeons to better understand which parts of the surgery are most likely to cause damage to the vestibulocochlear nerve. Electrocautery in the vicinity of the nerve results in loss of NAP amplitude. Consequently surgeons have greatly limited use of electrocautery when near the nerve.

Facial Nerve EMGs

The principal use of facial nerve EMGs in MVD surgery is for HFS. As discussed above, vascular compression causes hypersensitivity of the facial nerve resulting in the anomalous response (electrical stimulation of one branch of the facial nerve causes spasms of muscles supplied by other branches). By monitoring the anomalous response, the NIOM team can help determine when adequate decompression has been accomplished.

Technique

Facial nerve EMG monitoring involves recording compound muscle action potentials (CMAPs) from at least two muscles innervated by different branches of the facial nerve. When one branch is stimulated, instead of only the muscle innervated by that branch being activated, a CMAP is also seen in the other muscle. Two subdermal needle EMG electrodes are placed in the orbicularis oculi and mentalis muscles to obtain a bipolar recording. Another set of subdermal needle electrodes are placed along the temporal branch of the facial nerve to stimulate that nerve (5) (Figure 13.6). Filter and sensitivity settings are the same as for other types of EMG monitoring.

During surgery, the temporal branch of the facial nerve is stimulated periodically and responses observed in the orbicularis oculi and mentalis muscles. A short pulse duration of 100 μs is typically used and the intensity should be increased until a response is seen. The stimulation rate is between 1 and 5 Hz. The response is seen about 10 ms after stimulation.

Effects of Anesthetics

Inhalation and intravenous anesthetics have little effect on facial nerve EMGs. Even

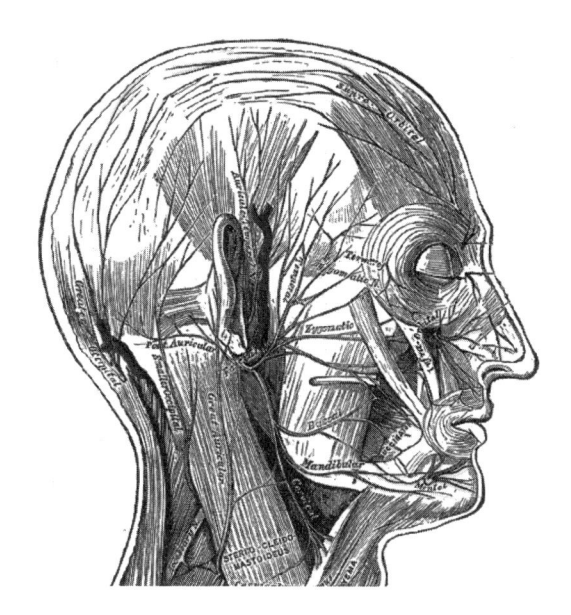

FIGURE 13.6 Schematic showing the terminal branches of the facial nerve. Subdermal needle electrodes are placed over the temporal branch most often (black circles). [Figure in public domain. Reproduced from reference (5).]

though motor evoked potentials (CMAPs in this case) are obtained, intravenous anesthesia is not necessary, since stimulation is distal to the anterior horn cells, the location of most sensitivity to anesthetics. Neuromuscular blocking agents, however, can significantly impair this type of monitoring. Ideally patients should have no neuromuscular blocking agents during this type of surgery. Blood pressure and temperature have minimal effects on facial nerve EMGs.

Interpretation

When the temporal branch of the facial nerve is stimulated in patients with HFS, the typical response consists of a delayed CMAP after 10 ms in the orbicularis oculi and mentalis muscles. Recurrent CMAPs may also be seen. When decompression has been adequately accomplished, this response disappears. Occasionally other branches of the facial nerve, such as the mandibular, can also be stimulated to obtain a CMAP. However, the reliability of the other branches in eliciting this type of response is inconsistent.

Occasionally, as soon as the dura mater is opened, the abnormal EMG response disappears. This is most often due to the vessel falling away from the nerve because of reduced CSF pressure. Stimulation ath a rate of 50 Hz can temporarily facilitate the return of the response. Thereafter, stimulation rates of 1 to 5 Hz will again elicit a response.

Once adequate decompression has been achieved, stimulation of the temporal branch of the facial nerve does not show a delayed EMG response. Thus this type of NIOM can be used to determine when adequate decompression has been achieved. When the offending vessel is removed from the facial nerve but the abnormal EMG response persists, there is most likely a second vessel also causing compression. This second vessel should also be separated from the nerve for best postoperative results.

Median Nerve Somatic Evoked Potentials

Whereas the types of NIOM discussed above are used to monitor various cranial nerves, median nerve SEPs have been used in MVD surgeries to monitor brainstem function. It is possible to have injury of the midbrain due to ischemia or excessive manipulation of the brainstem, and this has resulted in postoperative deficits (2). Since BAEPs evaluate the auditory pathways only up to the rostral pons, they are unable to detect such injuries. Median nerve SEPs would most likely demonstrate significant changes if such a problem occurred.

In most MVD surgeries, manipulation of the brainstem is minimal and the risk of injury is very low. Consequently most laboratories do not routinely perform median nerve SEPs in these procedures. These SEPs are more often performed in CPA tumor surgeries, as then the risk to the brainstem is much greater.

Details of median nerve SEP monitoring are discussed in other chapters and are not presented here. The technique, effect of anesthetics, and interpretation are much the same as in other types of monitoring.

UTILITY OF NIOM IN MVD SURGERIES

Hearing loss is a common complication of MVD and other surgeries in the vicinity of the CPA. Reviews have shown that as surgeons gain more experience with MVD surgery, all complications except hearing loss decline (6). Over the last few decades, several studies have documented reduction of hearing loss with BAEP monitoring.

Historically, the incidence of hearing loss with MVD surgeries was about 6% to 10% prior to the use of NIOM. In a report of 143 consecutive patients undergoing MVD surgery for TN or HFS using BAEP monitoring, the incidence of significant hearing loss was 2.8% (4). Another study compared the incidence of hearing loss before and after the initiation of BAEP monitoring (7). Prior to monitoring, the incidence of hearing loss was 6.6%, whereas after BAEP monitoring, no cases of hearing loss were seen. Other studies have also shown a similar reduction of hearing loss with the use of BAEP NIOM, clearly establishing the utility of this type of monitoring (6,8).

Vestibulocochlear NAP monitoring has been performed less than BAEP monitoring in patients undergoing CPA surgery. It offers the advantage of virtually instantaneous feedback to the surgeons. This has enabled neurophysiologists to help surgeons determine at which point during the surgery the vestibulocochlear nerve is at greatest risk. During electrocoagulation near the vestibulocochlear nerve, decrements in NAP amplitude have been noted, suggesting thermal trauma to the nerve (9). This has allowed surgeons to further refine the operative technique. Vestibular NAPs have also been obtained in patients with CPA tumors in whom BAEPs could not be obtained (10). This has enabled preservation of hearing in patients in whom BAEP NIOM could not be performed.

Facial nerve EMG is a unique type of NIOM, as it can confirm when adequate decompression has been achieved in patients undergoing HFS MVD surgery. In a series of 67 patients, the abnormal EMG activity disappeared or was significantly reduced in 60 (90%) patients with decompression of the facial nerve (11). Seven patients continued to have the same degree of EMG activity at the end of decompression. Of these seven, four (57%) did not have significant improvement in their symptoms and underwent reoperation. Hardly any of the patients who had resolution of their EMG activity had a recurrence of symptoms. These findings have been confirmed in another smaller series of 11 patients (12). In this series, facial nerve EMG was useful in deciding how much decompression was needed. Because of the value of facial nerve EMG monitoring in helping decide when decompression is adequate and its predictive nature as to whose symptoms will resolve, it has become a commonly used NIOM modality in HFS MVD surgery.

TECHNICAL CONSIDERATIONS

Preparation

Patients undergoing MVD surgery for various cranial neuralgias will need BAEP monitoring at a minimum. Depending on laboratory protocol, vestibulocochlear NAPs and median nerve SEPs may also be obtained. For HFS MVD surgery, facial nerve EMG monitoring is also useful. Consequently, when a patient is referred for NIOM for MVD surgery, it is important to determine which type of MVD surgery will be performed. This will dictate which electrodes will be needed and which modalities will be monitored.

It is may be helpful to evaluate patients in the outpatient laboratory a day or more before surgery. A routine BAEP study should be conducted to confirm that a BAEP response is present which can be obtained and followed in the operating room. Absence of BAEPs would prompt consideration for vestibulocochlear NAP monitoring if not done routinely. Additionally, if the BAEP response is absent, it may prompt the surgeon to evaluate other etiologies for the patient's symptoms, as BAEPs are not typically abnormal in patients with cranial neuralgias. If there is any hearing loss, formal audiologic evaluation should be considered to determine its extent. This information will be useful in evaluating postoperative hearing loss.

Preoperative facial nerve conduction studies (NCSs) and EMGs may be helpful in patients undergoing MVD surgery for HFS to demonstrate the anomalous response. Stimulation of the temporal branch may cause a CMAP in the mentalis muscle. Additionally, the patient's history of use of botulinum toxin for treatment of HFS is important to elicit. If it has been used, EMG responses may be difficult to obtain in the operating room.

The technologist should make certain that adequate numbers of electrodes are available for surgery. If subdermal needle electrodes are used, enough sets should be available to put one each at Cz and both mastoids (or earlobes) and two each for the orbicularis oculi and mentalis muscles (and any other muscle to be monitored). Stimulating subdermal needle electrodes will be needed to stimulate the branches of the facial nerve in surgeries for HFS.

For auditory stimulation, an acoustic stimulator capable of delivering broadband clicks should be used. Typically a transducer with plastic tubing ending in ear inserts is used. High-quality tubing should be used, so that it does not get kinked or clamped during positioning and draping.

Relatively few channels are required for NIOM in MVD surgeries. Four channels are needed for bilateral BAEP monitoring and two more for facial EMG in patients with HFS. If vestibulocochlear NAP is to be monitored, one additional channel will be needed. Almost all NIOM machines currently available will enable this type of monitoring. These machines also have built-in auditory stimulators that provide broadband clicks of adequate rate and intensity.

Procedure

The NIOM technologist should make an effort to meet the patient prior to the surgery to explain the role of monitoring. If EEG disc electrodes are used for monitoring, they can be applied in the induction room or preoperative holding area. However, if subdermal needle electrodes are being used, it is best to wait until after induction of anesthesia so that unnecessary pain can be avoided.

The auditory stimulator must be securely applied to the patient. Tubing from the transducer ends in specially designed ear inserts. These inserts must be secured in the external auditory canal and sealed with a waterproof seal. This seal is important, because if water or fluid seeps into the ear canal, adequate stimulation of the cochlea may not be possible. The tubing must also be secured, so that when the pinna is clamped forward it does not occlude the tubing.

Patients undergoing MVD surgery for HFS also require electrodes for monitoring facial nerve EMGs. Subdermal needle electrodes should be placed within 1 cm of each other without touching. The needles should point away from the sterile field to avoid contamination during skin retraction. Needles in the orbicularis oculi muscle should be placed such that the bony orbit protects the eyeball from the needle point. If needles are to be placed in the orbicularis oris muscle, they should be placed subdermally at a small angle of about 10 degrees to avoid punctures into the mouth. Subdermal needle electrodes should also be placed along the temporal branch of the facial nerve (Figure 13.6). These will serve to stimulate the nerve. Additional stimulating electrodes can be placed in the middle third of the lower margin of the mandible to stimulate the mandibular branch of the facial nerve.

The facial nerve branches should be stimulated with a duration of 100 μs and intensity gradually increased until a response is seen. For this a triggered EMG program should be used. This stimulation should be repeated periodically throughout the procedure until decompression has been achieved. After decompression, an attempt should be made to elicit the response again; if a response is seen, it is likely that adequate decompression has not been achieved. The surgeon may elect to look for other vessels that may be causing compression of the facial nerve. When the facial nerve branches are not being stimulated, a free-running EMG program should be viewed to look for abnormal spontaneous discharges.

If the vestibulocochlear NAP is to be recorded, special electrodes must be available. These can be either monopolar or bipolar as discussed above and will need to be secured on the vestibulocochlear nerve by the surgeon. If median nerve SEPs are to be recorded, stimulating electrodes must be applied to the wrist and recording electrodes to Erb's point and the scalp (C3, C4, and Fz at a minimum). Details of median nerve SEPs are presented elsewhere in this book.

The anesthesia team should be notified of necessary considerations for NIOM. If only BAEPs are to be monitored, the anesthesiologist can use an anesthetic of his or her choice. This applies to recording vestibulocochlear NAPs as well. However, if facial nerve EMG is to be recorded, neuromuscular blocking agents should not be used except during induction of anesthesia. Even in cases where EMG is to be monitored, the anesthesiologist is free to use an inhalation or intravenous anesthetic of his or her choice. The NIOM technologist should note the blood pressure and temperature, especially after the dura mater is opened; drops in blood pressure and temperature may cause prolongation of the absolute latencies of the BAEP waveforms.

Baselines of the BAEPs and facial nerve EMGs should be obtained as soon as setup and patient positioning is complete. BAEPs should be obtained constantly to ensure maximal patient safety. Electrocautery and drilling will prevent monitoring. BAEPs should be obtained before and after drilling of bone to detect a rare complication of vasospasm causing ischemic of the cochlea. Should wave I disappear during or immediately after drilling of bone, the blood pressure should be increased and technical problems quickly be ruled out. Once the dura mater is opened, baseline responses should be reset. Often the draining of CSF will cause a loss of wave II and a decrease in wave III and/or V responses. From this time until closing, BAEPs should be obtained constantly. With modern NIOM machines, BAEP responses from the left and right sides can be obtained simultaneously with interleaved stimulation. Neuromuscular blocking agents should have worn off by the time drilling is completed and constant real-time EMG monitoring should be performed until closing.

Whenever significant changes in BAEP waveforms are noted, the NIOM technologist should troubleshoot to ensure that the change is not due to artifact or nonsurgical causes. If averaging of BAEPs is continued during drilling, the noise from the drill will mask the broadband clicks and cause a drop in amplitude of the waveforms (Figure 13.7). This should be recognized so that an inappropriate alert is not raised. An increase in the EMG activity during surgery may suggest that the patient's anesthesia is light; this may prompt the anesthesiologist to reevaluate the anesthesia. High impedance of the electrodes can introduce significant artifact as well, which degrades the BAEP signal. Checking electrode impedances will alert the NIOM technologist to this problem. The electrodes should be regelled or if possible replaced. If spare electrodes were applied during setup, they should be used instead. When significant change is

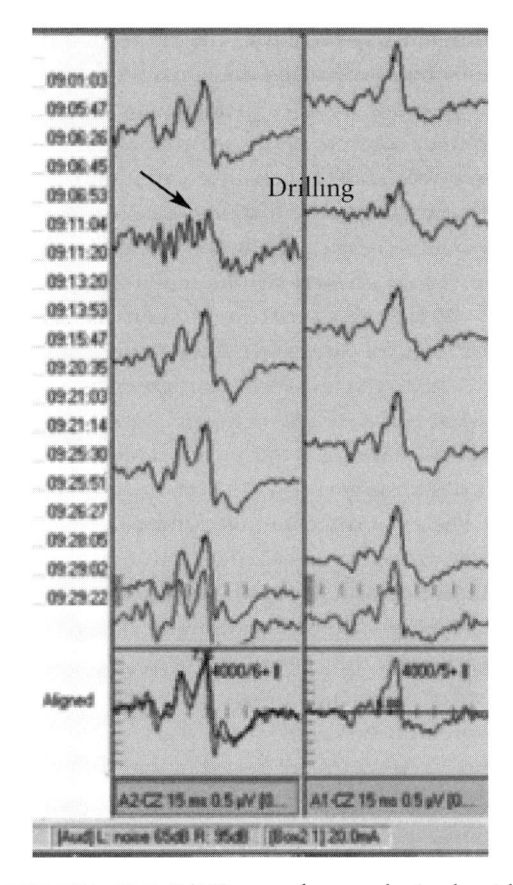

FIGURE 13.7 BAEP waveforms obtained with stimulation of the right ear during MVD surgery for TN. A robust BAEP waveform is seen initially. However, when averaging is continued during bone drilling (arrow), a loss of wave V amplitude is noted. This is not a clinically significant change. [Reproduced with permission from Husain (1).]

noted in the BAEPs, it is critical to average only as many repetitions as necessary to have a reliable response. Further repetitions may degrade the response, as with continuous traction on the nerve there is progressive prolongation of latency or drop in amplitude. When these progressive changes are averaged in a single response, the response becomes unreliable. Thus, responses should be repeated as frequently as possible.

The NIOM team must communicate frequently with the surgeon. Whereas some investigators suggest that the surgeon should be informed only when the latency shift of the wave V of the BAEP is greater than 1.0 ms or amplitude decrement is greater than 50%, others feel that a constant communication with the surgeon informing him or her of incremental latency changes is better. The surgeon is told of incremental changes in BAEP wave V latency so that he or she will have a better idea of which surgical manipulations have caused the most trauma to the vestibulocochlear nerve. When a critical change is seen, the surgeon is in a better position to undo that part of the surgery.

The NIOM technologist must keep accurate records during the surgery. Demographics about the patient should be recorded; in addition, type of surgery, anesthetics being used, temperature, and blood pressure should be recorded frequently. Most importantly, any communication with the surgeon must be recorded. If alerts are raised, these should be specifically recorded; if possible the surgeon's response to the alert should also be noted. Complete and thorough documentation is a critical part of any NIOM procedure.

Postprocedure

After termination of the surgery, all sites at which electrodes were placed should be meticulously cleaned. Tape, if used, should be carefully removed to avoid skin tears, especially in elderly patients with thin skin. Pressure should be applied with gauze to prevent excessive bleeding from electrode sites. Needle electrodes should be disposed of in a proper sharps container. All wires and extensions used should be cleaned according to laboratory protocol. Equipment and supplies are then replaced and restocked in preparation for the next case. Before leaving the operating room, any additional notes should be written in the log. All critical communications must be documented during the case, but notes can reviewed and any additional comments added. The NIOM data should be stored in paper or electronic format according to laboratory protocol. As well as daily maintenance, monitoring equipment is required to have an electrical safety check at least every 6 months.

The neurophysiologist should create a report of the procedure. This report should include the modalities monitored and any significant changes that occurred. Findings at the termination of the case should be noted. An interpretation of the significance of the findings should also be provided.

CONCLUSIONS

NIOM has markedly reduced the complications of MVD surgery for cranial neuralgias. BAEPs are used most often for these surgeries, however facial nerve EMGs, vestibulocochlear NAPs, and median nerve SEPs also have utility. The use of BAEPs has resulted in a significant reduction of the incidence of hearing loss postoperatively. Facial nerve EMG allows the neurophysiologist to direct the surgeon when adequate facial nerve decompression has been achieved. Vestibulocochlear NAP monitoring allows rapid feedback to the surgeons and helps him or her determine which part of the surgery is causing most damage to the nerve. Median nerve SEPs can detect injury to the brainstem in cases when excessive bleeding or manipulation occurs. Attention to detail and a collegial working relationship with the surgical and anesthesia teams allows for successful monitoring.

REFERENCES

1. Husain AM. Neurophysiologic intraoperative monitoring. In: Tatum WO, Husain AM, Benbadis SR, Kaplan PW, eds. *Handbook of EEG Interpretation*. New York: Demos, 2007:223–260.
2. Erwin CW, Erwin AC. The use of brain stem auditory evoked potentials in intraoperative monitoring. In: Russell GB, Rodichok LD, eds. *Primer of Intraoperative Neurophysiologic*

3. James ML, Husain AM. Brainstem auditory evoked potential monitoring: when is change in wave V significant? *Neurology* 2005;65: 1551–1555.
4. Moller MB, Moller AR. Loss of auditory function in microvascular decompression for hemifacial spasm. Results in 143 consecutive cases. *J Neurosurg* 1985;63:17–20.
5. Facial nerve [online]. In: Wikipedia. Available at: http://en.wikipedia.org/wiki/Facial_nerve. Accessed July 15, 2007.
6. Kakizawa T, Shimizu T, Fukushima T. [Monitoring of auditory brainstem response (ABR) during microvascular decompression (MVD): results in 400 cases]. *No To Shinkei* 1990;42:991–998.
7. Radtke RA, Erwin CW, Wilkins RH. Intraoperative brainstem auditory evoked potentials: significant decrease in postoperative morbidity. *Neurology* 1989;39:187–191.
8. Wiedemayer H, Fauser B, Sandalcioglu IE, et al. The impact of neurophysiological intraoperative monitoring on surgical decisions: a critical analysis of 423 cases. *J Neurosurg* 2002;96:255–262.
9. Moller AR, Jannetta PJ. Monitoring techniques for microvascular decompression procedures. In: Loftus CM, Traynelis VC, eds. *Intraoperative Monitoring Techniques in Neurosurgery*. New York: McGraw-Hill, 1994:163–174.
10. Roberson JB Jr, Jackson LE, McAuley JR. Acoustic neuroma surgery: absent auditory brainstem response does not contraindicate attempted hearing preservation. *Laryngoscope* 1999;109:904–910.
11. Moller AR, Jannetta PJ. Monitoring facial EMG responses during microvascular decompression operations for hemifacial spasm. *J Neurosurg* 1987;66:681–685.
12. Haines SJ, Torres F. Intraoperative monitoring of the facial nerve during decompressive surgery for hemifacial spasm. *J Neurosurg* 1991;74:254–257.

14 Cerebellopontine Angle Surgery: Tumor

Dileep R. Nair
James R. Brooks

Neurophysiologic intraoperative monitoring (NIOM) has seen a number of changes over the past 25 years. It has become an important component in many orthopedic, neurologic, and vascular surgeries. From its initial foundations of monitoring the somatosensory pathways and facial nerves, NIOM has evolved to evaluate the function of many brainstem structures and cranial nerves as well as other regions of the brain and spinal cord.

Cerebellopontine angle (CPA) tumors pose a number of unique challenges to neurosurgeons and head neck surgeons, not the least of which is preservation of adjacent neurologic structures such as cranial nerves and brainstem structures. NIOM of these cases is often challenging owing to the number of closely spaced important structures and compact tracts within the brainstem in which a slight error could lead to major deficits of function. Brainstem and cranial nerve monitoring may help preserve function during these surgeries. Early detection of changes noted during the intraoperative monitoring of pathways may allow the surgeon to recognize a potentially damaging maneuver and make corrections once the mechanism of injury is understood. Intrinsic to this technique is the ability to intervene early so that a potential injury can be identified early, prior to the complete loss of function. This method of making changes in the surgical procedure cannot occur without the presence of NIOM (Figure 14.1).

The prevention of neurologic deficits in CPA tumor surgeries is particularly important, since damage in this region can result in pain, functional disability, and cosmetic deformities. The cranial nerves are particularly prone to injury because of their small size and circuitous path. Tumors in this region can distort the normal anatomy and result in difficulty in the identification of neural structures owing to distortion of normal anatomic relationships.

ANATOMY AND PATHOLOGY

The CPA is a region in the subarachnoid space in the posterior fossa. Its borders include the posterior surface of the temporal bone anteriorly, the cerebellum posteriorly, the brainstem medially, and the cerebellar tonsil inferiorly. The surgical approach through the middle cranial fossa to the internal auditory canal was first described in 1904. The middle cranial fossa approach is considered one of the most difficult approaches in skull base surgery. It includes removal of the petrous bone from its subtem-

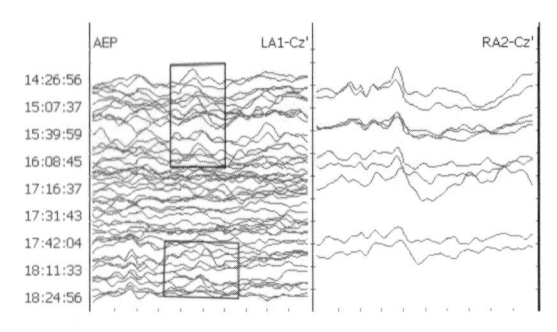

FIGURE 14.1 BAEP monitoring data from a 4-year-old girl undergoing resection of a posterior fossa ependymoma. During surgery there was a sudden loss of the left BAEP. This information was immediately discussed with the surgeon. With more careful dissection of tumor and change in position of the retractor, the responses returned by the end of the case. There was no noticeable change in hearing function following surgery.

poral surface in order to expose the internal auditory canal and posterior fossa dura while preserving all the important closely related anatomic structures.

The difficulties in surgical resection of CPA tumors can be attributed in part to the great anatomic variations in the locations of cranial nerves and vascular structures even among normal individuals. These relationships may then become even more distorted in the presence of tumors. The trigeminal nerve courses above the cerebellopontine space, while the glossopharyngeal, vagus, and hypoglossal nerves travel below it. The vetibulocochlear and facial nerves travel through this space in the superoanterolateral course from the brainstem toward the temporal bone, where they enter the internal auditory canal.

The facial nerve is responsible for facial expression. The pathways for the facial nerve are variable. It is composed of nearly 10,000 neurons, of which 7,000 are myelinated and innervate muscles of facial expression. The course of the facial nerve can be roughly divided into six segments: supranuclear, brainstem, meatal, labyrinthine, tympanic, mastoid, and extratemporal. The course up to the internal auditory canal is discussed below. The supranuclear or cortical/internal capsule segment arises from efferent discharges from motor face regions, which then are carried through corticobulbar tracts to the internal capsule. They continue through midbrain and lower brainstem, where they synapse with the pontine facial nerve nucleus. The facial motor nucleus is located in the lower third of the pons beneath the fourth ventricle. The neurons leave the nucleus to pass around the abducens nucleus before emerging from the brainstem. The facial nerve emerges from the brainstem along with the nervus intermedius (which conveys afferent taste fibers from the chorda tympani nerve, which comes from the anterior two thirds of the tongue), which lies between the facial nerve and vestibulocochlear nerve. The average distance from where the facial nerve exits the brainstem to where it enters the internal auditory canal is approximately 15.8 mm. The close anatomic relationships between the facial nerve, nervus intermedius, and vestibulocochlear nerve at the level of the CPA and internal auditory canal can result in disturbances in taste, hearing, balance, salivary gland flow, and facial function by a lesion in this region. The facial nerve courses superior and anterior to the vestibulocochlear nerve as a tubular structure throughout the length of the internal auditory canal.

The vestibulocochlear nerve is a sensory nerve that functions to impart hearing and equilibrium arising from the inner ear. The vestibular nerve conveys sensation from the semicircular canals, the sacculus, and the utriculus. The cochlear nerve conveys auditory sensations from the cochlea. The vestibulocochlear nerve arises from the medulla, where the trapezoid body passes beneath the cerebellum. It enters the internal auditory canal as a tubular structure but becomes crescent-shaped in cross section in the middle portion of the canal and is separated into individual nerves only in the most lateral portion of the canal.

The relationship between facial and vestibulocochlear nerves shows variation among individuals. Near the brainstem, almost half of the vestibulocochlear nerves are partially segmented on magnetic resonance imaging (MRI), whereas others are completely divided into separate nerves only in the most lateral portion of the internal auditory canal. The facial and cochlear nerves are of similar size in a third of cases.

CPA tumors represent about 10% of all intracranial tumors. Vestibular schwannomas (acoustic neuromas) account for nearly 75% of these lesions, with the remainder including meningiomas, arachnoid cysts, epidermoids, lipomas, metastatic tumors, or vascular lesions (Table 14.1). Vestibular schwannomas arise from the vestibulocochlear nerve at the entrance to the internal auditory canal. These tumors are usually unilateral; however, about 5% are bilateral and associated with neurofibromatosis type II. Patients with these tumors typically present in middle age with progressive unilateral sensorineural hearing loss. The typical MRI findings include a pear-shaped mass centered on the internal auditory canal. Small tumors (up to 1.5 cm) appear as a tubular mass in the internal auditory canal. Medium-sized tumors (3 cm) resemble an ice cream cone on MRI. These tumors enhance intensely with contrast. The internal auditory canal may be eroded or enlarged by the tumor expansion.

Meningiomas usually present in patients aged 30 to 60 years and are derived from the arachnoid villi of the meninges. The clinical symptoms depend on the precise location of the tumor and may overlap significantly with vestibular schwannomas. CPA meningiomas appear typically as a broad, dural-based sessile mass often with an extension of the dura or dural tail.

SURGICAL PROCEDURES OF THE CEREBELLOPONTINE ANGLE

The middle cranial fossa approach (transtemporal approach) provides a broad, atraumatic access to the basal portion of the middle cranial fossa, the anterior surface of the petrous pyramid, the internal auditory canal, and the CPA. The patient is positioned supine under general anesthesia with the head turned to the opposite side. The surgeon sits at the head of the operating table. A curvilinear postauricular incision is made with the apex 3 to 4 cm posterior to the postauricular crease. The primary incision divides the skin and subcutaneous tissue but not the temporalis muscle. The temporalis muscle is exposed and opened with a triradiate incision and reflected from the bone. Alternatively, a temporalis muscle flap can be created and reflected with the scalp flap. Complete cortical mastiodectomy is performed, the sigmoid sinus is skeletonized, and the facial nerve is identified anteriorly but left covered with bone in its vertical segment. Next a labyrinthectomy is performed and all the internal auditory canal bone is removed. If the vestibular schwannomas is small, it is exposed by opening the dura of the internal auditory canal. For large tumors, CPA exposure is necessary. Intracapsular tumor debulking is completed before tumor is dissected directly from the facial nerve. After the tumor is removed, the Eustachian tubes are packed with the temporalis muscle. The dural defect is loosely approximated with sutures, and the mastoidectomy defect is filled with strips of abdominal fat.

TABLE 14.1 Pathology of Tumors in the CPA

Vestibular schwannomas (acoustic neuromas)
Meningiomas
Globus tumors (paragangliomas)
Epidermoids
Arachnoid cysts
Dural sinus thrombosis
Lipomas
Vascular tumors
Facial nerve schwannomas

The pathology of the CPA cistern is primarily that of nervous and vascular structures as well as the meninges that line it. Prior to the advent of modern imaging and microsurgical techniques, the incidence of facial paralysis following removal of CPA tumors was as high as 30%, with many of the patients also losing hearing on the side of tumor. With the advances in imaging, microsurgery, and NIOM in the past 20 years, the rates at which the facial and vestibulocochlear nerves are preserved has improved steadily. A study in which a group of patients (n = 48) who underwent acoustic neuroma resection with facial nerve monitoring was compared to historical controls matched for age, tumor size, type of surgical procedure, and surgical team found that the rates of facial nerve function sparing was higher in the monitored group as compared to controls (67% vs. 33%) (1). Similar findings were seen in cases in which brainstem auditory evoked potential (BAEP) monitoring was performed to preserve function of the vestibulocochlear nerve. The efficacy of BAEP monitoring was particularly noticeable for acoustic neuromas less than 2.5 cm in diameter.

TIMING OF NEURAL INJURY IN SURGERIES OF THE CEREBELLOPONTINE ANGLE

The anatomic proximity of the facial nerve to the vestibulocochlear nerve puts the facial nerve at great risk during resection of tumors in the CPA. As the tumor size increases, the facial nerve may become involved within the tumor. In particular, with tumors with a diameter greater than 3 cm, there is the possibility that the facial nerve will have been spread apart by the tumor or enveloped in the tumor capsule and thus have been damaged by the tumor. The timing of cranial nerve injury depends on the nature of the injury. Injury can occur as a result of the underlying pathology that has necessitated surgery, or it can occur during the operation itself (2) (Figure 14.2). Damage during sur-

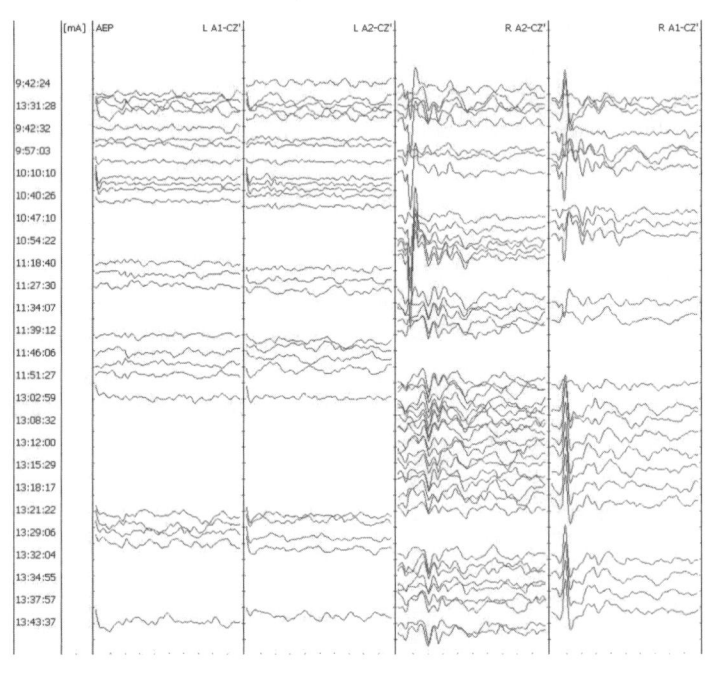

FIGURE 14.2 BAEP data from a patient with left-sided hearing loss undergoing resection of a large CPA tumor. The BAEP waterfall shows a lack of any BAEP response from the left ear. The right BAEP shows presence of all waveforms.

gery can occur from a mechanical injury, a thermal injury, or as a result of ischemia to the neural structures.

In situations where the tumor is greater than 3 cm in diameter, there is a risk of severing the facial nerve during tumor debulking. Direct electrical stimulation helps identify and distinguish trigeminal and facial nerves and creates a map of these nerves in relation to the tumor. A monopolar stimulator is generally used in cranial nerve monitoring and mapping of the surface of the tumor. Triggered electromyographic (EMG) responses are sought during this time to indicate whether the facial nerve is in close proximity to the stimulating electrode; if so, more careful dissection can be used. A smaller bipolar electrode can be used, if needed once the nerve is seen, to evaluate whether motor nerve function is intact. A monopolar stimulator can also be used with appropriate stimulation intensity. It delivers focal stimulation and performs a function similar to that of a bipolar stimulator.

Being able to identify areas of tumor where there are no facial nerve fibers allows for larger parts of the tumor to be debulked with minimal injury to the facial nerve. This also allows for considerable amount of time to be saved in surgery once mapping of the tumor is completed. It is necessary to probe all regions of the tumor to ensure that the entire nerve has been identified, particularly in large tumors where the nerve may have been splayed by the tumor into separate fascicles. In situations where the facial nerve is involved in the tumor, nerve tissue can be identified from the surrounding tumor tissue so that a nerve-sparing dissection can be attempted. However, this is an extremely delicate and exacting process. Sometimes it is accomplished by scraping the tumor mass off the facial nerve.

A sustained neurotonic discharge during electrocautery may indicate that the nerve is at risk of damage by thermal energy. In this situation, the electrocautery can be used at lower current intensities and for shorter time intervals. In the case of surgeries in the CPA, only high-quality bipolar electrocautery should be used, as there is a high risk for injury to the facial nerve with monopolar electrocautery. The issue of thermal injury can also apply during the drilling of bone in the internal auditory canal. Cool irrigation during the time of drilling may help decrease the injury to neural structures from the heat given off by the drill. Once there is a complete injury to the facial nerve, it may no longer produce neurotonic discharges when manipulated. It may, however, produce triggered EMG responses when the distal end of the sectioned nerve is electrically stimulated. Therefore, prior to beginning debulking, it is important that all regions of the tumor be probed and mapped with direct electrical stimulation using a monopolar stimulator.

NIOM TECHNIQUES IN CPA SURGERY

Various structures are at risk during CPA surgery. Most important are the facial and vestibulocochlear nerves. The integrity of the facial nerve is monitored by using continuous and triggered EMG recordings. The vestibulocochlear nerve is monitored with BAEPs, with close attention to changes in wave I and the interpeak latency (IPL) of waves I to III. In the case of large tumors, there may be risk associated with manipulation of the brainstem, which can result in tragic complications. For these scenarios, changes noted in BAEP waves III to V IPL can give information as to brainstem function. Thus BAEP monitoring can give information about not only changes in auditory nerve function but also brainstem manipulation. Additionally, monitoring median nerve somatosensory evoked potentials (SEPs) can also give information as to brainstem function. Early signs of brainstem manipulation should also be evaluated and can be monitored using BAEPs and median nerve SEPs (Figure 14.3). However, the monitoring of brainstem function is less crucial

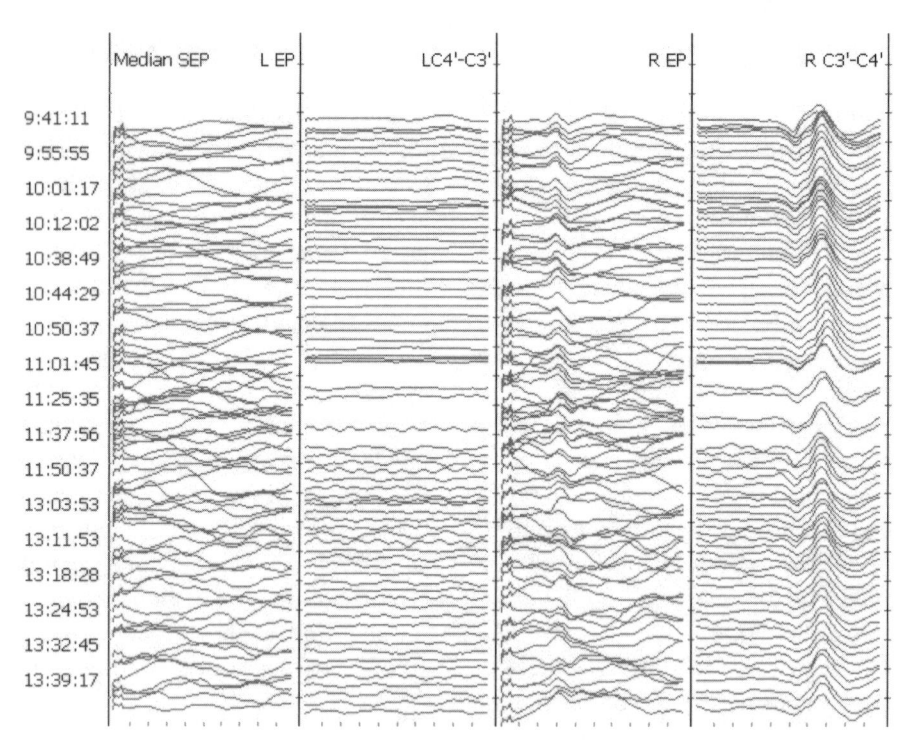

FIGURE 14.3 Median nerve SEP data from a 57-year-old patient with left hemiparesis undergoing surgery for a recurrent left epidermoid cyst in the CPA. There is absence of waveforms from the left median nerve from the beginning of the surgery. Recordings from Erb's point were also inconsistent in spite of clear twitches of the left thumb with stimulation. This was thought to be a result of suprascapular lesion from chronic shoulder dislocations.

than that of structures situated in the CPA, since they are at highest risk during surgery. The modalities commonly used for NIOM in CPA tumor surgeries are presented in Table 14.2.

Transcranial electrical motor evoked potentials (MEPs) can also potentially evaluate the facial nerve pathway much above the surgical site, thereby giving information on the integrity of the entire pathway. However, the use of MEPs brings up a number of technical problems. These include significant movement during transcranial electrical stimulation, which may cause damage during delicate microsurgical procedures. Additionally, there may be contamination of the MEP recordings from facial contraction by current spread of the stimulus across the scalp. This contamination can be differentiated from MEP activity by evaluating the latency of such responses. Transcranial electrical MEPs should have a latency of approximately 12 to 15 seconds, whereas facial contractions elicited by current spread will occur much sooner, close to the stimulus artifact. Finally, the large stimulus artifact from transcranial stimulation may make it difficult to accurately determine correct latency of the MEPs.

Trigeminal nerve SEPs in this type of surgery is another potential monitoring technique that has not been frequently used owing to difficulties associated with obtaining reliable recordings and lack of clear changes denoting that a pathologic deficit may be imminent (3).

Changes seen during the monitoring may also help predict postoperative deficits, which may be helpful in early rehabilitative measures, as well as providing patients with information about the nature of the deficit and

TABLE 14.2 Techniques of Monitoring Brainstem and Cranial Nerve Function during CPA Tumor Surgeries

---

Brainstem auditory evoked potentials
Facial nerve EMG monitoring
Trigeminal nerve EMG monitoring
Median nerve somatosensory evoked potentials
Posterior tibial nerve somatosensory evoked potentials
Motor evoked potentials

---

how it came about. In addition, the correlation of the timing of injury to the surgical events may help elucidate the mechanism of injury and provide a means to improve surgical techniques over time.

Electromyographic Recordings

Initially monitoring of neural structures consisted of evaluating a visible muscle twitch in response to direct nerve stimulation to assess whether there was integrity to the peripheral nerve being stimulated. EMG recordings as a continuous evaluation for peripheral nerve function were first used in the mid-1980s (4). Since that time, a number of advances in NIOM have occurred owing to improvements in technology and anesthetic regimens. Cranial nerves can be monitored using EMG, nerve conduction studies (NCSs), and EPs triggered from electrical stimulation. Using direct nerve stimulation, compound muscle action potentials (CMAPs) and nerve action potentials (NAPs) can be recorded. Spontaneous motor unit potentials can warn surgeons of mechanical or thermal irritation of cranial nerves. These modalities are designed to provide immediate feedback to the surgeon as to the location and status of particular cranial nerves.

The intraoperative use of EMG recordings consists of continuous monitoring for spontaneous motor unit potentials. Standard EMG settings for sensitivity are used for cranial nerve muscle monitoring (sensitivities 50 to 200 µV per division, filters 20 to 20,000 Hz, time window 5 to 10 ms per division). There are a number of differences from the techniques used in routine outpatient needle EMG. The activity of interest in the intraoperative setting is the neurotonic discharges. These changes consists of high-frequency EMG bursts or trains that may be continuous and occur in response to mechanical or metabolic stimulation (4). Things that need to be differentiated from neurotonic discharges include movement artifact, EMG activity due to light anesthetic levels, and electrode artifact. Neurotonic discharges usually last 1 to 20 seconds, whereas motor unit potentials have a duration of less than 200 ms (2). The appearance of neurotonic discharges in a single cranial nerve may indicated nerve irritation and allow feedback to the surgeon about the presence of the nerve near the surgical instrument being used. Sharp transection of the nerve is less likely to give rise to neurotonic discharges as compared to mechanical irritation, saline irrigation, or heat due to electrocautery.

Facial Nerve Monitoring

The facial nerve is one of the most frequently monitored cranial nerves. Monitoring of the facial nerve is accomplished by placing needle electrodes in facial nerve–innervated muscles, such as the orbicularis oris, mentalis, orbicularis oculi, frontalis, and rhizoris muscles. Free-running EMGs can be monitored while surgery around the vicinity of the facial nerve takes place. Stimulation with a monopolar electrode can also be used to localize the facial nerve within a tumor or identify various branches of the facial nerve by noting the muscles that are activated.

Trigeminal Nerve Monitoring

The trigeminal nerve can be monitored by placing two needle electrodes in the masseter or temporalis muscle to record EMG activity. Much like monitoring of the facial nerve, trigeminal nerve monitoring involves review of the free-running EMG obtained from the masseter or temporalis muscles. Additionally, the motor component of the trigeminal nerve can also be stimulated and CMAPs recorded from the muscles. Trigeminal nerve SEPs are technically difficult to record, as mentioned above.

BAEP Monitoring

Preservation of auditory function is possible during the removal of small acoustic tumors. BAEPs obtained with broadband clicks have been useful in NIOM of the vestibulocochlear nerve as well as brainstem structures for CPA surgeries. Intraoperative BAEPs differ from BAEPs obtained in an outpatient setting. Ear inserts are used in the operating room instead of headphones. Headphones are bulky and likely to fall off during surgery. When ear inserts are being used, additional tubing may be placed to extend from the ear inserts to the stimulators. This extra tubing adds an additional delay in the peak latencies of the BAEPs. For each inch of extra tubing, 1.0 ms will be incurred in latency prolongation. The time display on the outpatient BAEP is typically 10 or 15 ms. During NIOM a display window of 20 ms is often helpful, to not only to account delays in the peak latencies brought on by variable lengths of tubing but also to "compress the waveforms" so as to make the identification of wave V more clearly visible.

BAEPs are relatively resistant to the effects of anesthesia; however, like other EPs they can be affected by changes in temperature. Use of cold irrigation in the surgical field can cause delays in the BAEP waveforms and appear to prolong the peak latencies. In this instance the IPL will not change. This makes monitoring waves I to V and III to V IPL as well as waves I and V peak latencies useful during surgery.

Standard recording channels used for BAEP monitoring are a mastoid or ear electrode referenced to a vertex electrode. The ground electrode can be placed at FPz or Fz. A two-channel montage, A1 to Cz and A2 to Cz, is then used. Mastoid electrodes can be used instead of ear electrodes; they tend to offer more stable recordings, since movement artifact is often seen with the ear electrodes. Filter settings typically used are 30 Hz to 3 kHz. If this filter setting incorporates significant artifact because of the operating room environment, the bandpass can be narrowed to 100 Hz to 2 kHz. Stimulation rates of 11 Hz are typically used in the outpatient setting. Higher stimulation rates up to 20 Hz have been successfully used to monitor BAEPs in the operating room. Higher stimulation rates are desirable in this modality, as typically 1,000 to 2,000 response must be averaged for a good signal-to-noise ratio.

Because wave V has the largest amplitude, it is the waveform that is easiest to monitor (Figure 14.4). The wave I latency may also be useful to monitor during surgeries that place the vestibulocochlear nerve at risk. However, since wave I has low amplitude, using the standard ear or mastoid electrode may not allow for clear localization of this waveform. In these instances, placing an electrode on the surgically exposed vestibulocochlear nerve (either a ring electrode or a wick electrode) may allow for clearer interpretation of wave I (5). This technique provides for more clear responses from the vestibulocochlear nerve as well as more rapid interpretation of changes.

Mechanisms of injury that may be associated with BAEP changes include stretch, compression, ischemia, and transection of the vestibulocochlear nerve (6). The typical warning criteria used for BAEP changes is a 1.0-ms or greater prolongation of latency or greater than 50% reduction of amplitude of the wave V if the recordings have been stable and reliable (6,7) (Figure 14.5). If wave V is present at the end of surgery, this is a very good indicator that hearing will be preserved (8).

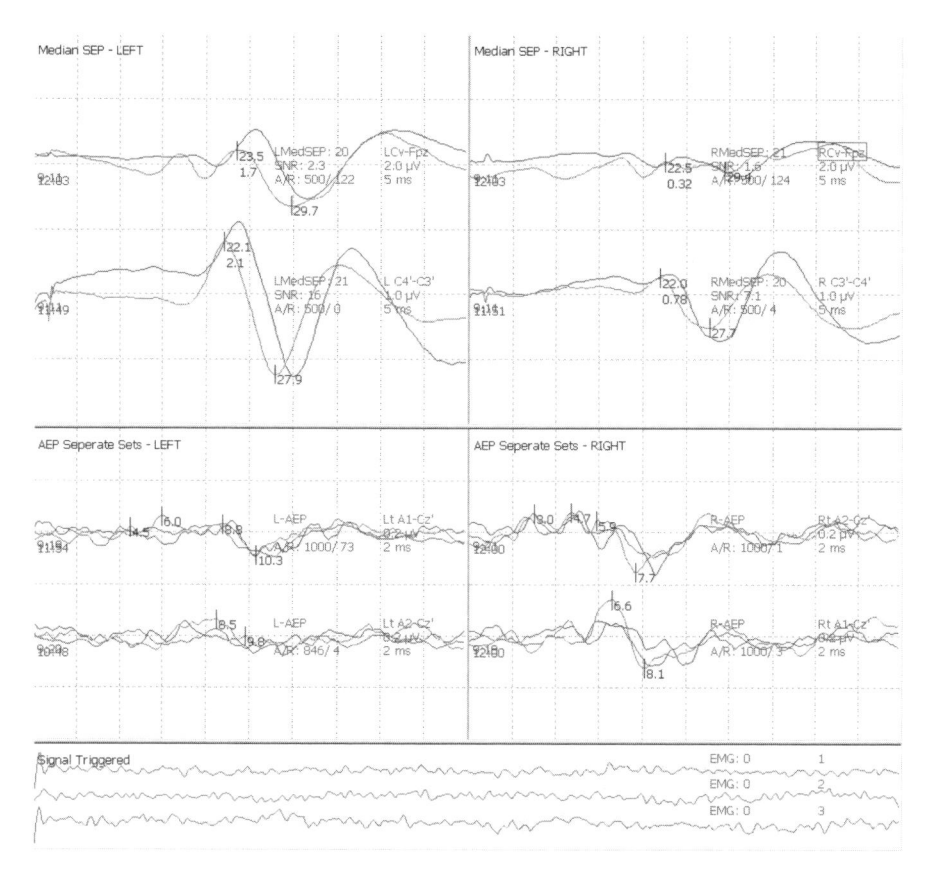

FIGURE 14.4 Multimodality monitoring (median nerve SEPs, BAEPs, and triggered EMGs) from a patient undergoing CPA tumor resection. This figure shows that in BAEP monitoring, wave V is clearly the easiest waveform to monitor. In this figure a prolongation of wave V latency obtained after stimulation of the left ear was seen from the beginning of surgery.

TECHNICAL CONSIDERATIONS

Preparation

Most important in preparing for a CPA tumor surgery is knowledge of the size of the tumor. Surgeries on large tumors can last more than 12 hours. In these situations, arrangements for relief of the primary NIOM technologist must be made so that he or she can take breaks. It is not reasonable to expect a single technologist to be present in the operating room for the whole duration of such a case.

Knowledge of the modalities to be monitored is important as that will determine which electrodes will be used. There may be laboratory protocols that dictate which modalities are monitored for various procedures. Even when such protocols are present, it behooves the NIOM team to confirm with the surgeon that additional monitoring will not be required. Sometimes, with very large tumors, monitoring of additional cranial nerves or other modalities may be requested. For most CPA tumor surgeries, at least BAEP and facial nerve monitoring will be needed. Median nerve SEP and trigeminal nerve monitoring may also be needed in special circumstances.

For facial and trigeminal nerve monitoring, EMG electrodes will be needed. They can be either surface of subcutaneous electrodes, both of which will capture discharges that emanate near to the location of the electrodes.

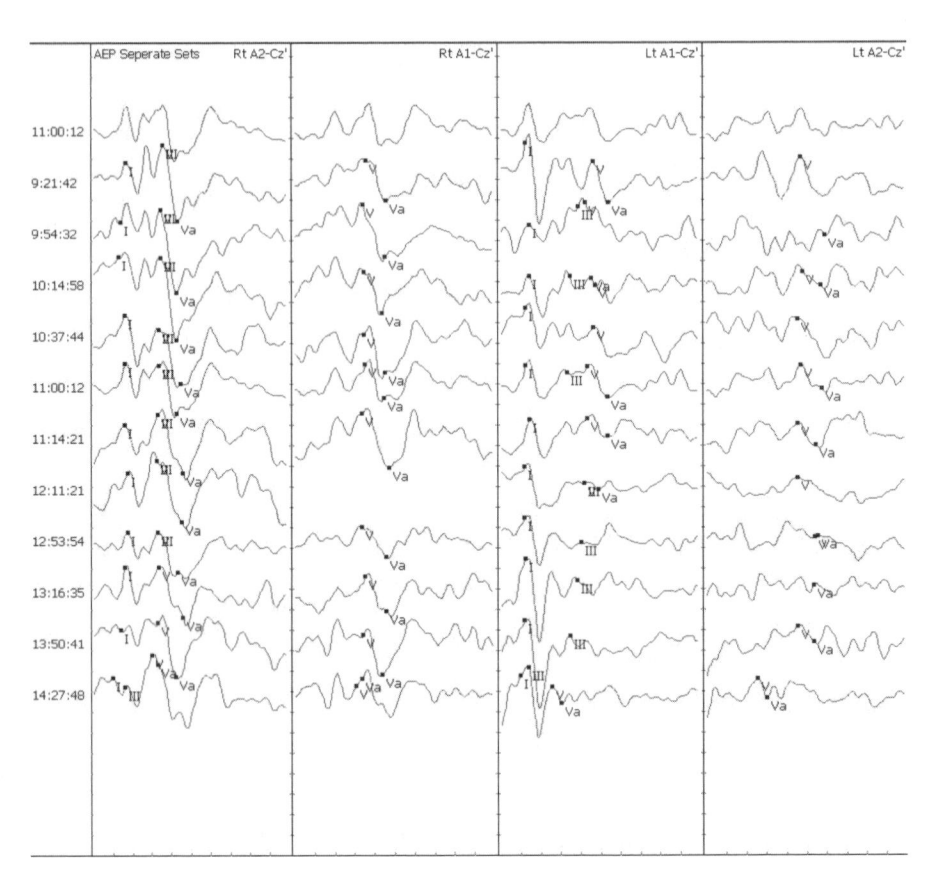

FIGURE 14.5 BAEP data from a 3-year-old girl undergoing resection of a laterally exophytic ganglioglioma arising from the lateral pons and medulla and extending into the left CPA. The surgeon debulked the tumor down to the level of the brainstem. Demarcation between tumor and brainstem was lost and dissection was continued until changes in the BAEPs with left ear stimulation were noted. At this point the tumor appeared to blend into normal brainstem and no further attempts at debulking were undertaken. In the BAEP waterfall, notice the initial significant loss of amplitude of wave V, which triggered the alert to the surgeon. By the end of the case, no wave V can be seen.

These electrodes will have trouble picking up discharges from the deep areas of the muscle. For purposes of recording deeper regions in the muscle, a concentric or monopolar needle electrode can be used. The size of the needle electrode is dependent on the depth and location of the muscle to be monitored; therefore, for most cranial nerve–innervated muscles, a small (10-mm, 0.3-mm diameter) stainless steel electrode is appropriate (2). Surface electrodes can give a quantitative measurement of amplitude of the activity recorded. Other types of electrodes which can work well in cranial nerve monitoring include malleable wire electrodes, in which a needle is used to insert the wire electrode, after which the needle can be removed. These electrodes produce stable and possibly more selective recordings with less movement artifact as well as producing less tissue injury.

BAEPs and median nerve SEPs are recorded with electroencephalography (EEG) electrodes. The technologist must make sure that enough EEG electrodes are available to do both BAEP and SEP monitoring. For short cases, the scalp electrodes can be applied with paste; however, for longer cases (such as those involving large CPA tumors), it is best to use collodion. An auditory stimulator with tubing extending to the external auditory canals will be needed. As noted earlier, this is differs from the headphones used to deliver the auditory stimulus in an outpatient setting. The latency of wave I will depend on the length of tubing used; however, in NIOM, this is not of major concern, as changes from baseline are more important than prolongation of peak waveforms. The ear plug at the end of the tubing must be securely inserted into the external auditory canal at the time of setup. The ear should then be sealed either with wax or Tegaderm. This prevents fluids from seeping into the external auditory canal and preventing adequate stimulation. Median nerves are stimulated at the wrist with either needle or surface electrodes. If needle electrodes are used, 1-cm needles work well. Disposable self-adhesive or reusable surface electrodes can also be used. Surface electrodes require higher stimulation intensity.

The NIOM technologist should also have a variety of handheld stimulating electrodes with which the surgeon can stimulate structures within the surgical field (i.e., the facial or trigeminal nerves). Handheld stimulators of various types are available and used intraoperatively based on certain factors such as size, location of the nerve, and ability to stimulate the nerve in isolation from surrounding tissue or fluid. The stimulation of cranial nerves typically requires small stimulators with tip exposures of 1 to 3 mm. This is to minimize the current spread that can occur with larger electrodes. Cranial nerve stimulators are best designed with a tip of 1 mm, as compared to the peripheral nerve stimulators with tips of 3 to 5 mm (6). The use of a bipolar stimulator allows for localized stimulus delivery, whereas monopolar stimulators increase the region of current spread, which also results in a larger stimulus artifact. There are various different shapes and sizes of nerve stimulators available commercially. Some are designed with hooks, which allow the nerve to be lifted away from the rest of the surgical field to minimize the possibility of shunting the stimulus. Lack of adequate stimulation can be tested by test-stimulating an exposed muscle. An excessive amount of fluid in the surgical field can cause shunting of the current, causing inadequate stimulation.

Obtaining baseline BAEP and median SEP responses the day before surgery can be very useful. When CPA tumors are very large, ipsilateral BAEP responses may be absent. If this is the case, when this response is not obtained in the operating room on the day of surgery, time does not have to be spent in troubleshooting. The preoperative baselines provide a guide to the technologist as to what to expect in the operating room.

The NIOM technologist should also try to meet the patient before the surgery and explain the role of the NIOM team. The patient must not be told that the NIOM team will prevent complications. Rather, it should be explained that NIOM helps alert the surgeon should complication may occur and helps decrease the probability of complications.

Procedure

At the start of the surgery, preferably before the incision is made, operative baselines for BAEPs (and median nerve SEPs) should be obtained. If preoperative baseline were obtained, the operative baselines should be compared to them to make certain that they are similar. Free-running EMG from facial (and trigeminal) nerve–innervated muscle should be viewed continuously. Throughout the case, except as noted below, BAEPs and free-running EMGs should be monitored. Modern NIOM machines allow BAEPs from both sides to be monitored independently and simultaneously in an interleaved manner. The EMG should be connected to a speaker, so that when EMG activity is present, it is not only seen but also heard. This will provide immediate auditory feedback to the surgeon as well.

When exposure is complete, the surgeon may request the nerve stimulator. During nerve stimulation, a triggered EMG program is most useful to monitor for CMAPs. A stimulation rate of 1 to 5 Hz, duration of 50 to 300 μs, and intensity of 0.5 to 4 mA (for constant current stimulators) or 3 to 15 V (for constant voltage stimulators) are used for cranial nerves. It has been suggested that by using constant voltage stimulation, the current that passes to the tissues is relatively resistant to electrical shunting by fluid in the operative field. Prior to stimulating the nerve of interest, a control nerve (one not involved in the pathology) should be stimulated to determine threshold of stimulation for a normal nerve. Once this is determined, this or an 0.5 mA increment in intensity can be used to search for nerves or nerve roots in the surgical field or within the tumor. Measurement of the stimulus threshold has been used to predict postoperative function. The typical stimulus intensity at which a healthy cranial nerve will produce a response is 0.5 mA or less. Higher thresholds may indicate some traction injury to the nerve, which may predict early postoperative deficits. It is not clear how these thresholds affect long-term functional status, however. A lack of a triggered CMAP to direct nerve stimulation is a poor prognostic finding.

Since the purpose of monitoring is to preserve all branches of the facial nerve, two groups of muscles innervated by two major branches of the facial nerve should be monitored. This can be accomplished by individually monitoring the mentalis/orbicularis oris and frontalis/orbicularis oculi muscle groups. With this montage, triggered responses can be individually recorded from muscles innervated by two major branches of the facial nerve. Monitoring the masseter muscle will differentiate when the motor part of trigeminal nerve is stimulated. At times, stimulation of the trigeminal nerve will result in CMAPs recorded from facial nerve–innervated muscles; this is due to volume conduction of the CMAP to these muscles (Figure 14.6). Such a volume-conducted response can easily be identified if the massester muscle is also being monitored. Another differentiating point is that stimulation of the trigeminal nerve gives rise to a CMAP at a latency of about 2 to 3 ms, whereas the latency of a CMAP obtained from facial nerve stimulation is about 5 ms.

It is also important to remember that cold irrigation can give risk to muscle activity that may be sustained for several seconds. Spontaneous activity seen with cold irrigation has not been associated with a functional deterioration of the nerve. However, fluids above the normal body temperature can pose risk to the nerve.

During periods when electrocautery, microscope, and head lamps are being used, significant noise is produced, so that EMG recordings may be obscured. An electronic circuit can be used to suppress the electrical artifact when EMG recordings are being made by means of a pulse generator, allowing the amplifier to be grounded during periods of stimulation. This allows for frequent use of electrocautery and direct nerve stimulation without large stimulation artifacts being displayed. It also prevents the loud audible artifact from being transmitted, which can be annoying in the surgical environment. BAEPs are difficult to average when the surgeon is drilling bone during exposure. There is considerable artifact produced, which prevents BAEP averaging. It is best to pause BAEP averaging during drill use. Similarly, during heavy electrocautery use, BAEP averaging should be paused. If averaging is not stopped during these times, the artifact contamination may give the appearance that BAEP responses have been lost; this would raise a false-positive surgical alarm.

BAEP and EMG recordings are quite robust to anesthetic influence. However, EMG recordings are influenced by the degree of neuromuscular blockade being used in the surgery. Recordings can be made using short-acting neuromuscular blocking agents that provide partial blockade, so that two out of a train of

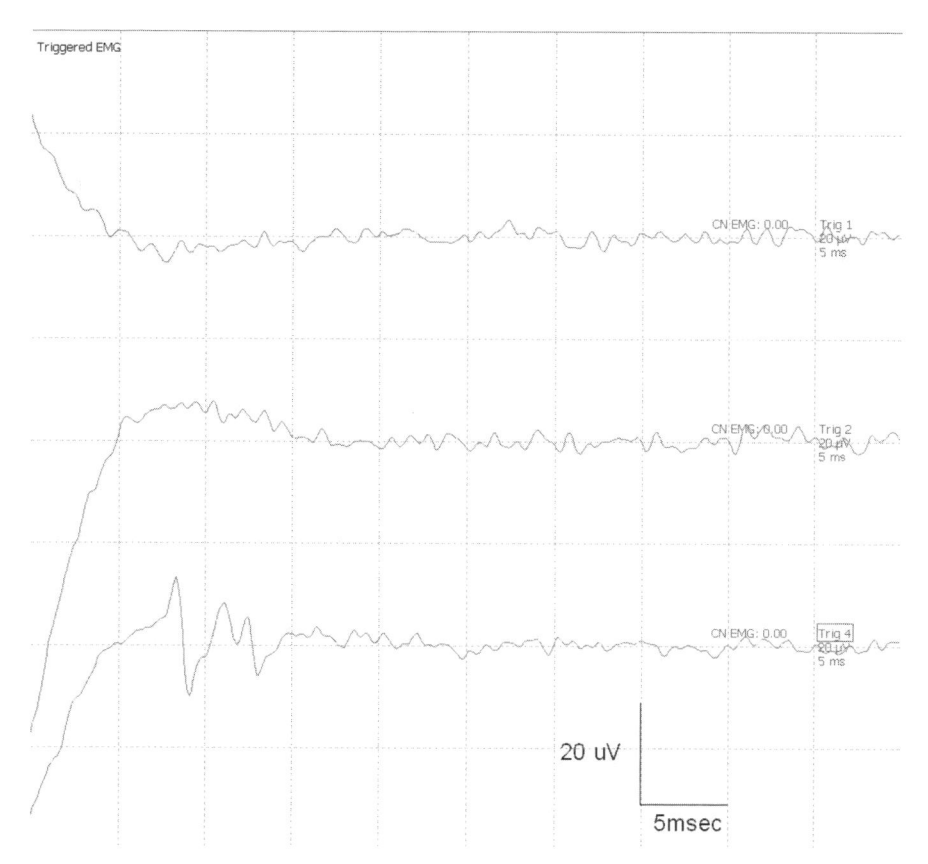

FIGURE 14.6 A triggered EMG response to direct nerve stimulation. The three muscles groups shown from top to bottom are orbicularis oculi, masseter, and orbicularis oris. The triggered EMG response is seen at 5 ms only in the orbicularis oris muscle, indicating that the nerve stimulated is a branch of the facial nerve. This case highlights the importance in monitoring two groups of facial muscles, as monitoring of only the orbicularis oculi muscle group would have led to a false-negative stimulation response.

four twitches are present. It is important that the muscle being used to record twitches is a cranial nerve–innervated muscle such as the orbicularis oculi, as the degree of blockade can differ based on the muscle being used to test the blockade. Ideally, avoiding the use of neuromuscular blocking agents is preferable when facial EMG is being monitored.

As noted previously, another method of monitoring the proximal vestibulocochlear nerve (BAEP wave I) is to place an electrode directly on the exposed nerve. Since the vestibulocochlear nerve is located underneath the CPA tumor, it is often not easy to place an electrode directly on the nerve. In some centers a transtympanic electrode is placed in order to record the cochlear microphonic and nerve action potential. This type of monitoring can determine whether cochlear vascular supply is being compromised. It is not capable of detecting more proximal lesions. Additionally, this type of electrode must be placed and secured by the surgeon. Consequently, BAEP monitoring is often used instead.

Postprocedure

NIOM should be continued until the end of surgery, until the skin has been closed. Once the surgery is completed, the NIOM technologist must quickly remove all electrodes before the patient wakes up from anesthesia. The needle electrodes placed in the facial muscles must be carefully removed so as not to leave hematomas. Disposable electrodes must be appropriately discarded (i.e., in sharps container if needles) and reuseable ones cleaned.

If possible, it is best for the NIOM technologist to wait until the patient has woken up from anesthesia to test neurologic functions that were monitored. In particular, facial movement should be checked to see if a facial palsy is present. Additionally, bedside testing of auditory function is also important. If deficits are noted, additional follow-up testing with EP, audiologic, or EMG testing may be warranted.

CONCLUSIONS

With improvements in neuroimaging, microsurgery, and cranial nerve NIOM, there have been extraordinary improvements in patient outcomes following CPA tumor surgeries. Up to 90% of patients have normal or near normal facial nerve function and 40% have preserved hearing after these surgeries. However, in spite of these great advances, a significant number of patients still develop postoperative cranial nerve dysfunction. Consequently there is still a need to improve operative technique and further refine NIOM protocols. Integral to the success NIOM during CPA tumor surgery is the experience of the surgical and NIOM team. The rapid and clear communication of NIOM findings is crucial to the early identification of a potential surgical injury. Only then can corrective surgical measures can be undertaken.

REFERENCES

1. Harner SG, Daube JR, Ebersold MJ, Beatty CW. Improved preservation of facial nerve function with use of electrical monitoring during removal of acoustic neuromas. *Mayo Clin Proc* 1987;62:92–102.
2. Harper CM. Intraoperative cranial nerve monitoring. *Muscle Nerve* 2004;29:339–351.
3. Stechison MT, Kralick FJ. The trigeminal evoked potential: Part I. Long-latency responses in awake or anesthetized subjects. *Neurosurgery* 1993;33:633–638.
4. Harner SG, Daube JR, Ebersold MJ. Electrophysiologic monitoring of facial nerve during temporal bone surgery. *Laryngoscope* 1986;96:65–69.
5. Moller AR, Jannetta PJ. Monitoring auditory functions during cranial nerve microvascular decompression operations by direct recording from the eighth nerve. *J Neurosurg* 1983;59: 493–499.
6. Harper CM, Daube JR. Facial nerve electromyography and other cranial nerve monitoring. *J Clin Neurophysiol* 1998;15:206–216.
7. Moller AR. *Evoked Potentials in Intraoperative Monitoring.* Baltimore: Williams & Wilkins, 1988.
8. Tator CH, Nedzelski JM. Preservation of hearing in patients undergoing excision of acoustic neuromas and other cerebellopontine angle tumors. *J Neurosurg* 1985;63:168–174.

15 Thoracic Aortic Surgery

Aatif M. Husain
Kristine H. Ashton
G. Chad Hughes

Among all surgical procedures, morbidity associated with surgery of the thoracic aorta is among the highest, with complication rates of up to 30% to 40%. Although virtually every organ system is at risk during aortic surgery, the brain and spinal cord are particularly vulnerable because of their low tolerance for ischemia. This is particularly significant, as injury to the nervous system may result in remarkable long-term morbidity. Over the last 50 years, many advances have helped reduce the morbidity of thoracic aortic surgery; among these is neurophysiologic intraoperative monitoring (NIOM). NIOM has been used increasingly in thoracic aortic surgery in an attempt to decrease neurologic morbidity.

Surgery on the ascending aorta and aortic arch frequently involves temporary suspension of blood flow in the cerebral vessels, whereas descending aortic surgery may be complicated by ischemia of not only the spinal cord but also the brain. Consequently NIOM may be useful during all types of thoracic aortic surgery. However, since different parts of the nervous system are at risk with different procedures, it is important to understand aortic anatomy as well as the procedure being performed in order to design the most appropriate NIOM paradigm. In this chapter, after a short overview of relevant anatomy, a brief description of the common thoracic aortic diseases and their surgical treatment is presented. Thereafter, various NIOM modalities commonly used during thoracic aortic surgery are discussed, followed by a review of available data regarding their utility.

CLINICAL ANATOMY

The aorta arises from the left ventricular outflow tract at the level of the aortic annulus and terminates where it divides into two common iliac arteries in the pelvis. The initial part of the aorta, called the aortic root, contains the aortic annulus and valve leaflets, the sinuses of Valsalva, and the origins of the left and right coronary arteries. Contiguous to the aortic root is the tubular ascending aorta, which begins at the sinotubular junction and ascends posterolaterally, forming the aortic arch. From right to left, the brachiocephalic (innominate), left common carotid, and left subclavian arteries arise directly from the arch. The brachiocephalic artery ascends and divides into the right common carotid and right subclavian arteries.

Distal to the left subclavian artery, the aorta progresses inferiorly to form the descending thoracic aorta. Once the descending thoracic aorta passes through the aortic hiatus in the diaphragm, it becomes the abdominal aorta. Together the thoracic and abdominal aortas are called the thoracoabdominal aorta. From the descending thoracic aorta arise esophageal, bronchial, and intercostal arteries. From the intercostal arteries arise radicular arteries that supply blood to the spinal cord. They are discussed below in relation to the blood supply of the spinal cord. The most important of the radicular arteries is the arteria radicularis magna (ARM), also known as the artery of Adamkiewicz. The ARM usually arises from a left-sided intercostal artery between the T8 and L2 levels and is responsible for supplying the lower part of the anterior spinal cord (see below).

The abdominal aorta provides the blood supply to the abdominal viscera. Branches of the abdominal aorta include (in order) the inferior phrenic, celiac, superior mesenteric, renal, gonadal, lumbar, inferior mesenteric, and the median sacral arteries. The abdominal aorta terminates at the L4 level by bifurcating into the left and right common iliac arteries. Usually, branches of the abdominal aorta do not contribute significantly to the blood supply of the spinal cord, although lumbar collaterals are important in some patients. The surgical obliteration of these lumbar collaterals during replacement of the infrarenal aorta accounts for the subsequent increased risk of spinal cord complications following descending thoracic aortic surgery in patients who have undergone abdominal aortic aneurysm repair (1).

Knowledge of the blood supply of the spinal cord is vital to understanding the mechanisms by which aortic surgery may result in neurologic morbidity. The spinal cord is supplied by single anterior and paired posterior spinal arteries. The anterior spinal artery is formed by the union of the left and right anterior spinal branches that arise from the vertebral arteries. The anterior spinal artery runs the entire length of the spinal cord in the midline, supplying the anterior two thirds (including the corticospinal tracts) of the cord.

Anterior radicular arteries supplement the blood supply to the anterior spinal artery throughout its length. In the embryo, there are left and right anterior radicular arteries corresponding to each vertebral segmental level; however, at birth, only two to eight of these radicular arteries remain. Two or three of these anterior radicular arteries arise from the subclavian arteries and supply the cervical portion of the spinal cord. Only one to three anterior radicular arteries arise from the intercostal arteries of the descending thoracic aorta and supply the corresponding segments of the spinal cord. Consequently, the midthoracic spinal cord is most vulnerable to ischemia. The lower part of the thoracic and lumbosacral spinal cord is supplied by a large radicular artery that usually arises from a left intercostal artery between segmental levels T8 and L2. The anterior branch of this important artery, the ARM, supplies up to 70% of the blood supply of the anterior spinal artery and is primarily responsible for perfusing the lumbar enlargement of the spinal cord.

The posterior spinal arteries are a paired group of arteries descending along the posterolateral aspect of the spinal cord, although at times they become discontinuous. These arteries arise from the vertebral arteries and supply the posterior one third of the spinal cord. Posterior radicular arteries supplement blood supply to the posterior spinal arteries and are more numerous than their anterior counterparts. In the cervical region, each level has one or two such arteries, while in the thoracic and lower levels, there is one posterior radicular artery at every other level.

There is a rich anastomotic network between the two posterior spinal arteries and the anterior spinal artery. When there is impaired perfusion in watershed zones of the anterior spinal artery, these anastomoses become important. Patients with chronic diseases of the thoracic aorta—such as atherosclerotic aneurysms, which restrict blood supply to the intercostal arteries via chronic occlusion—frequently develop collaterals via the lumbar arteries and other branches of the abdominal aorta to supply the anterior and posterior spinal arteries. Thus, in these patients, maintaining perfusion of the distal abdominal aorta during aortic cross-clamping is important in preventing spinal cord ischemia.

Much as in the brain, blood flow in the spinal cord is autoregulated when the perfusion pressure is between 50 and 150 mmHg above cerebrospinal fluid (CSF) pressure. When the pressure falls below this level, autoregulation is impaired and ischemia may result. Consequently, increasing blood pressure and reducing spinal fluid pressure are potentially therapeutic measures that can be implemented to minimize ischemia. As discussed later, these measures are often used during thoracic aortic surgery when the spinal cord is deemed to be ischemic based on NIOM.

THORACIC AORTIC DISEASES

Aneurysm and dissection are the commonest aortic diseases requiring surgical treatment. Other conditions such as tumors are rare and are not discussed in detail. The particulars of these conditions can be found in standard surgical texts; only a brief overview is presented here (2).

Aneurysmal Disease

An aortic aneurysm is a dilatation of the aorta beyond 50% of its normal diameter. Such dilatations occur for many reasons, but all have in common weakening of the aortic wall. Common etiologies include connective tissue disorders such as Marfan's syndrome or Ehlers-Danlos type IV disease. Hypertension, smoking, advanced age, aortic dissection, and atherosclerosis can also result in aneurysm formation. Aortic aneurysms are classified based on their extent and location. In general, aneurysms may be designated as fusiform or saccular. Fusiform aneurysms are the most common and represent a uniform dilation of the entire aortic segment. Saccular aneurysms, on the other hand, are aneurysms confined to one wall of the aorta and likely are the sequelae of a localized disease process of the aortic wall, most commonly a preexisting penetrating atherosclerotic ulcer. Saccular aneurysms are important surgically, as they are generally felt to pose a higher risk of rupture than fusiform aneurysms and are usually subjected to surgery at smaller sizes. No formal classification system exists for aneurysms of the ascending aorta, although different patterns clearly exist. For example, some aneurysms, typically those due to hypertension and atherosclerosis, involve only the tubular ascending aorta above the sinotubular junction, for which repair involves replacement of the supracoronary ascending aorta alone with sparing of the aortic root (Figure 15.1). Other ascending aneurysms, such as those seen in patients with the Marfan's syndrome, may involve the aortic root (sinus of Valsalva segment) and require formal aortic root replacement, including replacement of the aortic

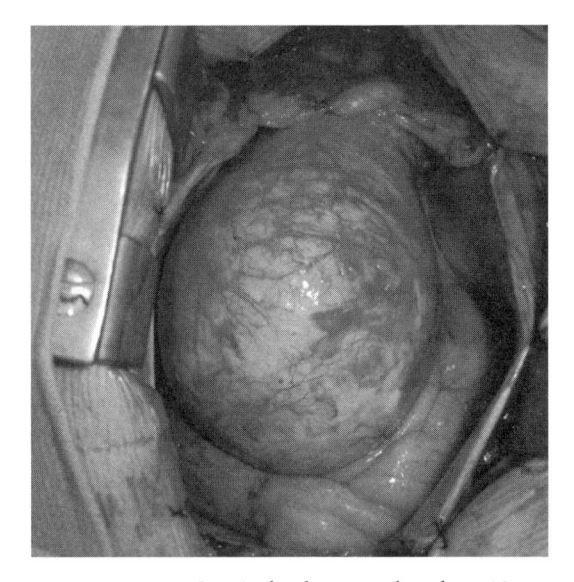

FIGURE 15.1 Surgical photograph of a 10-cm fusiform ascending aortic aneurysm. This aneurysm involved the tubular ascending aorta and proximal aortic arch. Repair involved replacement of the supracoronary ascending aorta and proximal arch using DHCA.

valve and coronary button reimplantation (Bentall procedure). Likewise, aneurysms of the transverse arch do not have their own classification scheme. Fusiform arch aneurysms are rarely found in isolation and usually coexist with either ascending or descending aneurysms or both as part of the "mega-aorta syndrome." A diagrammatic representation of the Crawford classification system for thoracoabdominal aortic aneurysms, which involve both the thoracic and abdominal aorta, is presented in Figure 15.2 and ranges from extent I to extent V (2). Likewise, descending thoracic aortic aneurysms limited to the chest can be classified based on their location and include types A to C (2) (Figure 15.3).

The clinical presentation of thoracic and thoracoabdominal aortic aneurysms can vary widely. Most often they are silent and detected incidentally (2). Nonspecific back pain is the most common symptom with aneurysms of the descending thoracic and thoracoabdominal aorta; however, this complaint is common and frequently difficult to differentiate from other more benign conditions. Aneurysms of the ascending aorta and arch may present with anterior chest pain. When an aneurysm becomes large enough to compress adjacent structures, other symptoms may occur. Examples include dyspnea due to compression of the bronchi, dysphagia from compression of the esophagus, and hoarseness from stretch injury to the recurrent laryngeal nerve. A fistula from the aorta to the airway or esophagus may occur, causing hemorrhage.

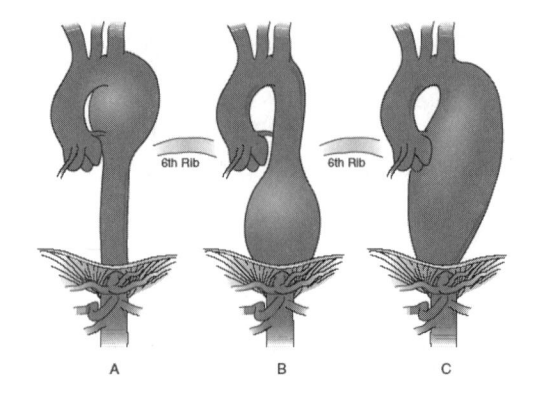

FIGURE 15.3 Diagram of the classification of aneurysms limited to the descending thoracic aorta. Type A is distal to the left subclavian artery to the sixth intercostal space; type B is from the sixth intercostal space to the diaphragm; and type C is distal to left subclavian artery to the diaphragm. [Reproduced with permission from Huynh et al. (2).]

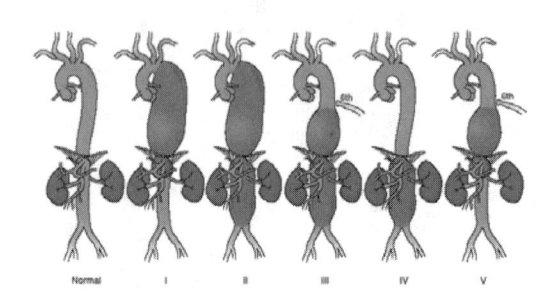

FIGURE 15.2 Diagram of the Crawford classification of thoracoabdominal aortic aneurysms. Extent I is distal to left subclavian artery to above renal arteries; extent II is distal to left subclavian artery to below the renal arteries; extent III extends from distal to the sixth intercostal space to below the renal arteries; extent IV extends from the twelfth intercostal space to below the renal arteries; and extent V is from distal to the sixth intercostal space to above the renal arteries. [Reproduced with permission from Huynh et al. (2).]

The decision to operate on thoracic and thoracoabdominal aneurysms involves weighing the risks of the procedure against the natural history of the underlying disease. Untreated, most thoracic aortic aneurysms will rupture. The risk of rupture is proportional to the size of the aneurysm and the underlying disease. Although many considerations go into the decision to operate, as a general rule, fusiform aneurysms 5 to 6 cm or greater are often considered for surgical repair. For saccular aneurysms, a protrusion of greater than 2 cm beyond the aortic wall for the saccular component is usually considered an indication for treatment in the absence of symptoms.

However, in patients with connective tissue diseases and those with symptomatic or rapidly expanding aneurysms, surgery on smaller aneurysms is often considered.

Aortic Dissection

Dissection of the layers of the aortic wall most often occurs due to a primary tear in the intima. This allows passage of blood between the layers of the wall, usually in the outer media; if the dissection ruptures back into the aortic lumen downstream, a false lumen is created within the wall of the aorta. Dissection can lead to progressive dilatation, aneurysm formation, and ultimately rupture. In addition, flow in the pressurized false lumen may compromise aortic branch vessel flow via compression of the true lumen feeding the branch vessel. Alternatively, the dissection may directly extend into the branch vessel, causing a reduction or cessation in flow. Either situation may result in ischemia of the end organ supplied by the vessel (malperfusion syndrome). Many of the same underlying conditions, such as hypertension and atherosclerosis, which predispose to aneurysm formation, can also lead to dissection. Dissections are classified based on the time from symptom onset and location. Within 14 days of the onset of symptoms, the dissection is classified as acute, whereas it is considered chronic thereafter.

Two systems of classification for aortic dissections are commonly used, DeBakey and Stanford (3) (Figure 15.4). Both are based on the segment of aorta involved and not the location of the primary tear. For example, a primary tear in the descending thoracic aorta with retrograde involvement of the ascending aorta is considered a Stanford type A dissection.

Aortic dissections most often present with sudden, severe pain, often described as tearing, although the spectrum of symptoms is quite varied and clinicians must remain vigilant for the protean signs and symptoms. The pain is frequently interscapular and radiates downward when the dissection involves the descending aorta. Dissection of the ascending aorta most often causes anterior chest pain; if it involves the aortic valve, with the subsequent acute onset of aortic insufficiency, it can also cause dyspnea or other symptoms of congestive heart failure. Stroke, paraplegia, syncope, myocardial ischemia, mesenteric ischemia, ischemic peripheral neuropathy, and renal failure can also occur, depending on which aortic branches are affected by the dissection (malperfusion syndrome). Patients surviving beyond the first 2 weeks are classified as having chronic dissections. Dissections that do not present with acute symptoms are frequently not detected until the chronic phase.

Acute type A dissections are considered surgical emergencies and require immediate surgical repair. However, exceptions to this rule occasionally exist, most frequently in the setting of a large concomitant stroke due to

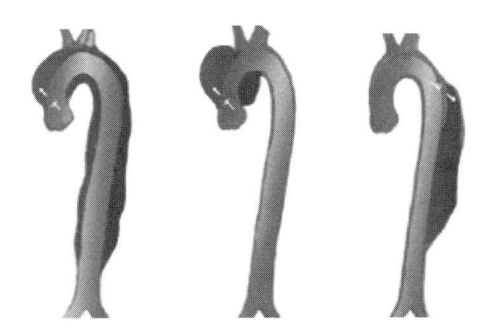

DeBakey I	DeBakey II	DeBakey III
Type A		Type B

FIGURE 15.4 Diagram of the DeBakey and Stanford classification systems for aortic dissection. DeBakey I involves dissection of the ascending aorta and extends to at least the arch and often beyond; in DeBakey II, the dissection is limited to the ascending aorta; and in DeBakey III the dissection involves the descending aorta and extends distally. Stanford Type A includes DeBakey I and II, and Stanford Type B is the same as DeBakey III. [Text reproduced with permission from Heuser (3).]

cerebral malperfusion, when surgical delay may be prudent if feasible. When type B dissections are associated with frank or impending rupture or end organ impairment (i.e., mesenteric ischemia, renal impairment, peripheral vascular compromise, etc.), they too must undergo immediate surgical treatment. Uncomplicated type B dissections, on the other hand, can be managed conservatively with antihypertensive medications. However, the extent of the dissection must be monitored closely, and the formation of an aneurysm or extension of the dissection may necessitate surgical intervention. The latter management strategy generally applies to chronic dissections as well.

SURGICAL TREATMENT

There are many different surgical procedures used for repair of aortic pathology; a review of all of them is beyond the scope of this chapter. The reader is referred to excellent texts on this subject (2). The purpose of the short review presented below is to acquaint the reader with some of the general principles of surgical repair of various segments of the aorta and how these procedures can cause neurologic morbidity.

Surgery on the Ascending Aorta and Aortic Arch

Surgery for aneurysm or dissection of the ascending aorta, especially when there is extension into the aortic arch, most commonly involves the open distal anastomosis technique. A dry surgical field affords the surgeon a clear view of the diseased aorta and allows a complete assessment of the extent of pathology so as to construct an adequate repair. For this, cardiopulmonary bypass (CPB) with deep hypothermia is instituted, followed by circulatory arrest. When adequate cooling has been achieved (see below), the distal ascending aorta or arch is opened during a period of temporary cessation of blood flow to the body and brain (circulatory arrest). Depending on the procedure to be performed, repair is carried out using Dacron grafts to replace the diseased segments of aorta (Figure 15.5). In general, adjunctive cerebral perfusion is carried out during the period of repair, while the remainder of the body, which has a greater tolerance to cold ischemia, is not perfused.

Neurologic morbidity in ascending aortic and arch procedures is generally due to cerebral ischemia. Because of the mandatory period of circulatory arrest, cerebral perfusion is impaired. Cerebral protection is provided by using deep hypothermic circulatory arrest (DHCA); the core body temperature is reduced to about 15°C, although one should not think of cooling to a specific temperature but rather to a physiologic endpoint indicative of maximal cerebral metabolic suppression, as

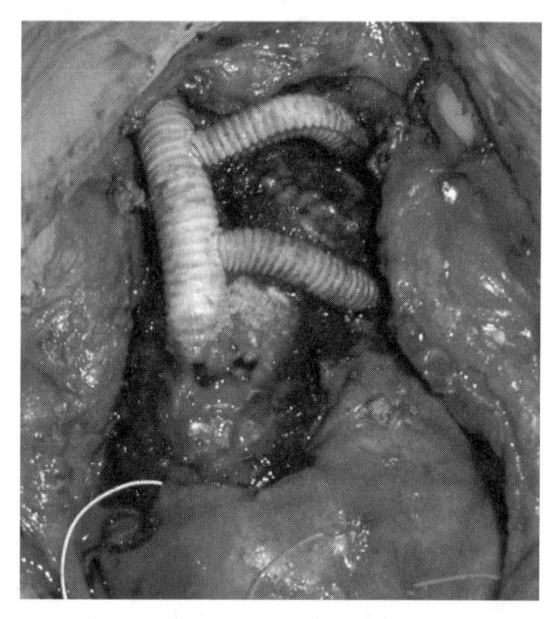

FIGURE 15.5 Surgical photograph of an ascending aorta and transverse arch aneurysm repaired with multiple Dacron grafts. The three-branched graft includes limbs to the left subclavian, left common carotid, and brachiocephalic arteries. This graft is anastomosed to the larger graft used to replace the ascending aorta and arch.

discussed below. This reduction in cerebral metabolism reduces the need for oxygenation and perfusion and provides time for safe repair to be carried out. Moreover, cerebral blood flow can be maintained despite circulatory arrest by providing retrograde cerebral perfusion through the superior vena cava or antegrade perfusion via the right axillary artery with a clamp on the proximal brachiocephalic and left common carotid arteries such that the left brain is supplied via an intact circle of Willis (4) (Figure 15.6). Alternatively, cerebral flow may be provided via cannulas placed directly into the ostia of the brachiocephalic and left common carotid arteries. These adjuncts to DHCA further reduce the potential for ischemic/hypoxic cerebral injury.

Surgery on the Descending Thoracic and Thoracoabdominal Aorta

Conventional open surgery on the descending aorta carries the potential for some of the highest morbidity in all of cardiovascular surgery. The chest cavity is opened via a lateral thoracotomy. The left lung is collapsed and ventilation continued to the right lung via a dual-lumen endotracheal tube. Historically, descending thoracic aortic repair involved the "clamp and sew" technique, whereby the aorta is clamped proximal and distal to the segment being replaced and a Dacron graft is sewn in proximally and distally while the aorta distal to the clamp is not perfused. Owing to the high complication rates reported with this method, it has generally fallen out of favor. Currently, descending aortic pathology is repaired using either distal aortic perfusion or DHCA. With the distal aortic perfusion technique, partial left heart bypass is instituted via cannulation of the left atrium in the chest for return of part of the oxygenated pulmonary venous effluent to the CPB pump (also known as the heart-lung machine), whereby it is pumped to the distal aorta or left femoral artery to supply the aorta distal to the clamp (5) (Figure 15.7). The pump, in addition to oxygenating the blood, serves as a heat exchanger and can cool or rewarm arterial inflow. With this technique, the heart supplies oxygenated blood to the aorta proximal to the cross clamp, whereas the pump supplies the distal aorta. The aortic cross clamp is then moved distally following each anastomosis (proximal aorta, intercostal patch, mesenteric segment, distal aorta), such that the pump provides less and less of the distal perfusion until the distal anastomosis is complete and the heart resumes the entire burden of the circulation.

Alternatively, the right atrium may be cannulated via the left femoral vein for pump

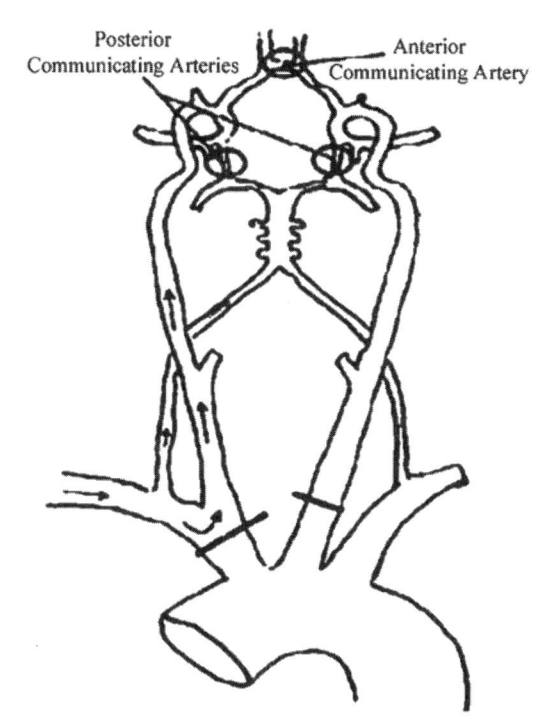

FIGURE 15.6 Diagram demonstrating antegrade cerebral perfusion via the right axillary artery during circulatory arrest. Cerebral blood flow is provided from the right axillary artery to the right common carotid and right vertebral arteries with cross filling to the left hemisphere via an intact circle of Willis. The proximal brachiocephalic and left common carotid arteries are clamped during the period of antegrade cerebral perfusion such that flow is provided only to the brain. [Reproduced with permission from Karadeniz et al. (4).]

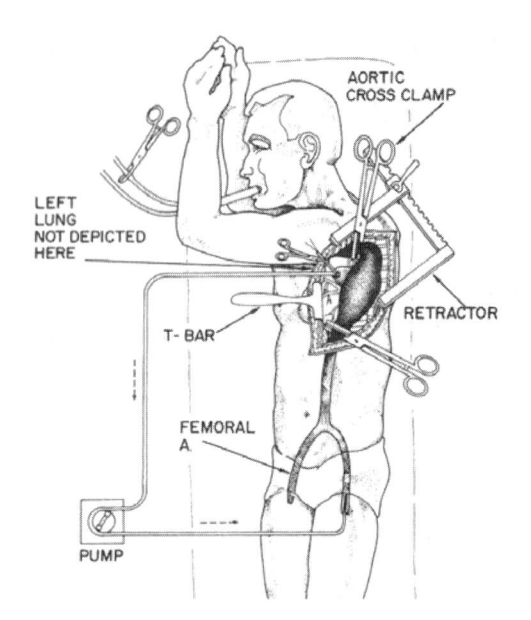

FIGURE 15.7 Diagram of the partial left heart bypass technique (left atrium to left femoral artery bypass) used for open descending thoracic aortic surgery. A portion of the pulmonary venous return to the heart is pumped from the left atrium to the femoral artery to supply the aorta distal to the distal cross clamp. [Reproduced with permission from Kern and Kron (5).]

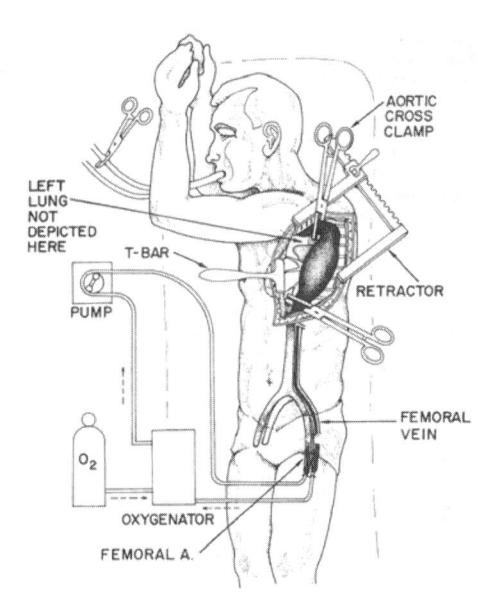

FIGURE 15.8 Diagram of the full CPB technique (right atrium via left femoral vein to left femoral artery bypass) used for open descending thoracic aortic surgery. Although not depicted in the drawing, the proximal anastomosis is typically performed in an open fashion, without the need for proximal cross clamping, under a brief period of DHCA. After completion of this proximal anastomosis, flow to the brain and upper body is resumed via cannulation of the proximal graft (not depicted) with a clamp placed distal to the inflow cannula. The distal anastomoses may then be performed during the period of rewarming, either with or without distal aortic perfusion. As mentioned in the text, distal perfusion is frequently unnecessary due to the prolonged period of protection of the spinal cord and viscera afforded by the use of hypothermia. [Reproduced with permission from Kern and Kron (5).]

inflow. With the DHCA technique, the right atrium via the left femoral vein is cannulated for venous return to the heart-lung machine and arterial inflow of oxygenated blood from the pump is returned to the patient, usually via the left femoral artery (5) (Figure 15.8). The patient is then placed on full CPB, such that the pump supports the entire circulation, and the patient is cooled for DHCA as described for ascending aortic surgery. When adequate cooling has been achieved, an open proximal anastomosis is performed under a brief period of circulatory arrest. The graft is then cannulated just distal to this proximal anastomosis and clamped distal to the cannula; then flow to the head and upper body is resumed (Figure 15.9). The distal anastomoses are then performed as described for the partial left heart bypass technique, either with or without distal aortic perfusion via the left femoral artery. Owing to the protection of the visceral organs (gut, liver, kidneys, etc.) provided by the hypothermia, distal perfusion is frequently unnecessary and each anastomosis may be performed in an open manner. As mentioned, an attempt is generally made to reimplant any large intercostal arteries, if patent, into the new Dacron graft. This is particularly important between the T8 to L2 levels as the ARM is in this location.

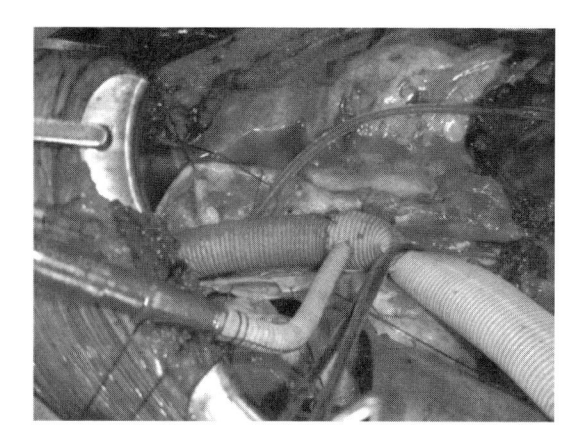

FIGURE 15.9 Surgical photograph of an open thoracoabdominal aortic aneurysm repair in a patient who had previously undergone total arch replacement with an "elephant trunk" procedure. The proximal graft (seen on the left in the photograph) is the elephant trunk graft, which was attached proximally in the arch with the distal end left hanging in the descending thoracic aorta at the original arch operation. At this second-stage repair, the graft used for replacement of the thoracoabdominal aorta (seen on the right in the photograph) has been anastomosed to the elephant trunk graft under a brief period of DHCA, as described in the text. The graft is then clamped distal to the side branch, providing inflow from the pump to reperfuse the brain and upper body. The distal anastomoses, including the intercostals and mesenteric segment, will be performed in an open fashion while the patient is being rewarmed. The clamp will be sequentially moved distally following each anastomosis to reperfuse each vascular bed after it has been reimplanted into the thoracoabdominal graft.

Cross clamping of the aorta results in a reduction of spinal perfusion pressure and an increase in CSF pressure. This may produce ischemia of the spinal cord, increasing the risk of paraplegia/paraparesis, the major neurologic morbidity of descending thoracic and thoracoabdominal aortic repair. This risk may potentially be mitigated by using distal aortic perfusion or DHCA in combination with CSF drainage via a lumbar CSF drain inserted prior to surgery. The CSF pressure is maintained below 10 to 12 mmHg. As mentioned above, the reimplantation of intercostal arteries may also be useful in maintaining spinal cord perfusion. Distal aortic perfusion using partial left heart bypass with mild hypothermia (32° to 34°C) preserves collateral flow to the spinal cord during the period of aortic cross clamping. The mild hypothermia provides additional protection via a reduction in spinal cord metabolism and oxygen demand, making it more tolerant of ischemia. In general, conventional open descending thoracic or thoracoabdominal repair in the current era should involve either partial left heart bypass or DHCA in conjunction with CSF drainage.(2) Exceptions may include emergent operations for rupture where there is insufficient time to allow implementation of these adjuncts or repair of extent IV thoracoabdominal aneurysms, which carry a low risk of paraplegia with clamp-and-sew techniques alone.

Endovascular Thoracic Aortic Repair

Because of the significant morbidity associated with conventional open repair, endovascular stent grafting procedures are being used more commonly for the treatment of aneurysms and dissections of the descending thoracic aorta. Although endovascular stent grafts (EVSG) are currently approved by the FDA only for the treatment of descending thoracic aortic aneurysms, in centers with expertise, there is frequent off-label use with application to the treatment of traumatic aortic transections; more extensive aneurysms, including those of the aortic arch and thoracoabdominal aorta; and acute and chronic descending aortic dissections (Figure 15.10). In a typical EVSG procedure, one femoral artery is surgically exposed through a small groin incision and cannulated with a large sheath through which the EVSG is introduced. The other femoral artery is cannulated percutaneously with a smaller sheath, which is used for introducing other catheters (i.e.,

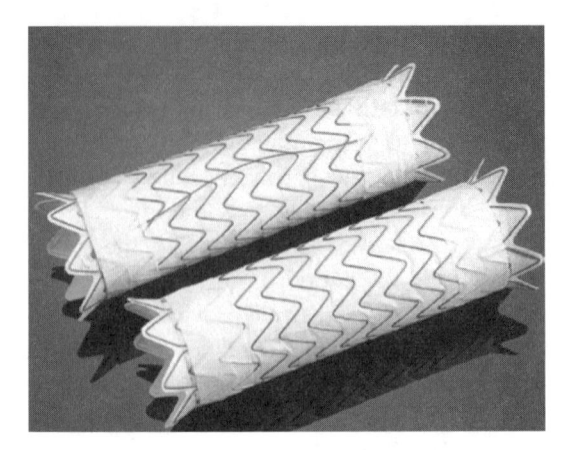

FIGURE 15.10 A picture of the Gore TAG EVSG (W. L. Gore and Associates, Flagstaff, AZ).

for radiologic contrast administration). A marker arteriogram is usually obtained to map the extent of pathology that will be treated and to determine adequacy of proximal and distal seal zones for the EVSG (6) (Figure 15.11A). The stent graft is then introduced through the large introducer sheath, correctly positioned, and deployed. In many patients more than one stent graft is needed to treat the entire aneurysm. After the EVSG is deployed, the seal zones are usually ballooned to facilitate seal to the outer aortic wall. A completion arteriogram is obtained to ensure complete exclusion of the aneurysm by the stent graft (Figure 15.11B). For routine procedures, the patient is typically extubated in the operating room.

In some patients, adequate seal zones are not present for conventional endovascular repair, yet EVSG seal could be obtained if the ostia of major aortic branch vessels were covered by the stent graft(s). If the patient is a suboptimal candidate for conventional open repair, a "hybrid procedure," which entails open surgical bypass of the artery or arteries to be covered by the EVSG followed by stent graft deployment across the ostia of the branch vessel(s), may be performed. Although still major surgery, these procedures avoid the need for CPB and aortic cross

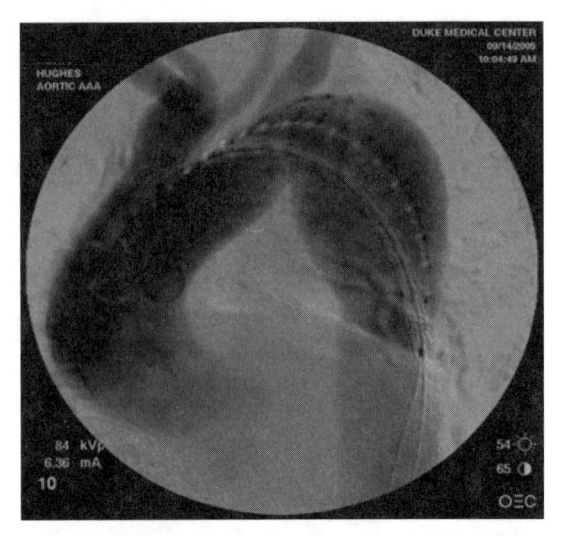

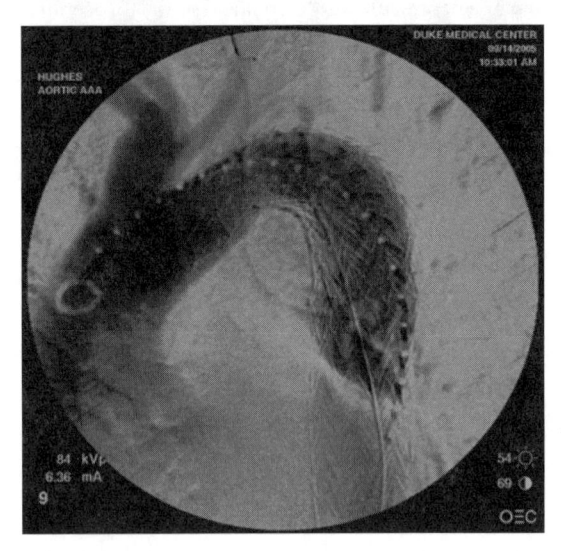

FIGURE 15.11 A. A marker arteriogram demonstrating a descending thoracic aortic aneurysm. B. A completion arteriogram, obtained after the aneurysm was treated with an EVSG, demonstrates complete exclusion of the aneurysm by the stent graft. Note that the left subclavian artery has been intentionally covered by the stent graft in this case. [Reproduced with permission from Husain (6).]

clamping and may be better tolerated by patients with multiple comorbidities. Proximally, these can involve bypass from right carotid to left carotid in the neck if the left common carotid artery is to be covered or may involve complete aortic arch debranching with bypass of both the brachiocephalic and left common carotid arteries from the ascending aorta if adequate proximal seal zone requires stent graft coverage of all of the arch vessels (7) (Figure 15.12). Coverage of the left subclavian artery alone is generally well tolerated by the majority of patients without the need for bypass. Similarly, debranching of the celiac axis, superior mesenteric artery, and renal arteries may be performed to allow EVSG treatment of thoracoabdominal aortic aneurysms.

Neurologic morbidity, particularly the risk of paraplegia, appears lower with EVSG repair of descending thoracic pathology as compared with conventional open repair (8). This is most likely because the aorta is not cross-clamped and blood pressure is well maintained throughout the procedure. However, adverse neurologic outcomes, including stroke and paraplegia, are still reported with these procedures. This may be due to covering of critical intercostal arteries with the stent graft, inadvertent positioning of the graft resulting in occlusion of critical vessels, or from dislodgement of emboli from the aorta by the catheters or guide wires. Spinal cord and brain ischemia, if either occurs, are most likely to begin during the time of graft deployment.

Cardiopulmonary Bypass

The CPB pump is commonly used in conventional open aortic surgery. By removing venous blood and reinfusing oxygenated arterial blood, the pump temporarily takes over function of the heart and lungs and fully supports the patient's circulation. It is important for NIOM personnel to become familiar with the CPB pump, as it can alter the patient's physiology and have a marked affect on NIOM.

The essential components of a CPB circuit include venous cannula(s) and reservoir, oxygenator, heat exchanger, roller pumps, blood filters, and arterial cannula(s). The circuitry is designed to cause minimal turbulence to blood flow so trauma to blood cells is minimized. There are numerous access points in this circuitry through which fluids and medications can be delivered or blood samples obtained for analysis. Oxygenated blood can also be cooled or rewarmed prior to being infused back into the patient. This is how patients are cooled and rewarmed before and after DHCA. Many CPB circuits incorporate other features, including a mechanism to collect and recycle shed blood from the surgical site. A separate pump is used to infuse a potassium-rich cardioplegia solution to the coronary arteries to protect the heart during induced cardiac arrest. Systemic heparinization is needed to prevent clotting of the CPB circuit.

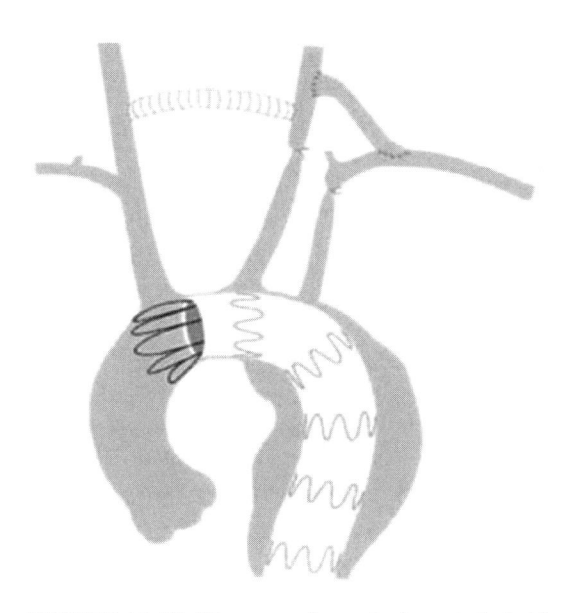

FIGURE 15.12 Diagram of a typical aortic hybrid EVSG procedure. The left common carotid and subclavian arteries have been "debranched" from the aortic arch via a bypass originating from the right common carotid artery, with a second bypass from the left common carotid to the left subclavian artery. This provides an adequate proximal seal zone for the EVSG for cases in which the aortic pathology extends to the origin of the left common carotid artery. [Reproduced with permission from Criado et al. (7).]

The venous cannula is typically inserted into the right atrium; occasionally the superior and inferior venae cavae are cannulated individually if it is necessary to divert all venous return from the heart (i.e., in surgery involving opening of the left or right atrium). The location of the arterial cannula depends on the site of surgery. In surgery of the ascending aorta or arch, the distal ascending aorta, right axillary artery, or femoral artery may be cannulated. Regardless of the cannulation site chosen, if antegrade cerebral perfusion is utilized for adjunctive cerebral protection during the period of DHCA, this may be accomplished by providing antegrade arterial flow to the brain via the brachiocephalic and, occasionally, left common carotid arteries, as described above. This may be performed most simply via initial cannulation of the right axillary artery for initiation of CPB. When adequate cooling has been achieved, antegrade cerebral perfusion is initiated via clamping of the innominate and left common carotid arteries, as described earlier. Alternatively, antegrade cerebral perfusion may be initiated by cannulating the brachiocephalic and left common carotid arteries directly, although this requires more cannulas in the surgical field and may carry an increased risk of stroke. If retrograde cerebral perfusion is used, the superior vena cava is cannulated and retrograde infusion of cold blood during the period of DHCA is carried out. Most authorities consider antegrade cerebral perfusion to be superior to retrograde perfusion for cerebral protection. For surgery of the descending or thoracoabdominal aorta requiring full CPB, the right atrium is typically cannulated via the left common femoral vein. Arterial cannulation in these cases is most often via the left femoral artery, although any uninvolved segment of the aorta may be used depending on the perfusion strategy to be utilized.

The CPB flow rate is adjusted depending on the oxygen requirement of the patient. With hypothermia, the oxygen requirement decreases and the flow rate can be reduced. The systemic blood pressure and distal aortic pressure can also be adjusted by manipulating the intravascular volume, administering vasoactive drugs (including inhalationalal and intravenous anesthetics), and changing the speed of the CPB pump. A basic knowledge of CPB physiology is important, as alterations in pump flow can profoundly affect the patient's hemodynamic status and consequently NIOM data.

NIOM PARADIGMS

The NIOM paradigm used depends on the site and type of aortic surgery that will be performed. Below is a description of the modalities that can be monitored, anesthetic considerations, and how they should be interpreted.

Ascending Aorta and Aortic Arch

Modalities to Monitor

Dissections and aneurysms involving the ascending aorta and arch are highly lethal conditions which often require urgent surgical repair. The neurologic morbidity of these procedures primarily relates to cerebral ischemia due to atheroemboli from the diseased aorta, direct involvement of the great vessels arising from the aortic arch in the disease process (i.e., dissection causing cerebral malperfusion) or from inadequate cerebral protection during DHCA. Although ischemia of any vascular bed may occur during CPB related to atheroemboli, regional vascular disease, or impaired autoregulation, the brain is particularly at risk during operations on the ascending aorta and arch.

As noted previously, several surgical innovations have greatly reduced the risk of cerebral ischemia during surgery on the ascending aorta and arch. Cerebral perfusion can be maintained during systemic circulatory arrest by continuing flow to the brain via the brachiocephalic and left common carotid arteries or superior vena cava. Additionally, the profound hypothermia used during DHCA significantly decreases cerebral metabolism to further help reduce neurologic morbidity. Provided adequate cooling such that maximal cerebral metabolic suppression has been achieved, DHCA alone with no cerebral adjunct safely allows up to 30 minutes of circulatory arrest time with a relatively low risk of neurologic injury. With antegrade cerebral perfusion this time may be extended even longer, although the actual safe duration of DHCA with antegrade cerebral perfusion is unknown.

The exact temperature at which DHCA should be instituted remains a topic of debate. Although both nasopharyngeal and core temperatures are measured during surgery, neither is an accurate reflection of brain temperature. Inadequate cooling prior to the institution of circulatory arrest can cause obvious complications; however, excessive cooling may lead to denaturation of cellular proteins, also potentially leading to deleterious effects. Consequently, a major use for NIOM in thoracic aortic procedures requiring DHCA is to serve as a "brain thermometer" to guide the surgical team as to when it is safe to institute circulatory arrest.

Electroencephalography (EEG) has been used most often to monitor the degree of hypothermia and determine when adequate cooling has been achieved. Cooling is considered adequate for circulatory arrest when no discernible activity is seen on the EEG (i.e., electrocerebral inactivity). EEG electrodes are applied according to the international 10/20 system; sometimes Fp1 and Fp2 electrodes cannot be placed because of prior placement of other anesthetic probes. Analysis of the EEG in an anterior-posterior bipolar montage is recommended, and the sensitivity must be increased to 2 μV/mm to ensure that no low-amplitude activity is present. When electrocerebral activity has been absent for at least 3 minutes, circulatory arrest can be instituted.

Median nerve somatosensory evoked potentials (SEPs) have also been used to monitor cooling. These responses can be easily obtained in most patients, and cortical (N20), subcortical (P13/14 and N18), and peripheral (EP) responses should be monitored. Cortical responses are lost prior to the other waveforms. Disappearance of the subcortical responses occurs after loss of the cortical responses; when these responses are lost, circulatory arrest can be instituted. The cervicomedullary (N13) and peripheral responses may not disappear at all despite cooling to about 15°C.

EEG and median nerve SEPs have been used to monitor other aspects of surgery on the ascending aorta and arch. Prior to inducing hypothermia, the EEG and median nerve SEPs can be used to determine presurgical asymmetry which may not have been evident previously; this may influence the counseling to families both before and after surgery. EEG and median nerve SEPs have also been used during the rewarming phase of surgery to determine prognosis after circulatory arrest. Since the spinal cord is not at significant risk during these procedures, tibial nerve SEPs and MEPs are not obtained.

Anesthetic Considerations

Since EEG is the main component of NIOM in surgeries on the ascending aorta and arch, it is important to use an anesthetic regimen that has minimal impact on this modality. Although all anesthetics in high doses can affect the EEG, some are more problematic than others. A good choice of anesthetics, especially since the monitoring of motor evoked potentials (MEPs) is not needed in these cases, is a low dose of a halogenated inhalationalal agent with narcotics used for analgesia. At doses less than 0.5 minimum alveolar concentration (MAC), halogenated inhalationalal agents have only a minimal effect on the EEG. Intravenous agents such as propofol, benzodiazepines, and barbiturates can have a profound effect on the EEG. These agents induce a burst-suppression pattern even in low doses, making interpretation difficult. They should be avoided; if they are used, their use should be suspended by the time the temperature reaches 30° to 33°C. Continued use of these agents beyond this temperature may make the EEG less reliable as a "brain thermometer," as recordings will reflect the effects of not only temperature but also the intravenous anesthetics. The use of low-dose halogenated inhalationalal agents and narcotics is also compatible with SEPs. Once again, use of high doses of these inhalational agents (greater than 0.5 MAC) may suppress the cortical responses of the median nerve SEPs, making interpretation difficult. Muscle relaxants can be used during these cases, as they will not affect either the EEG or median nerve SEPs adversely.

Interpretation of NIOM Changes

Predictable changes occur in the EEG and median nerve SEPs as the temperature decreases. These changes can be affected by the anesthetics used, as noted above. Additionally, a number of other factors, such as the patient's hematocrit, age, prior history of cooling, and the rate of cooling can also affect the changes seen on EEG. Despite all the variables that can affect the EEG, it is useful to have an understanding of the pattern of changes that occur as a patient is cooled (9).

As the patient is cooled, the EEG remains continuous until about 30.0°C, at which point generalized periodic epileptiform discharges (GPEDs) appear (Figure 15.13). In some cases, periodic lateralized epileptiform discharges (PLEDs) or bilateral, independent periodic lateralized epileptiform discharges (BiPLEDs) may appear before the appearance of GPEDs. It is important to realize that these discharges do not represent an "epileptiform" pattern and do not predict the development of epilepsy. At a temperature of about 24°C, the GPED pattern gives way to a burst-suppression pattern (Figure 15.14). Around 17°C, electrocerebral inactivity is noted (Figure 15.15). It should be remembered that the exact temperature at which a given patient will reach electrocerebral inactivity varies depending on other patient factors noted

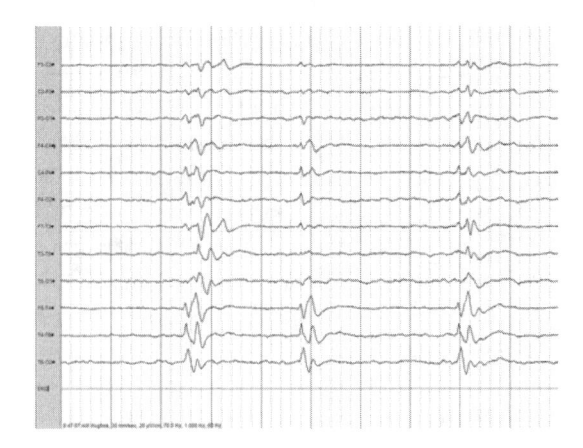

FIGURE 15.13 EEG of a patient being cooled for DHCA. The EEG shows a GPED pattern; the patient's temperature was 30°C.

above. As noted above, circulatory arrest can be instituted once electrocerebral inactivity has been present for 3 minutes. A summary of the temperatures and time from onset of cooling at which various electrographic features were noted in a large study is presented in Table 15.1 (9).

Median nerve SEPs also change predictably with cooling (10). At a temperature of about 21°C, the N20 response disappears, and the P14 response disappears at about 16°C. When both cortical and subcortical responses disappear, circulatory arrest can be instituted. Another study demonstrated that the N13 response disappeared at 17°C (9).

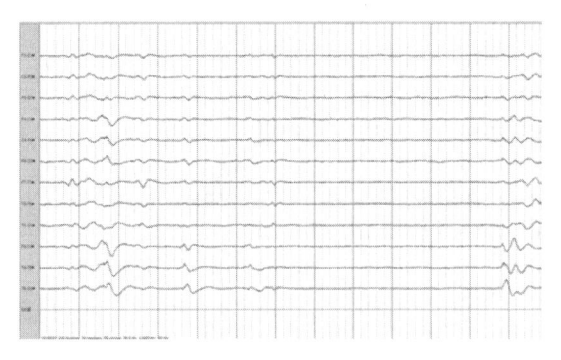

FIGURE 15.14 EEG of a patient being cooled for DHCA. The EEG shows a burst-suppression pattern; the patient's temperature was 22°C.

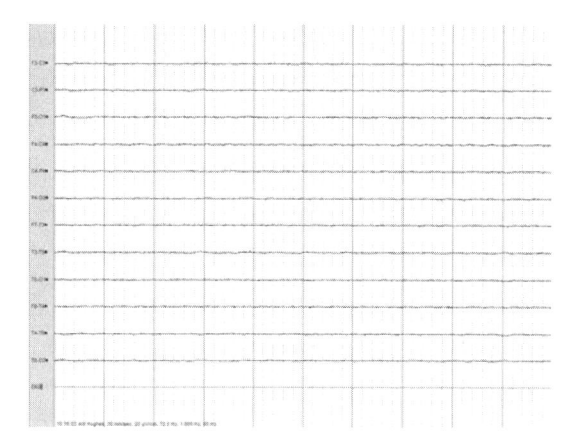

FIGURE 15.15 EEG of a patient being cooled for DHCA. The EEG shows electrocerebral inactivity; the patient's temperature was 15°C.

The N13 and EP responses may persist even at a temperature at which electrocerebral inactivity is noted on the EEG (see Table 15.1).

As predictable changes in NIOM occur with cooling, similarly predictable changes occur during rewarming (11). These can be helpful in prognosticating outcome. If recovery of the EEG or SEPs is not as quick as expected, the chances of subsequent neurologic morbidity are higher. Alternatively, if lateralized changes are seen during rewarming that were not present during cooling, the surgeon should be notified so that any flow related causes may be ruled out. A summary of the changes expected in EEG and median nerve SEPs during rewarming as seen in one large study is presented in Table 15.1 (11).

EEG patterns do not reappear at the same temperature during rewarming as they initially occurred during cooling. A burst-suppression pattern appears at about 21°C and after about 19 minutes of starting rewarming. The EEG becomes continuous at about 30°C and after 47 minutes of rewarming. The N13 of the median nerve SEPs reappears at about 17°C, whereas the N20 reappears at about 19°C (Table 15.1).

Descending Aorta

Modalities to Monitor

Thoracotomy for open surgery on the descending aorta most often involves cross

TABLE 15.1 NIOM Changes Associated with Deep Hypothermic Circulatory Arrest (Cooling and Rewarming)

Nasopharyngeal temperature (°C) ± SD	Time since cooling or rewarming (min) ± SD	Changes in EEG	Changes in median nerve SEP
Cooling			
Above 29.6 ± 3	7.9 ± 3	Continuous	Present
29.6 ± 3	7.9 ± 3	PLED/GPED	
24.4 ± 4	12.7 ± 6	Burst suppression	
21.4 ± 4	17.7 ± 9		N20 disappears
17.8 ± 4	27.5 ± 10	Electrocerebral inactivity	
17.3 ± 4	28.6 ± 15		N13 disappears*
Rewarming			
17.2 ± 2	12.6 ± 6		N13 reappears
18.6 ± 3	14.2 ± 7		N20 reappears
21.2 ± 5	19.0 ± 9	Burst suppression	
30.1 ± 5	47.1 ± 26	Continuous	

*The disappearance of the N13 is not required for the onset of circulatory arrest.
Sources: From Stecker et al. (9) and Ghariani et al. (11), with permission.

clamping the aorta. When the pathology is in the proximal descending aorta, perfusion to the spinal cord may be affected, especially if distal aortic perfusion is not performed. This ischemia may persist despite distal aortic perfusion if critical intercostal arteries supplying the spinal cord are sacrificed. Additionally, clamping of the aorta may cause elevation of blood pressure proximal to the clamp, which in turn can elevate CSF pressure; this elevation in CSF pressure can reduce spinal cord perfusion further. The gray matter has less tolerance for ischemia than the white matter tracts and is likely to infarct first. Additionally, since the anterior spinal artery circulation is more dependent on feeding intercostal arteries than the posterior spinal arterial system, ischemia to the anterior two thirds of the spinal cord is more likely. Since the aortic cross clamp is typically applied distal to the left common carotid artery, cerebral perfusion is not usually affected in these procedures. However, if retrograde aortic perfusion from the distal aorta or femoral artery is used for arterial inflow during CPB, cerebral atheroemboli may result from retrograde flow within the diseased thoracoabdominal aorta or arch.

Since it is the spinal cord and not the brain which is primarily at risk during open surgical procedures on the descending thoracic aorta, NIOM paradigms are designed to determine when the degree of ischemia to the spinal cord is significant and the risk of paraplegia high. Such alerts can guide the surgeon in the management of distal aortic perfusion as well as suggest the need for reimplantation of intercostal arteries. Additionally, adequacy of other measures to ensure adequate spinal cord perfusion, such as CSF drainage and maintenance of adequate systemic or distal aortic blood pressure, can be assessed by NIOM.

As noted above, the anterior two thirds of the spinal cord and its gray matter are at highest risk during open surgical procedures on the descending thoracic aorta. Consequently, transcranial motor evoked potentials (MEPs) are commonly used in these procedures. MEPs assess not only the anterior two thirds of the spinal cord (corticospinal tract) but also the gray matter, since the corticospinal tract synapses on the anterior horn cells in the gray matter. Details of MEP monitoring are presented in Chapter 2. For descending thoracic aortic surgery, monitoring one or two muscles in each upper and lower extremity is satisfactory. In the upper extremities, needle electrodes are placed in the abductor digiti quinti and abductor pollicis brevis, which are referenced to each other. In the lower extremities, needle electrodes are places in the abductor hallucis and tibialis anterior, which are referenced to each other. Additional needle electrodes can be placed in the lower extremities to provide redundancy. Neuromuscular blockade must be minimized or not used at all when MEP monitoring is performed. Because of this, when the transcranial electrical stimulus is applied, there may be considerable patient movement. The surgical team must be warned of this potential movement so that appropriate precautions can be taken. It is very important to obtain MEPs at frequent intervals during aortic cross clamping and when intercostal arteries are ligated. If changes in responses are noted, the surgeon must be informed immediately, as these findings may prompt alterations in the surgical procedure, such as institution of distal aortic perfusion if not already being utilized, reimplantation of intercostal arteries, increasing distal aortic pressure, increasing systemic blood pressure, or CSF drainage.

Along with MEPs, monitoring of SEPs is also performed in open descending thoracic aortic surgery. Although SEP monitoring assesses the dorsal aspect of the spinal cord, which is at less risk, it still provides useful complementary information to MEP monitoring and helps in the interpretation of changes when they occur. Tibial nerve SEP monitoring is performed most often, since it evaluates the spinal cord in its entirety, including the thoracic part, which is at most risk. Ulnar nerve SEP monitoring is also often performed, as it serves as a control to help evaluate systemic from localized changes. Additionally, at times positioning of the upper limbs can cause traction on the inferior trunk of the brachial plexus. If this is not detected in a timely manner, a postoperative brachial plexopathy may occur. Ulnar nerve SEP changes have been noted with inappropriate positioning of the upper limb, allowing correction of the positioning during surgery. Thus the monitoring paradigm for open descending thoracic aortic surgery includes MEP recorded from all four extremities and ulnar and tibial nerve SEPs. In addition, if DHCA is being used for descending thoracic aortic repair, EEG, as described previously, is used as well to guide the duration of cooling.

Most patients are not awake enough for a thorough neurologic examination for at least several hours after conventional open surgery on the descending thoracic aorta. During this time as well as later in the postoperative period, delayed postoperative paraplegia can still occur in these patients due to spinal cord ischemia, even if they have left the operating room neurologically intact. If detected and treated immediately, delayed postoperative paraplegia can often be corrected by increasing CSF drainage, commonly to a pressure of less than 10 mmHg, and increasing blood pressure to mean arterial pressure (MAP) of 90 mmHg or higher. The latter intervention can be associated with complications such increased bleeding from the suture lines of the aortic graft, and this may limit the utility of this intervention in certain situations. Nevertheless, augmentation of MAP is the mainstay of therapy for delayed paraplegia and should not be avoided over theoretical concerns for bleeding. Because of this "neurologic blind spot" between the cessation of NIOM in the operating room and the patient's emergence from anesthesia to a degree that a reliable neurologic exam is obtainable, NIOM has been used postoperatively in the intensive care unit (ICU) to detect spinal cord ischemia. Tibial nerve SEPs can be obtained in the ICU at periodic intervals to determine if adequate spinal cord perfusion is present; MEPs cannot be obtained, as the procedure is painful in a nonanesthetized patient (12). Monitoring tibial nerve SEPs postoperatively requires extensive resources, as the duration of monitoring may be hours to days. Moreover, the intervals at which tibial nerve SEPs should be obtained are not known. Performing tibial nerve SEP every 30 to 60 minutes has been proposed, but this is empiric; obviously spinal cord ischemia may develop between trials and intervention may be ineffective by the time it is detected. Most centers do not perform postoperative tibial nerve SEP monitoring because of these logistic difficulties.

Anesthetic Considerations

As with other types of surgeries in which MEP monitoring is needed, total intravenous anesthesia (TIVA) with propofol and an intravenous narcotic analgesic (such as fentanyl) is preferred when NIOM is to be used for open descending thoracic aortic repair. Neuromuscular blocking agents and inhalational anesthetics are not used, as they affect MEPs. Whereas this regimen allows reliable, reproducible NIOM data to be recorded, it poses challenges for the surgeon. For an open thoracotomy to be done quickly and safely, muscle atonia is preferred. Similarly, during closing approximation of the wound, monitoring becomes difficult if the patient is not given neuromuscular blocking agents. Additionally, blood pressure control in patients undergoing descending thoracic aortic surgery is much easier with inhalationalal agents than with TIVA. Consequently anesthesiologists may object to use of TIVA in these surgeries.

Keeping these opposing perspectives in mind, a compromise involves the use of TIVA during the period of vascular exposure and aortic cross clamping. Meanwhile, during opening of the chest cavity and closure, inhalational and neuromuscular blocking agents can be used. Consequently baseline

MEP responses frequently cannot be obtained until well into the surgical exposure. Open communication between the neurophysiologist, anesthesiologist, and the surgeon ensures that each team member is aware of what the others are doing.

Since TIVA is used during the main portions of these surgeries, the recording of SEPs also becomes easier. Without the amplitude suppression of the cortical response seen with inhalationalal agents, these responses are of high amplitude and easily reproduced. Recording subcortical potentials becomes less important. Depending on the number of channels available on the NIOM equipment, if some channels must be sacrificed due to lack of space, the subcortical channels are not recorded. If, however, extra channels are available, subcortical channels should be recorded, as they provide useful redundant information.

Interpretation of NIOM Changes

Many different patterns of loss of MEPs and SEPs can occur during open surgery on the descending thoracic aorta. The neurophysiologist must be able to recognize these patterns and provide the surgeon with the correct localization for the problem. Whereas it is imperative for the NIOM team to alert the surgeon when compromise to neural tissue is occurring, it is also important not to raise false alarms that will slow the surgery and potentially lead to more complications. Many changes in NIOM during these surgeries are due to reversible peripheral ischemia. A summary of the NIOM changes that may be seen with these procedures is presented in Table 15.2.

Loss of MEP responses from both lower extremities with preservation of responses in the upper extremities often implies spinal cord ischemia. Such a pattern often occurs within a few minutes of clamping the aorta if distal aortic perfusion has not been instituted. Alternatively, if distal perfusion has been instituted, such a pattern can still occur from spinal cord ischemia due to insufficient distal aortic perfusion pressure by the pump, ligation of critical intercostal arteries, or from excessively high CSF or central venous pressure. These changes must be immediately conveyed to the surgeon so that corrective action—such as increasing the distal aortic pressure, draining more CSF, or reimplanting intercostal arteries—can be undertaken. If

TABLE 15.2 Interpretation of Changes in NIOM during Descending Thoracic Aortic Surgery

	SEP				MEP	
	Ulnar		Tibial		Upper	Lower
	EP	N20	PF	P37		
Technical	−	−	−	−	−	−
Cerebral ischemia	+	−	+	−	−	−
Hypotension	+	−	+	−	−	−
Inhalational anesthetics	+	−	+	−	−	−
Neuromuscular blocking agents	+	+	+	+	−	−
Spinal cord ischemia	+	+	+	−	+	−
Lower limb ischemia	+	+	−	−	+	±
Upper limb ischemia	−	−	+	+	±	+
Brachial plexus injury	−	−	+	+	−	+
Scalp edema	+	+	+	+	−	−

ischemia of the spinal cord is reversed within 15 to 30 minutes, MEP responses often return (13). The vast majority of patients in whom the MEP responses from the lower extremities are present at the conclusion of surgery will not have paraparesis. It should be pointed out, however, that there are animal data suggesting that presence of MEP responses from the lower extremities does not guarantee a lack of paraparesis (14). On the other hand, if MEP responses to the lower extremities do not return despite corrective measures, the likelihood of postoperative paraparesis or paraplegia is very high.

Loss of the cortical and subcortical tibial nerve SEPs with preservation of the peripheral responses—along with preservation of ulnar nerve SEPs—is highly suggestive of spinal cord ischemia as well. Since SEPs are transmitted primarily by the dorsal column pathways, which are in the posterior aspect of the spinal cord, they are affected less often and later than MEPs. Because the blood supply to the posterior spinal arteries is primarily from the vertebral arteries, it is affected later than the anterior spinal artery system. Whereas MEP changes are seen within a few minutes of experimentally induced spinal cord ischemia, SEP changes lag by about 15 to 25 minutes. If the decrement in cortical SEP amplitude occurs in less than 15 minutes, it is more likely due spinal cord ischemia. If the amplitude loss is more gradual and extends beyond 15 minutes, it is likely due to peripheral ischemia of the tibial nerve (15). The ability of tibial nerve SEPs to predict postoperative paraparesis is less precise than that of MEPs, with a false-positive rate of about 50% and a false-negative rate of 13% (16).

Unilateral loss of all tibial nerve SEP responses (including peripheral ones) followed by loss of MEPs from the same lower extremity is suggestive of limb ischemia. This often occurs on the side of the femoral artery in which the bypass cannula is inserted. Adjusting the cannula, redirecting blood flow, or removing the cannula results in return of these responses. Whereas the surgeon must be alerted to these changes, his or her response does not need to be as urgent as when ischemia to the spinal cord is suspected. Several hours of ischemia to the limb can be tolerated without long-term adverse consequences.

Loss of MEPs from all four extremities as well as ulnar and tibial cortical SEPs is suggestive of systemic changes, such as low blood pressure or a change in the anesthetic regimen (i.e., addition of an inhalational agent). These changes can also occur from global cerebral hypoperfusion; however, this scenario is less likely to occur in open surgery on the descending thoracic aorta. The neurophysiologist should attempt to determine the etiology of this change and ask that it be corrected if possible. At times raising the blood pressure, though likely to improve the NIOM, may be detrimental (i.e., a low blood pressure may be preferred to minimize perioperative bleeding).

Selective loss of all ulnar nerve SEP waveforms, including peripheral, is suggestive of technical problems with ulnar nerve stimulation or brachial plexus trauma from positioning. After technical issues have been excluded, an attempt should be made to reposition the patient's arm to see whether the responses return. MEPs to the same arm are seldom affected in this situation, and responses from other limbs are also not affected.

As noted above, tibial nerve SEPs can be obtained postoperatively in the ICU to monitor for spinal cord ischemia. Loss of cortical and/or subcortical responses with preserved peripheral responses should raise concern for spinal cord ischemia. Elevation of the blood pressure or increased drainage of CSF can be instituted if this occurs. Caveats regarding this type of monitoring include the fact that SEPs assess the dorsal columns, and the more susceptible motor pathways are not being assessed. By the time changes are seen in SEPs, irreversible spinal cord ischemia may already have occurred. Also, as mentioned previously, the intervals at which tibial nerve SEPs should be monitored remain unknown.

EVSG Repair of the Descending Thoracic Aorta

Modalities to Monitor

EVSG repair of the descending thoracic aorta does not involve aortic cross clamping; however, paraplegia does occur with this type of surgery as well. The longer the length of aorta covered by the EVSG, the greater the possibility that spinal cord ischemia may occur. The exact mechanism by which the EVSG causes spinal cord ischemia is not known, but it most likely involves occlusion of critical intercostal arteries by the stent graft. As with open descending aortic surgery, NIOM can be of utility in determining whether spinal cord ischemia is occurring. If such a finding is noted, alternative measures—such as increasing the blood pressure and draining CSF—can be attempted to restore blood supply to the spinal cord. If the EVSG is removable, which is generally not the case, that should be attempted as well.

Since the greatest risk during EVSG surgery is to the spinal cord, monitoring modalities for this type of surgery are similar to those employed in open descending aortic surgery. MEPs provide assessment of the ventral aspect of the spinal cord, the part at most risk when intercostal arteries are occluded. Although MEPs must be obtained at short intervals, particularly when the EVSG is being positioned, care must be taken not to stimulate when the surgeon is about to deploy the device. Sudden movement of the patient may cause misplacement of the stent graft. Tibial nerve SEPs provide assessment of the dorsal spinal cord as well as complementary information. Since the patient is generally supine for EVSG surgery, unlike the lateral decubitus position necessary for left thoracotomy, the risk of brachial plexopathy is greatly reduced. Thus it is not critical to perform ulnar nerve SEPs for this indication. However, they do allow more precise localization of changes when they are seen. In addition, ulnar nerve SEPs may detect peripheral ischemia of the left arm in cases where the left subclavian artery is intentionally covered by the stent graft and collateral flow is inadequate. This may alert the surgeon to the need for adjunctive left carotid–subclavian bypass to prevent arm ischemia. TIVA is often used in EVSG cases to allow reliable MEP monitoring. Consequently only cortical SEP responses need to be monitored, because they are not significantly affected by TIVA and their large amplitudes have a better signal-to-noise ratio than subcortical responses. This allows recording of a reproducible response with fewer repetitions. Peripheral SEP responses should also be monitored to help localize changes to the limb or central nervous system.

Tibial nerve SEPs generally do not need to be monitored postoperatively in these surgeries, since patients are typically awake and extubated immediately postoperatively and can thus participate in the neurologic assessment.

Anesthetic Considerations

The anesthetic protocol for EVSG surgery is similar to that for open descending aortic surgery. Because MEPs are difficult to record with inhalational anesthetics and neuromuscular blocking agents, these drugs are avoided except at induction and at the end of surgery, when no more MEP monitoring is to be done. Patients can be induced with inhalationalal agents and neuromuscular blocking agents; however, after positioning, these drugs are discontinued and the patient is transitioned to TIVA with propofol and fentanyl. If excessive muscle movement is noted with transcranial electrical stimulation, low levels of neuromuscular blocking agents can be used as a continuous infusion. If this is done, at least two twitches in a train of four must be present to ensure adequate MEP monitoring. As noted above, toward the end of surgery, when MEP monitoring has been terminated, TIVA is transitioned back to inhalationalal agents to facilitate quick awakening.

Interpretation of NIOM Changes

NIOM changes that occur with aortic EVSG surgery are similar to those seen with open descending aortic repair (Table 15.2). Loss of MEP responses to the lower extremities with preservation of upper extremity responses is suggestive of spinal cord ischemia. When this is seen, increasing the blood pressure (MAP greater than 90 to 110 mmHg) or increasing CSF drainage (goal pressure less than 10 mmHg) may help improve MEP responses and reduce spinal cord ischemia (Figure 15.16). Loss of cortical (and subcortical) tibial nerve SEP responses is also suggestive of spinal cord ischemia, especially if associated with loss of MEPs to the lower extremities. With spinal cord ischemia, loss of MEPs occurs within a few minutes, whereas loss of tibial nerve SEPs can be delayed up to 15 minutes.

Although it is uncommon, cerebral hypoperfusion can occur with EVSG aortic surgeries. Sudden loss of MEPs from all four extremities with loss of cortical (and subcortical) ulnar and tibial nerve SEP responses should make one consider cerebral hypoperfusion (Figure 15.17). Peripheral ulnar and tibial nerve SEP responses are preserved, making it unlikely that the change is due to technical problems or peripheral ischemia. Such a change may be noted if an iatrogenic aortic dissection involving the arch vessels is created during stent graft deployment, if the EVSG inadvertently covers the great vessels of the arch of aorta, or with thromboembolism from the aorta to the cerebral circula-

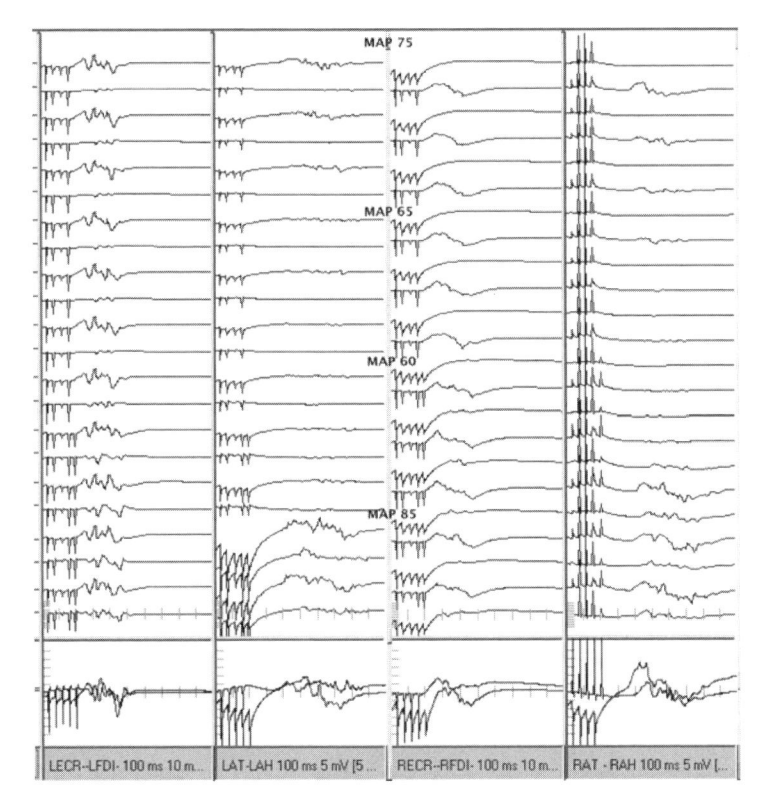

FIGURE 15.16 MEP responses obtained in a patient undergoing EVSG surgery. Displayed are MEP responses from the left upper extremity, left lower extremity, right upper extremity, and right lower extremity (from left to right). A drop in MAPs resulted in loss of MEPs from the lower extremities due to impaired spinal cord perfusion; after increasing the MAPs, the MEPs returned. Upper extremity MEPs remained unchanged.

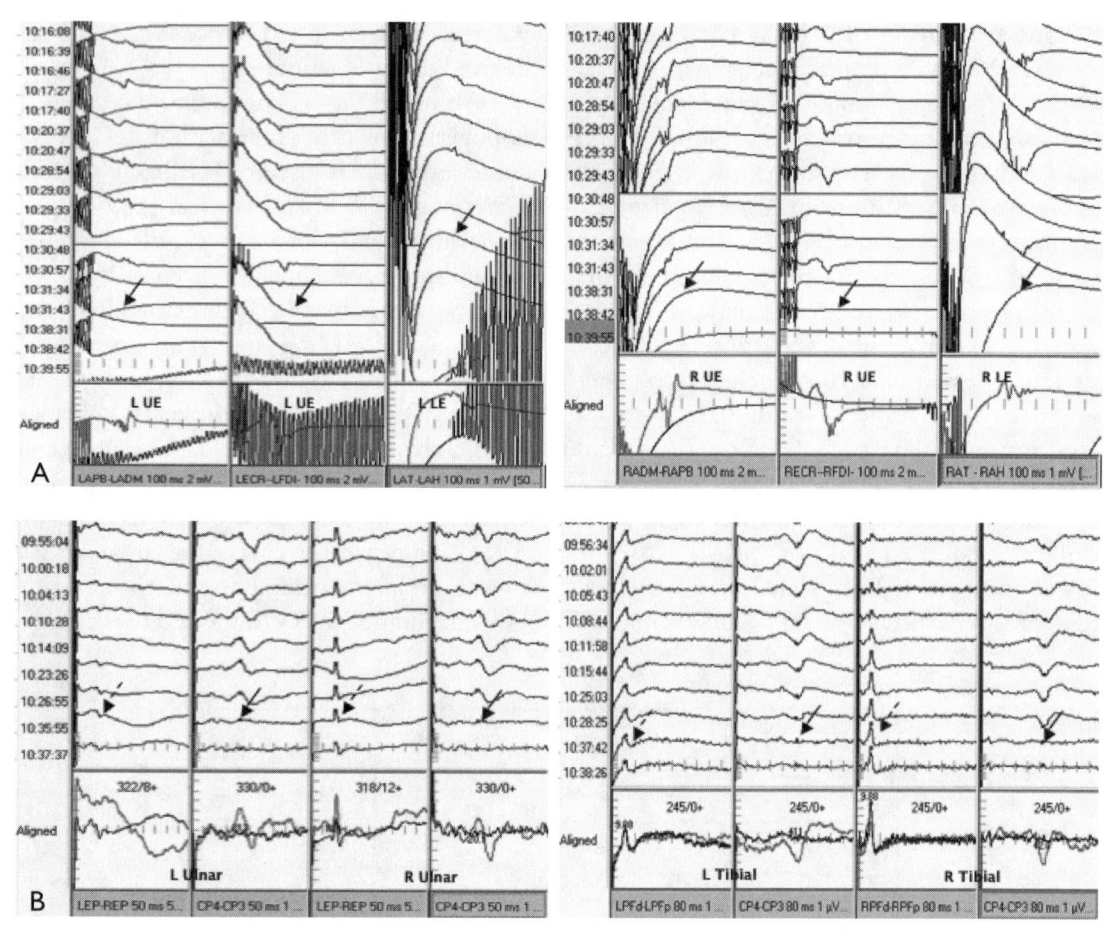

FIGURE 15.17 A. MEP responses in a patient undergoing EVSG surgery. Sudden loss of upper and lower extremity MEP responses (arrows) occurred. B. A few minutes later, loss of ulnar and tibial nerve cortical SEPs was noted (solid arrows). Peripheral responses were preserved (dashed arrows). These changes were thought to be due to cerebral ischemia. Further evaluation revealed that the EVSG had inadvertently moved to cover all the great vessels arising from the aortic arch, causing global cerebral ischemia.

tion. It should be noted that similar findings may occur with global hypotension and/or change of anesthetics, especially with the introduction of inhalationalal agents. The surgeon must be notified immediately of these findings, and if they indeed are due to cerebral hypoperfusion, corrective measures must be undertaken immediately.

A common NIOM change seen during EVSG surgeries is loss of the peripheral and cortical tibial nerve SEPs obtained after stimulating the side with the large (20 to 24 Fr) sheath used for stent graft introduction into the aorta. The introducer sheath causes ischemia to the leg, decreasing blood supply to the tibial nerve. Loss of the peripheral response confirms its peripheral localization. After about 10 to 15 minutes, there is typically loss of the MEPs to the lower extremity with the sheath as well. After the sheath is removed, the responses return to baseline (Figure 15.18). Although the surgeon should be apprised of this change, it is not one that necessitates a modification in the surgical procedure. The limb can withstand ischemia for at least 6 hours (a period longer than most

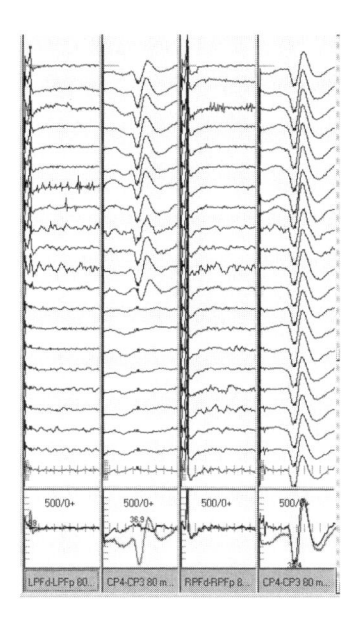

FIGURE 15.18 Tibial nerve SEPs in a patient undergoing EVSG surgery. The PF and P37 responses from the left and right tibial nerve stimulation are displayed from left to right. Loss of the peripheral and cortical SEP responses after left tibial nerve stimulation indicates ischemia to the leg. The responses recovered once the EVSG introducer sheath was removed from the left femoral artery.

EVSG surgeries), and withdrawal of the sheath typically results in the rapid return of responses, depending on the duration of the limb ischemia. However, this frequently observed loss of SEP and MEP responses from one limb can make detection of spinal cord ischemia more difficult.

Loss of MEPs from all extremities with preserved cortical tibial nerve SEP responses is most likely due to technical problems with the MEP, introduction of neuromuscular blocking agents, or even inhalationalal anesthetics. Although the latter often cause loss of cortical SEPs, loss of MEPs at moderate doses may be noted without much effect on cortical SEPs. Isolated loss of ulnar peripheral and cortical SEP responses suggests stretch injury to the inferior trunk of the brachial plexus or ischemia to the upper limb. As mentioned, stretch injury to the brachial plexus is uncommon in these procedures, as arm positioning is not the same as for thoracotomies. Ischemia to the upper limb can also occur if a sheath or catheter is introduced from the upper extremity or, as mentioned above, from EVSG coverage of the left subclavian artery.

UTILITY OF NIOM IN AORTIC SURGERY

NIOM with SEPs has been used during aortic surgery for many decades. More recently, the addition of EEG and MEP monitoring has increased the effectiveness of NIOM in warning the surgeon when neural tissue is at risk. In this section, an overview of the data supporting the use NIOM in various types of aortic surgery is presented.

Ascending Aorta and Arch Surgery

There are few outcomes data comparing patients who received NIOM with those who did not during ascending aortic and arch surgery. However, it is well known from neurosurgical as well as cardiothoracic literature that nasopharyngeal or core body temperature measurements do not necessarily reflect brain temperature. Similarly, the time required to reach electrocerebral inactivity varies among patients and depends on not only the rate of cooling but also on physiologic parameters such as hematocrit. Thus, it is not unreasonable to assume that a neurophysiologic assessment of the brain during cooling should be helpful in determining when electrocerebral inactivity occurs and when circulatory arrest may be safely instituted.

Studies that have evaluated the utility of EEG monitoring during ascending aortic and arch surgery involving DHCA support the need for NIOM in determining the optimal duration of cooling prior to institution of circulatory arrest. In patients undergoing DHCA, the rectal temperature at which electrocerebral inactivity was achieved varied anywhere between 12.8° to 28.6°C; the nasopharyngeal temperature at which similar EEG suppression was noted varied between 10.1° to 27.2°C (9,17). The time to electrocerebral inactivity also varied between 12.0 to 50.0 minutes (9). These studies suggest that cooling to a preset temperature or for a specified duration may not be adequate for some patients, whereas in others it may excessive, potentially leading to other complications.

Data from median nerve SEP studies also suggest that a fixed temperature cannot be used to predict the onset of electrocerebral inactivity. The cortical response (N20) was lost between 14.5° to 29.2°C and after 4 to 41 minutes from the start of cooling (9). The subcortical (P14) response disappeared between 16.7° and 19.7°C (18). As with EEG, a fixed target temperature for cooling is likely to be inappropriate for many patients.

Continuation of EEG monitoring during the rewarming phase has been useful in adults in predicting postoperative neurologic deficits (11). Longer recovery time to a continuous EEG was associated with a greater risk for postoperative neurologic complications. Similarly, longer time to return of the cortical response (N20) of the median nerve SEPs was associated with worse outcomes. Asymmetric return of EEG activity due to malperfusion of the great vessels has led to changes in intraoperative circulation management (19). This has potentially prevented perioperative strokes.

Descending Aorta

NIOM with SEP monitoring has been used for several decades to help improve outcomes in descending aortic surgery. Early studies showed that loss of cortical potentials occurred with cross clamping of the aorta if the distal aortic pressure dropped below 40 mmHg (20). This demonstrated inadequate perfusion to the spinal cord, and increasing the distal aortic pressure or reimplanting intercostal arteries resulted in improvement of the waveforms within 10 minutes. If the cortical potentials were present at the termination of the surgery, paraplegia was not seen. Additionally, the longer the cortical responses were lost (usually 40 to 60 minutes), the greater the chance of postoperative paraplegia. However, other studies have shown that SEP changes do not always correlate with postoperative outcome. In one study, the false-positive rate of the loss of cortical potentials was 67%, whereas the false-negative rate was 13% (21). These data suggest that even though SEP monitoring can detect most cases of spinal cord ischemia, it is slow in raising an alert and has a low sensitivity and specificity.

More recently, data have been accumulating that document the utility of MEP in detecting early spinal cord ischemia. Animal studies have shown that experimental clamping of the aorta resulted in loss of MEPs within 2 minutes; if the responses recovered after the clamp was released, the animals were less likely to have weakness than if the responses did not recover (14). Human studies have documented similar findings. In a large study of 210 patients undergoing descending thoracic aortic aneurysm repair, MEPs suggested spinal cord ischemia in 23% of patients after aortic cross clamping. Increasing distal aortic pressure or reattaching intercostal arteries resulted in improvement of MEPs in most patients. Persistent loss of MEPs at the end of surgery was seen in only one patient, who was the only patient with immediate postoperative paraplegia (22). Another study with 72 patients undergoing descending thoracic aortic aneurysm surgery with MEP monitoring found that if the amplitude of these responses was at least 75% of the baseline, patients had normal lower extremity function. On the other hand, 8 of 9 patients in whom MEP amplitude was less than 75% of baseline had paraparesis. In this study, the MEP sensitivity was 100% and specificity was 98.4% (23). There are numerous other smaller studies documenting the utility of MEP monitoring in descending aortic surgery (24).

EVSG Surgery on the Descending Thoracic Aorta

EVSG repair of the descending thoracic aorta is a relatively new procedure; only one large series has been reported in which NIOM was used (25). In this series, 31 patients underwent NIOM with MEPs and tibial nerve SEPs. In 11 patients, NIOM changes occurred that prompted alteration in hemodynamic management or CSF drainage. These alterations corrected spinal cord ischemia in almost all patients in whom changes were noted, likely preventing paraparesis. To date there are no reports comparing outcomes in patients undergoing EVSG surgery with and without NIOM.

TECHNICAL CONSIDERATIONS

Preparation

Many NIOM modalities are used in thoracic aortic surgery. It is is important to determine whether the surgery will involve the ascending aorta and/or arch or the descending thoracic aorta, as that will dictate what type of NIOM is performed.

Ascending Aorta and Aortic Arch

EEG and median nerve SEPs are often used during ascending aorta and aortic arch surgery to determine when electrocerebral inactivity is reached so that circulatory arrest can be safely instituted. Although there are no contraindications to EEG monitoring, it may be useful to know whether a patient has a preexisting abnormality that may be evident on the EEG. These include a prior stroke, head injury, neurosurgery, epilepsy, brain tumor, etc. If these conditions are present, the monitoring does not need to be altered; however, they may affect the interpretation of the EEG. Many of these conditions can also affect median nerve SEPs.

It is helpful if a preoperative baseline EEG and median nerve SEPs are obtained. This will determine whether there are focal findings that can affect interpretation in the operating room. If this is done the day prior to surgery, the electrodes can also be left on the patient, so that setup on the day of surgery will be quicker. It also gives the technologist time to meet the patient and answer any questions about the monitoring.

If a preoperative EEG is obtained, a full set of EEG electrodes should be applied according to the international 10/20 system with an electrocardiogram (ECG) lead as well. Application with collodion ensures that the electrodes are secure and will stay in place overnight and during the surgery. The electrodes should be braided for artifact reduction and labeled at both ends for ease of placement. As with all EEGs, the electrodes should be of the same metal type, wires of the same length for ease of use, and leads in excellent condition. Jumpers, lead extenders, and adapters can contribute to artifact and so should be avoided if possible. The same principles apply to preoperative median nerve SEPs.

If the patient is going home with the electrodes glued on, he or she should be reminded not to smoke or wash his or her hair. On the day of surgery, the electrodes should be inspected to make sure that they are not loose. They should be regelled and the impedances checked to ensure they are below 5,000 ohms.

Any NIOM machine capable of running a 16-channel EEG can be used to perform this type of monitoring. In the experience of the authors, EEG machines produce better recordings with fewer artifacts than NIOM machines, which are capable of also monitoring other modalities. If multimodality monitoring with EEG and median nerve SEPs needs to be performed, using two machines with one for EEG and one for SEPs, may be best. This, of course, will necessitate two NIOM technologists to be present during the surgery.

Descending Thoracic and Thoracoabdominal Aorta

The NIOM modalities used for open surgical and endovascular repair of the descending thoracic and thoracoabdominal aorta are the same and are discussed together. Where there are differences they are noted. Modalities that are important to monitor during these surgeries include MEPs from all four extremities and ulnar and tibial nerve SEPs. Patients should be evaluated for preexisting medical conditions that would affect MEP or SEP monitoring. These conditions include spinal cord injury or disease, prior strokes, neuromuscular disorders, and orthopedic issues (such as amputations). Also important to evaluate are conditions that may be contraindications to MEP monitoring. These include the presence of cardiac pacemakers or other implanted devices, epilepsy, prior craniotomy, etc. Many of these are not absolute contraindications and should be discussed with the neurophysiologist.

Preoperative SEP studies should be obtained if possible. This will alert the NIOM team to preexisting problems that might affect NIOM. Of course preoperative MEPs cannot be obtained. If preoperative studies are obtained, the electrodes should be left on the patient, if possible, to expedite hookup on the day of surgery.

An NIOM machine capable of recording MEPs and SEPs and delivering transcortical electrical stimulation should be used for monitoring surgeries on the descending thoracic and thoracoabdominal aorta. Many of the newer machines have 16 channels; some even have 32. Enough channels should be available to record MEPs from at least one set of muscles from each extremity as well cortical and peripheral SEP responses. If there are extra channels, subcortical SEPs should also be obtained. The latter are not critical, as in most cases TIVA is used, resulting in robust cortical responses. If the NIOM machine is not able to deliver a high-intensity transcranial electrical stimulus, a separate transcranial stimulator, such as the Digitimer, should be used.

Procedure

The NIOM requirements are very different depending on the surgery, as noted previously. When surgery involves the descending thoracic aorta, it is important to know whether it is an open surgical or endovascular repair. The duration of these surgeries is significantly different, which has implications for the technologist.

Ascending Aorta and Aortic Arch

If the EEG is to be monitored, the electrodes should be placed on the patient a day prior to the surgery. This will ensure more meticulous application and save time during preoperative setup. However, if necessary, electrodes can be applied on the day of surgery in the preoperative holding area or induction room.

An operation of this kind is typically a long procedure, and the anesthesia team has a lot of preparation to do before such a case. In addition, the patient's body, especially the head, will be moved around when different types of monitoring devices are being applied. Because of this, it is recommended that the EEG electrodes be applied with collodion. A full set of leads using the standard 10/20 system of electrode placement should be used. It is not necessary to apply A1 or A2 electrodes and Fp1 and Fp2 may not be applied either, as the forehead is often used by various anesthesia monitors. Ground and reference electrodes can usually be placed on the midline without interfering with any other electrodes or equipment. Braiding all electrodes together helps reduce artifact. Electrode impedances should be 5,000 ohms or less and equal. The ECG electrodes should be placed on the left side to stay out of the way of the central line. They should be placed high enough so that they are not in the surgical field. Electrode application can take up to 30 to 40 minutes, even when done by an experienced technologist. This should be discussed with the surgery and anesthesia teams so that they are aware of the time issues.

Standard EEG recording parameters (sensitivity of 7 µV/mm, low-frequency filter of 1 Hz, high-frequency filter of 70 Hz, page speed of 10 seconds per page) are adequate to begin the recording. Each technologist should discuss with his or her neurophysiologist which montages will be viewed during the case to be sure all necessary electrodes are placed. Typically, an anterior-posterior bipolar montage is used. As cooling of the patient progresses, the sensitivity will need to be changed; prior to informing the surgeon of electrocerebral inactivity, the EEG should be viewed at a sensitivity of 2 µV/mm.

Once the patient is in the operating room, electrodes are plugged into the EEG machine and a baseline tracing is obtained. The duration of this portion of the recording should be determined by each individual laboratory's protocols. It is important to note the patient's temperature, blood pressure, and anesthetic agents used during induction. Any artifact should be removed, if possible, by troubleshooting. The NIOM team should communicate findings of the baseline portion of the recording to the surgeon, especially if focal abnormalities are noted.

It is usually not necessary for the NIOM technologist to remain in the room during exposure. The EEG should be "paused" in the absence of the technologist. The technologist should return before the patient is placed on CPB, and the EEG recording should be restarted. When the tracing is restarted, the temperature, blood pressure, and anesthetics are again noted. Once again, if new focal findings are noted in the EEG, these should be communicated to the surgeon.

Shortly after the patient is placed on CPB, cooling begins. The patient's temperature should be annotated frequently on the EEG. Anesthetic doses should be noted as well, since these will be changing (see below). As cooling proceeds, the EEG will undergo predictable changes and drop in amplitude (as discussed earlier). This will necessitate gradually increasing the sensitivity, eventually up to 2 µV/mm. When electrocerebral inactivity is reached (often between 13° to 18°C) for at least 3 minutes, the NIOM team should inform the surgeon as such. The surgeon waits for this alert prior to instituting DHCA. During circulatory arrest, there is relatively little for the NIOM team to do as there are no signals to monitor.

After the circulation has been restarted and the patient is being rewarmed, EEG monitoring again becomes important. As the temperature increases, the sensitivity will have to be adjusted. As with cooling, a predictable pattern of EEG changes is noted with rewarming. The times when anesthetics are reintroduced should be noted by the technologist, as there will be a diffuse change in the EEG. The time it takes for the EEG to return to baseline and whether any new focal findings are present are important to note and communicate to the surgeon. Once the patient is taken off CPB, monitoring is complete, and the surgeon is given a final verbal report as to the return and symmetry of the EEG.

The operating room is an electrically hostile environment and the EEG is recorded at very high sensitivity. Consequently, artifacts can often become a problem, making troubleshooting critical. The most important factor in reducing artifact is electrode impedance. All electrode impedances should be below 5000 ohms and equal. Braiding the electrodes also reduces artifact. The electrode leads should be no longer than necessary to reach the headbox. Electrical cords should be plugged all the way into the outlet. Often the CPB pump produces a high-frequency artifact; attaching a ground electrode to this machine may also reduce artifact. There may be other sources of artifact as well that are amplified due to the high sensitivity of the recording. The technologist must troubleshoot each piece of equipment one at a time to see if it makes a difference in the NIOM tracing. If the artifact is not eliminated, it can make EEG interpretation very difficult.

If median nerve SEPs are being recorded, recording electrodes are placed on the scalp and Erb's point. Stimulating electrodes can be surface or subdermal needles, depending on the laboratory's preference. These electrodes are applied as they would be for any other median nerve SEP monitoring. Monitoring progresses as it does for EEG, with a predictable pattern of SEP changes during cooling and rewarming. Monitoring is stopped, as it is with EEG.

Anesthetics can have a profound effect on EEG and SEP monitoring in ascending aorta and aortic arch surgeries. The anesthesiologist can induce the patient with inhalational and intravenous agents; however, once cooling is initiated, anesthetics with the least effect on NIOM should be used. The various possibilities are discussed earlier in the chapter. Regardless of the method used, consideration should be given to discontinuing the anesthetic when the patient's temperature reaches about 25°C. Discontinuing anesthetics allows the neurophysiologist to confidently determine that the suppression of the EEG is due to hypothermia and not anesthetics. Depending on the anesthetic used, changes noted in EEG during cooling may vary as discussed earlier. Of course, during circulatory arrest anesthetics are not and cannot be used. Once rewarming starts, anesthetics will need to be restarted at about 25°C. Narcotics and paralytics have little affect on the EEG. However, SEP can be affected by anesthetics; inhalationalal agents have a greater effect than intravenous agents. Regardless of which agents are used, consideration should be given to discontinuing them as noted above. It is critical that the NIOM technologist document the anesthetic dose on the EEG record. The patient's MAP should also be recorded on the EEG. It should be remembered that anesthetics can be administered through the CPB pump, and the technologist should check with the perfusionist regarding the status of any drugs administered via that route.

Descending Thoracic and Thoracoabdominal Aorta

Both conventional open and endovascular surgery on the descending thoracic and thoracoabdominal aorta are monitored with MEPs obtained from all four extremities and ulnar and tibial SEPs. The NIOM technologist must quickly determine if there are any contraindications to performing MEP monitoring. If none exist, setup for MEPs and SEPs should proceed. Conditions that may affect SEP, such as a peripheral neuropathy, should also be noted. If preoperative SEP studies were done the previous day, electrodes may still be attached but will need to be reassessed and regelled. Since applying SEP electrodes is not as time-consuming as applying EEG electrodes, these can be applied in the preoperative holding area or induction room.

For SEP recordings, reusable EEG electrodes are used on the scalp, Erb's points, and popliteal fossae. Braiding and labeling the electrodes at both ends helps with artifact reduction and ease of placement. Disposable subdermal needle electrodes are best for recording MEPs from muscles and for stimulating the motor cortex at the scalp. They are also used for stimulating peripheral nerves. Corkscrew electrodes can also be used for scalp stimulation, just as self-adhesive pads can be used to stimulate peripheral nerves for SEPs. Which electrodes are used depends on the NIOM team's preference.

Once the electrodes are placed, they are plugged into the NIOM machine and the wires draped out of the view of any fluoroscopy equipment and secured. For open descending aortic surgery, a large thoracotomy will be needed for exposure. Most surgeons prefer to have the patient atonic with neuromuscular blocking agents during exposure. This may prevent obtaining MEP baseline responses until after the exposure is nearly complete and the use of neuromuscular blocking agents discontinued. SEP responses can be acquired during opening and exposure even while the patient is paralyzed. Once the use of neuromuscular blocking agents is discontinued, MEPs and SEPs should be acquired continuously. MEP and tibial nerve SEP acquisition should be alternated. Ulnar nerve SEPs are acquired less frequently. The most critical time during these surgeries is when the aorta is cross-clamped. MEPs should be obtained frequently during this time. The MAP and anesthetics must be observed closely because if changes are noted in MEPs or tibial nerve SEPs, the NIOM team should tell the surgeon whether either of those issues may be responsible. The surgical procedure may change if NIOM changes are noted, with the surgeon deciding to institute distal aortic perfusion (if not already being done), reimplant intercostals arteries, etc. Even after the surgical repair is complete and the cross clamp released, it is important to continue NIOM. Blood pressure fluctuations are common, and if a drop in MAP results in changes in MEPs or tibial nerve SEPs, the surgeon must be immediately notified. Consequently, monitoring is continued until the surgery is complete, making these cases very long. Other technologists should be available to provide short breaks in such cases.

For endovascular aortic repair, neuromuscular blocking agents are not needed after induction, and both MEPs and SEPs can be obtained continuously throughout the procedure. As with open surgical repair, acquisition of MEPs and tibial nerve SEPs should be alternated and ulnar nerve SEPs acquired less frequently. Significant changes are most likely to occur during and after the EVSG is deployed. MEPs should be obtained frequently during this time. It is very important to inform the surgeon and anesthesiologist when the MEP stimulus is delivered. Sudden movement of the patient during EVSG deployment may result in suboptimal placement of the graft. The anesthesiologists frequently perform transesophageal echocardiography (TEE) during these procedures, and their fingers are often close to the patient's teeth. An unexpected MEP stimulus may result in the anesthesiologist's fingers being injured due to jaw contraction. Monitoring for these cases should also be continued until the end of the surgery.

During EVSG surgeries, a large introducer sheath is placed in one femoral artery. Tibial nerve SEP responses (both cortical and peripheral) may be lost on the side of the sheath due to ischemia of the tibial nerve. Less often, MEP responses from that leg are also lost. These responses typically return once the sheath is removed. It is important for the technologist to document the leg in which the sheath and other catheters are placed.

Troubleshooting is an essential part of the duties of the NIOM technologist. Many of the issues discussed above for ascending aortic surgery apply to descending cases as well. Additionally, in descending cases, from time to time, all MEP responses will be lost. Often, this is due to one of two problems: the anesthesiologist has administered a bolus of a neuromuscular blocking drug or the MEP stimulating needles have been dislodged. This must be quickly resolved and the surgeon notified accordingly.

Anesthetic management is complex when NIOM is performed during surgery involving the descending thoracic and thoracoabdominal aorta. From the NIOM team's perspective, TIVA without neuromuscular blocking drugs is ideal, since both MEPs and SEPs must be obtained. However, as noted previously, during open surgical repairs, neuromuscular blockade is needed during exposure and closing. Thus, in these cases, TIVA or inhalational anesthesia with neuromuscular blocking drugs is often used until exposure is nearly complete, with the anesthetic regimen then transitioned to TIVA without neuromuscular blocking drugs. Similarly, during closing, neuromuscular blocking agents are reintroduced to facilitate wound approximation. Of course, when neuromuscular blocking drugs are being used, there will be an impact on MEPs. During EVSG surgery, neuromuscular blocking agents are not needed beyond induction and a TIVA protocol works well. Toward the end of an endovascular surgery, when MEP monitoring is no longer critical, patients can be transitioned to inhalational agents to expedite awakening.

At times, surgery is performed on all levels of the thoracic aorta. Hybrid endovascular cases that require debranching of the aortic arch followed by stent graft placement into the arch and descending thoracic aorta are examples of such cases. NIOM in these cases is even more complex. Often DHCA with EEG monitoring is combined with MEP and SEP monitoring, depending on the region of the aorta on to be repaired. The principles of monitoring remain the same as discussed above, only they are combined.

Postprocedure

The main responsibility of the NIOM technologist after an aortic surgery has been completed is to remove the electrodes safely. Unlike many other types of surgery in which patients are awake soon after surgery, in aortic surgery patients often remain intubated and sedated. Consequently, an examination to ensure that no new neurologic deficits have occurred cannot be conducted.

Ascending Aorta and Aortic Arch

NIOM is often terminated in surgeries of the ascending aorta and aortic arch after the patient is off CPB. This is considerably before the skin is closed and surgery terminated. Thus, electrodes are removed while surgery is ongoing. The technologist must accomplish this task with great care. The anesthesiologists are still working near the patient's head and should be asked if it is acceptable to remove the electrodes. Extra care should be exercised when removing electrodes that are near central lines or other intravenous or arterial lines. Of course the surgical field should not be contaminated during electrode removal. If the technologist is not comfortable removing electrodes in this environment, he or she should return to remove them once the surgery is completed.

Documentation must be completed after the surgery. Interactions with the surgeon should be clearly annotated on the record. The most critical communication is when the surgeon was informed of electrocerebral inactivity. Physiologic parameters, such as temperature, should also be noted. A procedure report should also be completed by the neurophysiologist describing the significant events during monitoring. Each laboratory must develop protocols for storing data. If possible, the entire intraoperative tracing should be retained. If that is not possible, screen shots of at least the critical times of the surgery should be kept.

The equipment must be thoroughly cleaned after surgery. The computer cart, headbox, cables, and surfaces should be cleaned with disinfectant wipes. Reusable surface electrodes should be disinfected using laboratory protocols. Computer equipment should be maintained by the hospital's biomedical engineering department. It is the responsibility of the NIOM technologist to ensure that equipment inspections are up to date.

Descending Thoracic and Thoracoabdominal Aorta

NIOM continues until skin closure for surgeries on the descending thoracic and thoracoabdominal aorta, so electrodes are removed after termination of surgery. Caution should be exercised when removing electrodes around the head and Erb's point so as not to disturb any central lines. Needle electrode sites should be checked for bleeding; if bleeding is present, it should be stopped and/or cleaned with an alcohol pad. Additionally, one should confirm that the needle is intact and has not broken off into skin. Any stimulating sites should be checked for burns. If burns occur, they should be reported to the surgeon and neurophysiologist and an incident report completed.

In certain circumstances, monitoring may not end with the termination of surgery. Patients who undergo open surgical repair of the descending thoracic and thoracoabdominal aorta are frequently not awake for several hours to days after surgery. Consequently, they cannot participate in a neurologic examination and remain susceptible to spinal cord ischemia. Monitoring can be continued in the ICU until the patient is awake. However, in these situations, only tibial nerve SEP monitoring is performed. As discussed previously, MEP monitoring is too painful in a patient who is not anesthetized. Ulnar nerve SEPs are not needed as there should be no risk of a brachial plexopathy in the ICU. Peripheral, subcortical, and cortical waveforms of the tibial SEPs should be recorded. A significant change should be immediately brought to the attention of the surgeon or intensivist. Often, increasing the blood pressure or draining additional CSF results in an improvement of the waveforms. How often tibial nerve SEPs should be obtained is unclear; however, on average, this step should be repeated at least every 30 minutes. When the patient is awake enough to reliably participate in a neurologic examination, monitoring is discontinued. ICU monitoring requires a wealth of resources, as it may be several hours and occasionally days before the patient is awake. Consequently such monitoring is seldom performed. Patients undergoing EVSG surgery are typically awake immediately after surgery and do not need ICU monitoring.

As with other types of NIOM, documentation during descending thoracic and thoracoabdominal aortic surgery is very important. All alerts raised should be noted. If possible, the surgeon's response to them should also be recorded. Physiologic parameters, such as temperature and blood pressure, should be noted frequently, especially when an alert is raised. The neurophysiologist should write a report noting the significant events of the surgery.

Many of the electrodes used in descending thoracic and thoracoabdominal aortic surgery are disposable and should be appropriately discarded after surgery. If snap-on lead wires are used, they are cleaned with disinfectant wipes. The NIOM machine should undergo routine maintenance, as discussed above.

FUTURE DIRECTIONS

There remains a need for improvement of current NIOM techniques as well as new monitoring modalities to further decrease the neurologic morbidity of aortic surgery. With the use of EEG, the temperature for DHCA can be tailored for each individual patient. However, the effect of anesthetics on the brain during DHCA remains unclear. Whether the EEG or median nerve SEP is a better "brain thermometer" is not known.

With MEP and SEP NIOM, assessment of the anterior and posterior aspects of the spinal cord can be performed during aortic surgery and ischemia can be detected within minutes. However, standards for interpretation of MEPs have not been established. Whereas many authors consider complete or near complete loss of responses as an abnormality, some have reported a 25% decrement in amplitude as significant. Further research into what is a true abnormality will help improve outcomes and prevent unnecessary interventions, such as increasing blood pressure or draining CSF for a false-positive MEP change, either of which may themselves cause serious complications.

Extending NIOM with SEPs or transcranial magnetic MEPs, which are painless, into the ICU may be useful in monitoring for spinal cord ischemia postoperatively in patients who have undergone open surgical repair of the descending thoracic aorta. Many patients cannot participate in their neurologic examination early after surgery; with this monitoring, the spinal cord can be assessed neurophysiologically. Paradigms for how frequently the monitoring should be performed and staffing arrangements will need to be determined.

With all types of aortic surgery, especially EVSG surgery, more data are needed comparing outcomes of patients undergoing NIOM with those not receiving this monitoring. These types of studies can conclusively establish the need for NIOM.

CONCLUSIONS

Surgery on the thoracic aorta carries a high risk of nervous system injury, including the brain, spinal cord, and peripheral nerves. NIOM with EEG and/or median nerve SEPs can help guide the degree of cooling needed prior to institution of DHCA for aortic repair. This monitoring can also determine prognosis during rewarming. MEP and SEP NIOM may help in minimizing spinal cord ischemia and paraplegia in both open and endovascular surgery on the descending thoracic and thoracoabdominal aorta. Peripheral ischemia and nerve injury are both seen during various types of aortic repair, the risk of which can be reduced with ulnar nerve SEP monitoring. Consequently, NIOM has a definite role in almost all surgeries involving the thoracic aorta.

REFERENCES

1. Cheung AT, Pochettino A, McGarvey ML, , et al. Strategies to manage paraplegia risk after endovascular stent repair of descending thoracic aortic aneurysms. *Ann Thorac Surg* 2005;80:1280–1288.
2. Huynh TTT, Estrera AL, Miller CC, Safi HJ. Thoracic vasculature (with emphasis on the thoracic aorta). In: Townsend CM, ed. *Sabiston Textbook of Surgery: The Biological Basis of Modern Surgical Practice*, 17th ed. Philadelphia: Elsevier Saunders, 2004: 1905–1951.
3. Heuser J. Aortic dissection [online]. Available at: http://en.wikipedia.org/wiki/Aortic_dissection#DeBakey_classification_system. Accessed July 17, 2007.
4. Karadeniz U, Erdemli O, Ozatik MA, et al. Assessment of cerebral blood flow with transcranial Doppler in right brachial artery perfusion patients. *Ann Thorac Surg* 2005;79: 139–146.
5. Kern JA, Kron IL. Descending thoracic and thoracoabdominal aneurysms. In: Kaiser LR, Kron IL, Spray TL, eds. *Mastery of Cardiothoracic Surgery*, 2nd ed. Philadelphia: Lippincott Williams & Wilkins, 2007:545–555.
6. Husain AM. Neurophysiologic intraoperative monitoring. In: Tatum WO, Husain AM, Benbadis SR, Kaplan PW, eds. *Handbook of EEG Interpretation*. New York: Demos, 2007:223–260.
7. Criado FJ, Barnatan MF, Rizk Y, et al. Technical strategies to expand stent-graft applicability in the aortic arch and proximal descending thoracic aorta. *J Endovasc Ther* 2002;9(Suppl 2):II32–II38.
8. Lee JT, White RA. Current status of thoracic aortic endograft repair. *Surg Clin North Am* 2004;84:1295–1318, vi–vii.
9. Stecker MM, Cheung AT, Pochettino A, et al. Deep hypothermic circulatory arrest: I. Effects of cooling on electroencephalogram and evoked potentials. *Ann Thorac Surg* 2001;71: 14–21.
10. Ghariani S, Matta A, Dion R, Guerit JM. Intra- and postoperative factors determining neurological complications after surgery under deep hypothermic circulatory arrest: a retrospective somatosensory evoked potential study. *Clin Neurophysiol* 2000;111:1082–1094.
11. Stecker MM, Cheung AT, Pochettino A, et al. Deep hypothermic circulatory arrest: II. Changes in electroencephalogram and evoked potentials during rewarming. *Ann Thorac Surg* 2001;71:22–28.
12. Guerit JM, Dion RA. State-of-the-art of neuromonitoring for prevention of immediate and delayed paraplegia in thoracic and thoracoabdominal aorta surgery. *Ann Thorac Surg* 2002;74:S1867–1869.
13. Lips J, de Haan P, de Jager SW, et al. The role of transcranial motor evoked potentials in predicting neurologic and histopathologic outcome after experimental spinal cord ischemia. *Anesthesiology* 2002;97:183–191.
14. Qayumi KA, Janusz MT, Jamieson EW, et al. Transcranial magnetic stimulation: use of motor evoked potentials in the evaluation of surgically induced spinal cord ischemia. *J Spinal Cord Med* 1997;20:395–401.
15. Laschinger JC, Cunningham JN Jr, Catinella FP, et al. Detection and prevention of intraoperative spinal cord ischemia after cross-clamping of the thoracic aorta: use of somatosensory evoked potentials. *Surgery* 1982;92: 1109–1117.
16. Crawford ES, Mizrahi EM, Hess KR, et al. The impact of distal aortic perfusion and somatosensory evoked potential monitoring on prevention of paraplegia after aortic

aneurysm operation. *J Thorac Cardiovasc Surg* 1988;95:357–367.
17. Mizrahi EM, Patel VM, Crawford ES, et al. Hypothermic-induced electrocerebral silence, prolonged circulatory arrest, and cerebral protection during cardiovascular surgery. *Electroencephalogr Clin Neurophysiol* 1989; 72:81–85.
18. Guerit JM, Soveges L, Baele P, Dion R. Median nerve somatosensory evoked potentials in profound hypothermia for ascending aorta repair. *Electroencephalogr Clin Neurophysiol* 1990; 77:163–173.
19. Bavaria JE, Pochettino A, Brinster DR, et al. New paradigms and improved results for the surgical treatment of acute type A dissection. *Ann Surg* 2001;234:336–342.
20. Laschinger JC, Cunningham JN Jr, Isom OW, et al. Definition of the safe lower limits of aortic resection during surgical procedures on the thoracoabdominal aorta: use of somatosensory evoked potentials. *J Am Coll Cardiol* 1983;2:959–965.
21. de Haan P, Kalkman CJ. Spinal cord monitoring: somatosensory- and motor-evoked potentials. *Anesthesiol Clin North Am* 2001;19: 923–945.
22. Jacobs MJ, Elenbaas TW, Schurink GW, et al. Assessment of spinal cord integrity during thoracoabdominal aortic aneurysm repair. *Ann Thorac Surg* 2002;74:S1864–1866.
23. Kawanishi Y, Munakata H, Matsumori M, et al. Usefulness of transcranial motor evoked potentials during thoracoabdominal aortic surgery. *Ann Thorac Surg* 2007;83:456–461.
24. Sloan TB. Electrophysiologic monitoring during surgery to repair the thoracoabdominal aorta. *Semin Cardiothorac Vasc Anesth* 2004;8:113–125.
25. Weigang E, Hartert M, Siegenthaler MP, et al. Perioperative management to improve neurologic outcome in thoracic or thoracoabdominal aortic stent-grafting. *Ann Thorac Surg* 2006;82:1679–1687.

Carotid Surgery

Jehuda P. Sepkuty
Sergio Gutierrez

Carotid endarterectomy (CEA) is a surgical procedure designed to prevent ischemic stroke by removing an atheromatous lesion at the carotid bifurcation and restoring the patency of the carotid vessels to an almost normal level. Stroke is the third leading cause of mortality in the United States, following heart disease and cancer. Neurophysiologic intraoperative monitoring (NIOM) is carried out during this prophylactic intervention in order to reduce the risk of stroke as a complication of the procedure. In this chapter, the use of NIOM in CEA is discussed in detail. Brief references are made to other types of carotid surgery, such as aneurysm clipping and endovascular carotid surgery.

ANATOMY AND PATHOLOGY

Ischemic stroke occurs secondary to thromboembolism from atherosclerotic large extracranial or intracranial arteries, embolism from cardiac sources, and atherosclerotic disease of small vessels in the brain. Carotid artery atherosclerosis is the most common etiology and has been the focus of several studies comparing surgical versus medical therapy. The goal of a surgical procedure in patients with atherosclerotic carotid disease is to prevent ischemic stroke and minimize distal embolization of atheromatous material. The carotid bifurcation with the proximal internal carotid artery (ICA) is the most common location involved in carotid atherosclerosis (1) (Figure 16.1). Both ICAs supply approximately 90% of the cerebral blood supply, whereas the posterior cerebral arteries provide roughly 10%. Loss of blood supply to neural tissue can result in cell death within a few minutes, reflecting the high oxygen and metabolic needs of the brain. Endarterectomy addresses lesions located in the internal and common carotid arteries.

Understanding the anatomy of the ICA is crucial to understanding the physiologic consequences of occlusion. The ophthalmic artery is the first branch arising from the intracranial ICA as it emerges from the cavernous sinus. Cholesterol emboli to the ophthalmic artery can cause amaurosis fugax, or the sudden loss of vision in one eye. Terminal branches of the internal carotid include the middle and anterior cerebral arteries perfusing the brain. Communicating branches among the anterior, middle, and posterior cerebral arteries form the circle of Willis.

Several collateral pathways and anastomotic vascular beds connect between various portions of the carotid system. These can provide important sources of blood supply if a

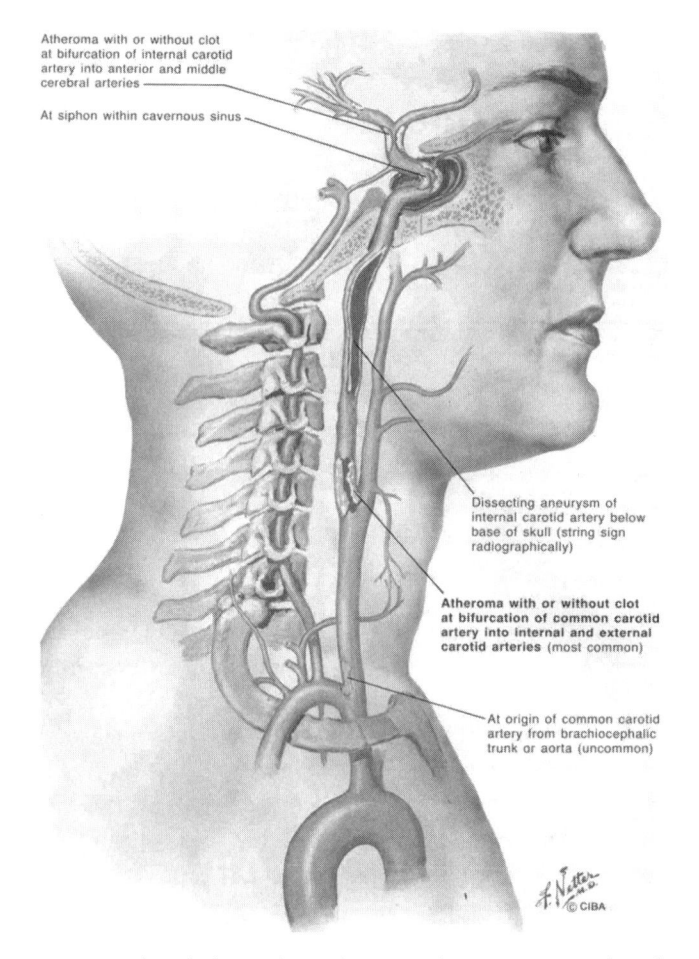

FIGURE 16.1 Common sites of pathology along the carotid artery. [Reproduced with permission from Netter (1).]

hemodynamically significant stenosis occurs at the carotid bifurcation. The most significant of these is the communication between the external carotid and ophthalmic arteries. Angiographic identification of these pathways may be a useful part of the preoperative evaluation of patients with occlusive disease (1) (Figure 16.2).

The neurovascular structures close to the area of operative dissection are important considerations in CEA. Cranial nerves—such as the hypoglossal, vagus, recurrent laryngeal branch of the vagus, and marginal mandibular branch of the facial—can be injured during CEA (2) (Figure 16.3A and B). Precise documentation of a preoperative neurologic examination with special attention to cranial nerve function and consideration for monitoring intraoperatively is therefore important.

Local hemodynamic conditions along the arterial tree create an environment that fosters plaque formation in the carotid artery, most commonly near the bifurcation of the common carotid in the region of the bulb. At the carotid bulb, areas of flow separation with stasis and nonlaminar flow—along with low shear stress along the wall of the bulb—creates an area where bloodstream particles have more time to interact with the vessel wall. Plaque formation is enhanced as a result of this increased contact between blood-borne lipid particles and the vessel wall. The athero-

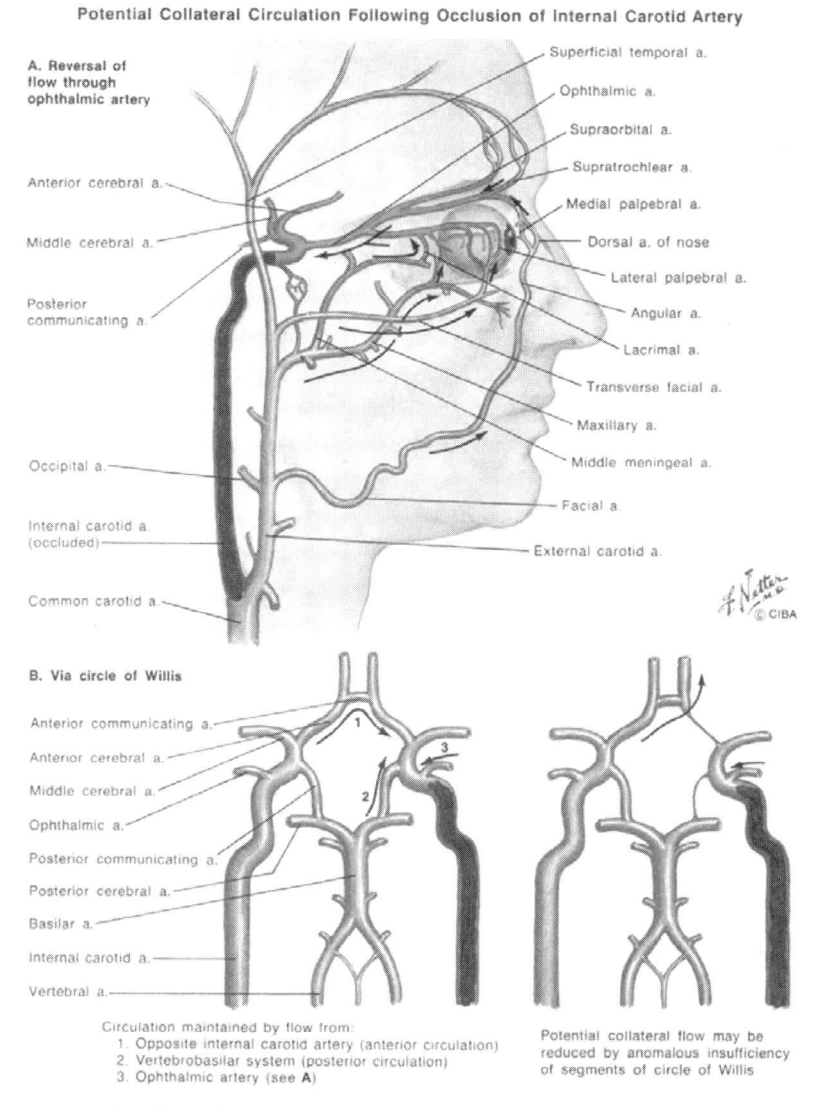

FIGURE 16.2 Potential collateral circulation in the carotid system. [Reproduced with permission from Netter (1).]

sclerotic plaque is created by the formation of a fatty streak with mononuclear and foam cell infiltration.

The development of unstable plaques with subsequent embolization leads to the symptoms of stroke and transient ischemic attack (TIA). In a complex plaque, the intimal proliferation is accompanied by lipid accumulation, calcification, and a necrotic core that becomes covered with a fibrous cap (1) (Figure 16.4). A plaque alone may not suffice to cause a hemodynamically significant alteration in carotid blood flow, but the exposure of the necrotic core of a complex plaque with subsequent platelet deposition may convert an asymptomatic lesion to a symptomatic one. Plaque disruption may be secondary to intraplaque hemorrhage or mechanical forces that create an ulcerated, thrombogenic surface. Symptoms of ischemic stroke may result from distal embolization of atheromatous material or platelet–fibrin aggregates.

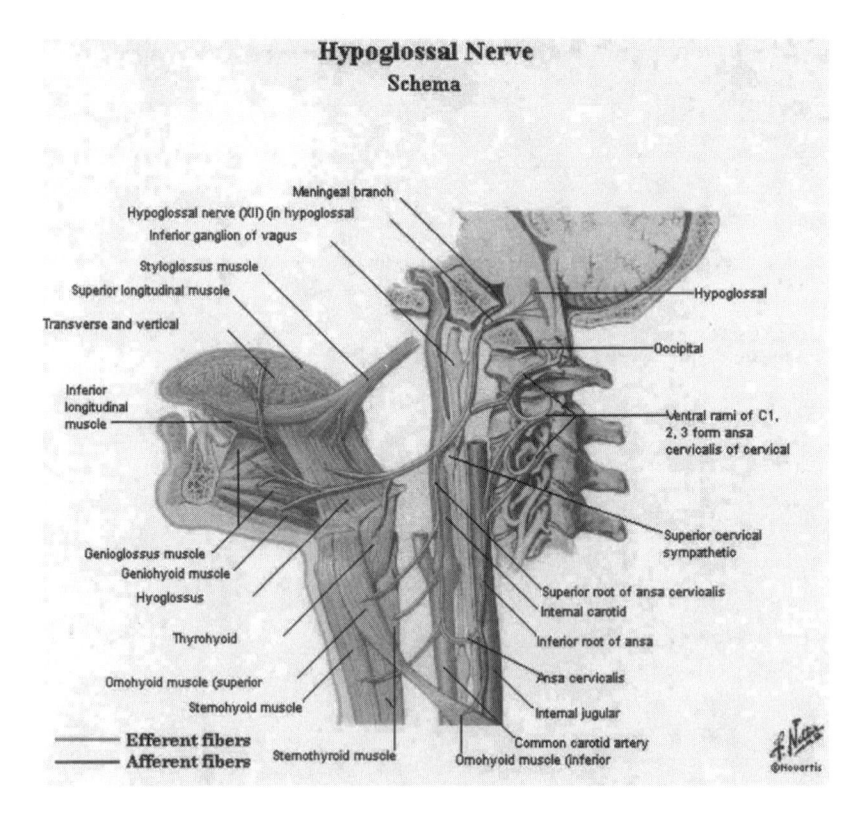

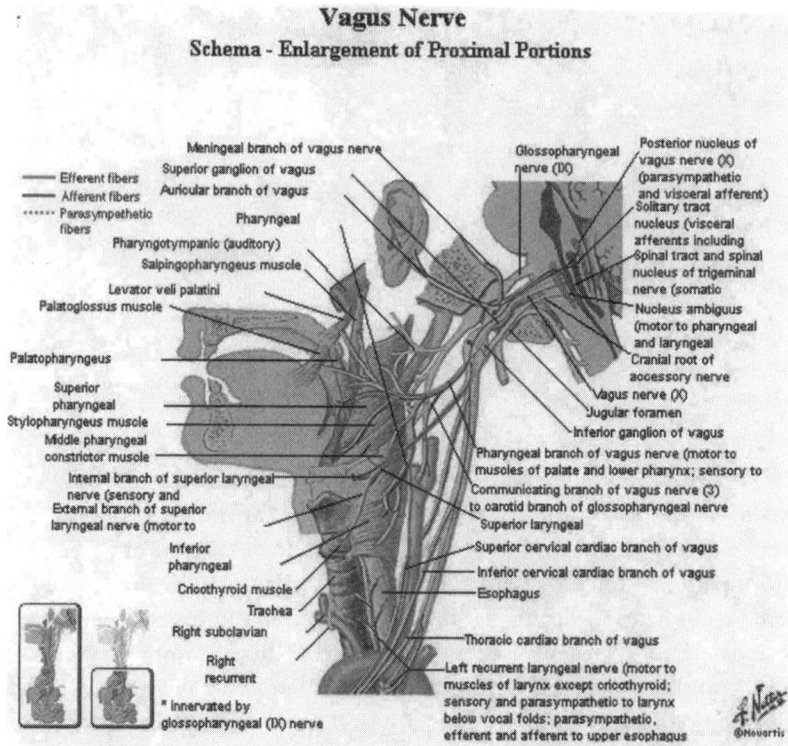

FIGURE 16.3 A. Schema of hypoglossal nerve in the carotid region. B. Schema of vagus nerve in the carotid region. [Reproduced with permission from Netter (2).]

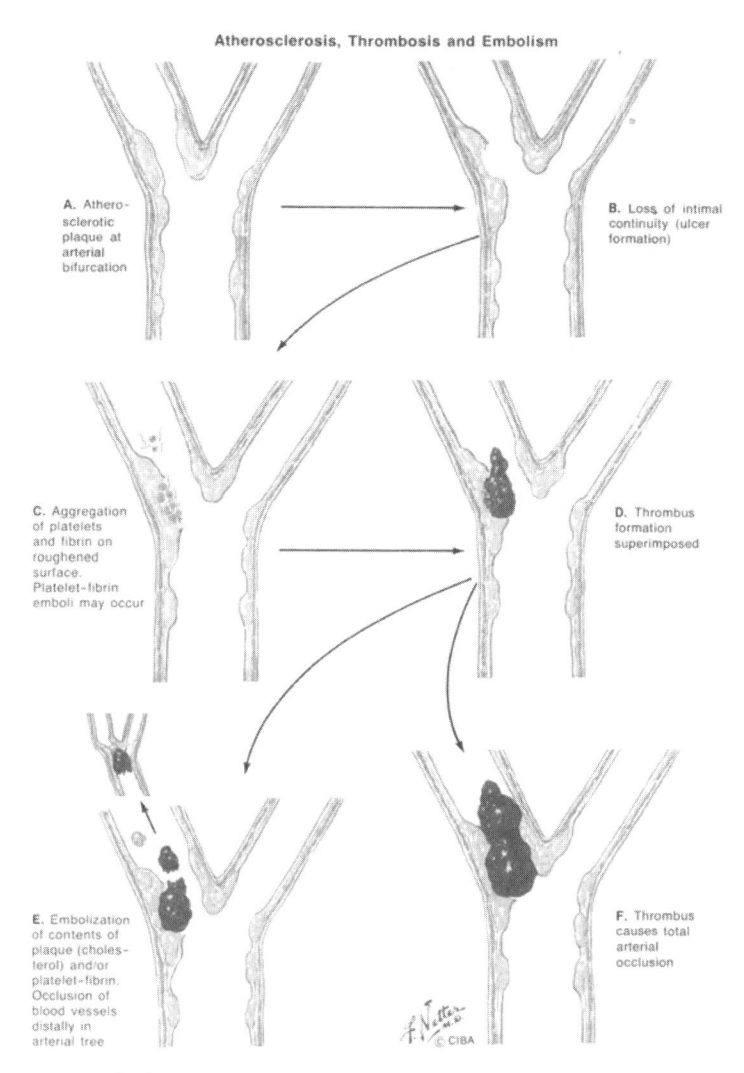

FIGURE 16.4 Formation of atherosclerosis, thrombosis and embolism. [Reproduced with permission from Netter (1).]

Thrombosis of the artery itself can result in symptoms if there are no adequate collateral pathways. This tends to occur only if multiple cerebral arteries in a vascular territory have significant stenosis affecting hemodynamic stability.

CLINICAL SYMPTOMATOLOGY AND PRESENTATION

Atherosclerotic disease of the carotid system declares itself in a variety of ways, depending on the site of stenosis and location of the distal embolization. It is important to remember that atherosclerosis is a systemic disease often affecting the coronary, peripheral, and cerebral circulation concomitantly; thus patients presenting for the evaluation of other conditions should be specifically screened for carotid disease as well. Screening for carotid disease during preoperative evaluation for coronary or lower extremity revascularization is the route whereby many asymptomatic patients declare themselves. Symptomatic patients are those who have sustained a TIA, reversible ischemic neurologic deficit (RIND), or stroke with a fixed neurologic deficit. Patients with TIA experience the sudden onset of a focal neurologic deficit that resolves within 24 hours of onset of the initial symptoms. TIA often consist of contralateral motor and/or sensory deficits or amaurosis fugax. RIND result in neurologic dysfunction lasting greater than 24 hours but less than 2 weeks (1) (Figure 16.5). It is important to distinguish symptoms resulting from vertebrobasilar insufficiency from those secondary to a diseased carotid circulation. Posterior circulatory symptoms are more commonly characterized by "drop attacks," vertigo, and binocular visual loss.

The evaluation of a TIA should carefully exclude other potential causes of similar symptoms, such as heart disease causing neurologic symptoms (i.e., atrial fibrillation, valvular heart disease, dilated cardiomyopathy), intracranial lesions, or metabolic encephalopathy (i.e., hypoglycemia). The physical examination—with close attention to the cardiac, vascular, and neurologic systems—is important in identifying and localizing the disease. The risk factors for atherosclerotic carotid disease include hyper-

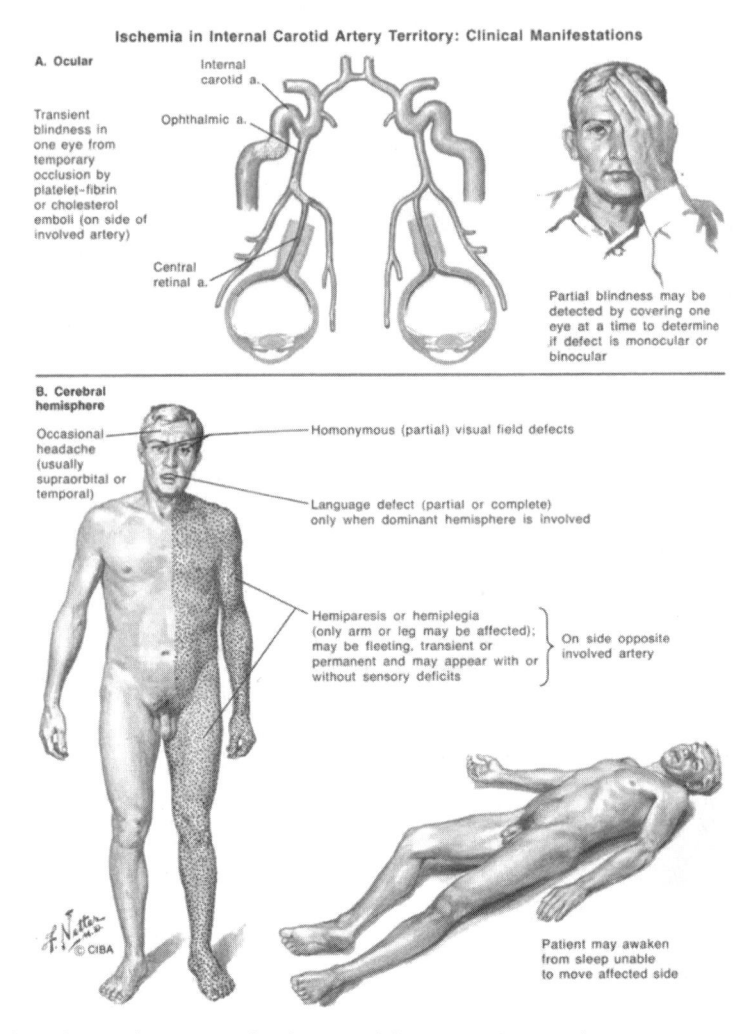

FIGURE 16.5 Clinical manifestations of ischemia of the internal carotid territory. [Reproduced with permission from Netter (1).]

tension, diabetes mellitus, hyperlipidemia, hypercoagulable states, advanced age, and smoking. Carotid bruits detected on physical examination should prompt further investigation; however, published data show no correlation between the presence of carotid bruits and stroke risk.

SURGICAL PROCEDURE

The patient is positioned supine on the operating table after establishment of adequate anesthesia. The head and neck are placed in slight extension, often with the aid of an axillary roll beneath the shoulder blades. The area of sterile preparation is extended to key landmarks, including the mastoid process, lower portion of the ear, mandible, clavicle, and suprasternal notch. The standard surgical approach involves creating a neck incision either along the anterior border of the sternocleidomastoid or a transverse incision at the level of the carotid bulb. A combination of sharp dissection and unipolar electrocautery is used to pass through the platysma muscle and subcutaneous tissues to enter the carotid sheath. The internal jugular vein is identified and mobilized laterally with ligation of vein branches crossing medially, including the facial vein. The common carotid, external, and internal carotid arteries are identified and isolated with vessel loops. The "no touch technique," which minimizes manipulation of the carotid bulb throughout the dissection, aids in the prevention of blood pressure lability and embolization of atheromatous debris. Adequate proximal and distal exposure of the common carotid and internal carotid arteries is necessary, especially if shunt placement and/or patch angioplasty is planned.

Several important nerves traverse the operative field and must be preserved carefully. The vagus nerve is located within the carotid sheath and may be injured in freeing the carotid artery from the internal jugular vein. The hypoglossal nerve is at risk in dissecting above the bifurcation, as is the marginal mandibular branch of the facial nerve, although this nerve more commonly sustains a retraction injury.

Sequential clamping of the internal, common, and external carotid arteries follows systemic heparinization. The area of disease and the normal portion of the vessel can be palpated to determine the appropriate length of the arteriotomy. A standard CEA is performed through a longitudinal arteriotomy starting below the bifurcation and is extended along the internal carotid artery distal to the diseased segment. Before proceeding with the endarterectomy, the surgeon must decide whether shunt placement is necessary based on the data from NIOM or the individual practice of routine shunting.

Endarterectomy is carried out in a plane between the diseased media and the adventitia such that the transition between the endarterectomy plane and the normal vessel proximal and distal to the plaque is smooth. The endarterectomized surface is inspected carefully for atheromatous debris and potential intimal flaps. Most vascular surgeons favor a patch angioplasty rather than primary closure of the arteriotomy based on data suggesting a decreased rate of restenosis (21% vs. 7%, respectively) and ipsilateral stroke with angioplasty. Data regarding the type of patch are more controversial. Polytetrafluoroethylene and Dacron are the two most common synthetic patches. Vein patch angioplasty avoids the use of a prosthetic material but may be associated with harvest site morbidity. The internal carotid artery must be unclamped distally and flushed with heparinized saline to ensure a clean endarterectomized surface before closure of the arteriotomy (1) (Figure 16.6). The common and external carotid arteries are unclamped before the internal carotid artery to provide a less morbid destination for atheromatous debris. Any loose intima distally within the internal carotid that cannot be successfully removed may be tacked

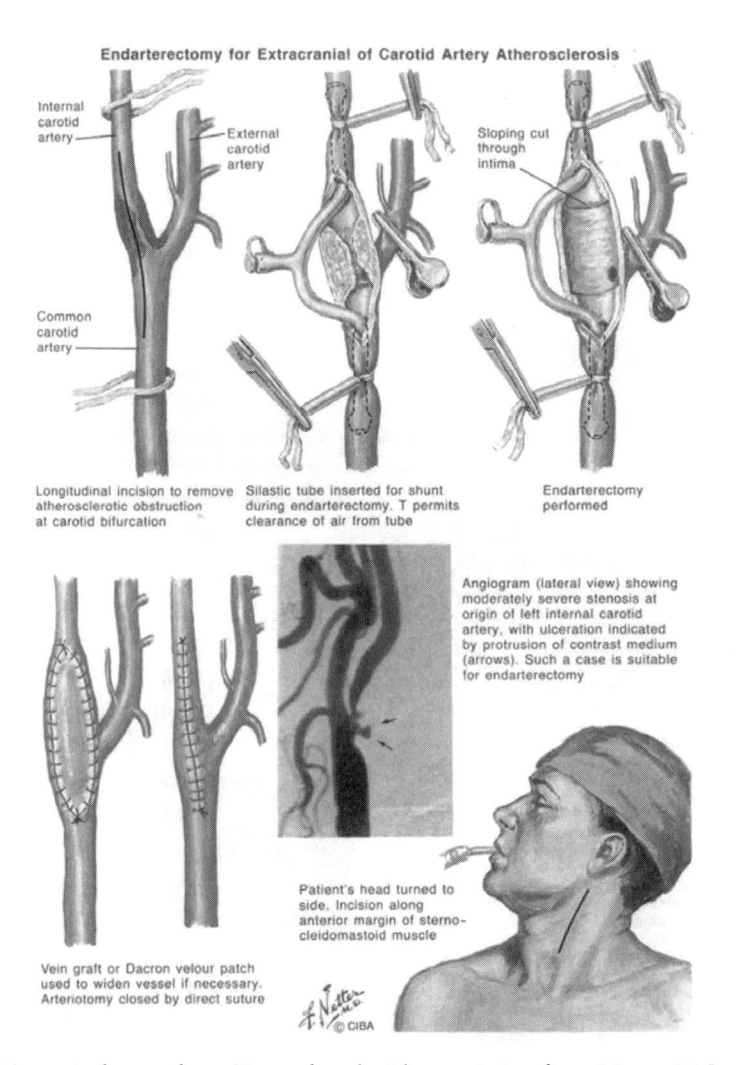

FIGURE 16.6 CEA surgical procedure. [Reproduced with permission from Netter (1).]

against the wall of the artery to prevent intimal flap formation. Some surgeons will perform intraoperative duplex scanning of the repaired artery to evaluate for flow abnormalities. This noninvasive, relatively quick method allows the surgeon to determine whether immediate reexploration of the vessel is required. Adequate hemostasis is obtained and the platysma muscle and skin are reapproximated. A drain may be left beneath the platysma muscle to herald bleeding if hemostasis is of concern.

Eversion endarterectomy is an alternative approach to conventional endarterectomy with primary closure or patch angioplasty. It involves transection of the internal carotid artery circumferentially from the bifurcation and everting the artery while removing the atherosclerotic plaque. Purported advantages to this technique include faster operative times and decreased restenosis. Carotid stenting is another technique that may play a role in select patients who would otherwise be difficult operative candidates. Patients with high extracranial lesions, irradiated necks, or prior neck dissections may be candidates for percutaneous approaches to the carotid artery. Recent randomized data indicate equal efficacy of carotid angioplasty and stenting compared with CEA; however, the stroke rate in the control group (standard CEA) was higher than currently acceptable (3). Angioplasty is still controversial because technical devices that trap atheromatous debris, protecting the distal cerebral circulation, are still undergoing research and improvement. In the future, carotid angioplasty and stenting may play an important role in the management of patients with prohibitive cardiac disease, hostile cervical anatomy, and early restenosis after CEA.

NIOM DURING CAROTIC ENDARTERECTOMY

Utility of NIOM

Endarterectomy is the process of stripping the artery of its inner lining (and with it all the atherosclerotic buildup that is blocking it). During CEA surgery, a cross clamp must be applied to the proximal and distal ends of the artery to be incised and repaired. In most patients there will be adequate collateral flow (from the contralateral internal carotid, external carotidand the basilar arteries via the circle of Willis) to prevent ischemia when the carotid artery is clamped (1) (Figure 16.2). In a minority of patients (approximately 20%), carotid clamping results in a significant cerebral ischemia with an associated high probability of ischemic stroke. The main use of NIOM is to identify these high-risk patients so that a carotid artery bypass shunt can be placed. Although in principle the routine use of shunting may eliminate the need for NIOM, the risk of iatrogenic problems associated with shunting is significant. The inherent risks associated with shunting may be attributed to the following factors: (a) intraoperative thrombosis formation; (b) technical problems that limit the surgeon's ability to expose and dissect the atheroma, especially the distal segment; (c) shunt kinking or occlusion due to improper placement, resulting in ischemia; (d) increased risk of cerebral embolization of atherosclerotic debris and air into the distal cerebral circulation; and (e) potential intimal damage resulting in postoperative thrombosis at the operative site. Therefore selective shunting is considered by many to offer the optimal surgical management of CEA, tailoring the technique to the needs of the individual patient and thus minimizing the above risks (4).

There are other possible benefits to monitoring, such as detecting thrombosis or shunt malfunction, but the most important reason is shunt prevention. In the case of carotid artery stenting procedures, the monitoring is aimed at detecting perfusion changes due to stenosis of the lumen along with the risk of thrombosis and/or embolization. In endovascular therapy of cerebral aneurysms, the rationale for monitoring is the same as in the case of the classic aneurysm clipping surgeries, where there is a risk of decreased perfusion of brain regions due to clipping or endovascular embolization of blood vessels supplying those regions (5). Early detection of a regional perfusion deficit through monitoring allows for changing the surgical procedure to prevent an ischemic stroke. Cerebral ischemia from arterial clipping may occur in several situations: (a) The surgeon may accidentally include a normal vessel within the clip on the aneurysm. An unexpected change in NIOM may alert him or her to any mistake and will usually result in adjustment of the clip. (b) The surgeon may need to deliberately occlude a major intracerebral vessel (usually upstream from the aneurysm) to reduce the blood pressure inside the aneurysm or test for collateral flow when the permanent clip will be placed in a similar location. Based on the findings of the NIOM, the surgeon may chose to protect cerebral function by increasing the blood pressure, cooling the patient, inducing burst suppression, working more expeditiously, or removing the clip.

In the awake patient undergoing CEA under regional anesthesia, repeated neurologic examination may be performed to assess the adequacy of cerebral blood flow (CBF).

During general anesthesia, indirect methods must be used to monitor the adequacy of cerebral blood flow during carotid cross clamping. No currently available monitor of CBF is as sensitive or specific as the awake patient. The monitoring modalities that have been commonly used are electroencephalography (EEG), somatosensory evoked potentials (SEPs), and transcranial Doppler (TCD).

NIOM Modalities

Both EEG and SEPs evaluate neural structures that are at risk for brain ischemia after carotid cross clamping (CCC). Therefore both are good tools for intraoperative detection of patients who require a shunt during CEA. EEG is more sensitive than SEPs, while SEPs are more specific owing to their lower sensitivity to anesthesia. Median nerve SEPs are used more often than tibial nerve SEPs for CEA NIOM. It should be kept in mind that, even if neurophysiologic techniques proved extremely sensitive to hemodynamic disturbances and macroembolism, TCD remains the method of choice for intraoperative detection of microembolism (6).

In this chapter only neurophysiologic monitoring techniques are discussed. The authors use both SEPs (from all four extremities; median and tibial nerves) and raw/processed EEG in these cases (CEA and carotid artery stenting, aneurysm clipping, and endovascular procedures) because they are complementary. EEG is sensitive for detecting cortical ischemia and assesses large areas of brain cortex. SEPs assess both the cortical and subcortical structures but are restricted to the sensory areas. Both EEG and SEPs have limitations: EEG does not detect subcortical ischemia well and is easily affected by confounding variables (routine anesthetic agents, cooling, iatrogenic burst suppression, etc.), while SEPs provide useful information only about sensory pathways.

EEG monitors the spontaneous electrical activity of cortical neurons and is widely used to monitor cerebral perfusion during CEA and endovascular procedures (7). Cortical ischemia is manifest as ipsilateral slowing, attenuation, or both. Normal mean CBF is approximately 50 mL/100 g/min. Mild hypoperfusion from the normal range to 22 mL/100 g/min is tolerated well and does not induce neuronal dysfunction. When flow decreases below the functional threshold, EEG and SEP alterations appear. As opposed to the lesion CBF threshold, the functional threshold does not depend on time. A decrease in EEG amplitude and/or EEG slowing become manifest when mean CBF falls below 22 mL/100 g/min (8) (Figure 16.7). A further decrease in perfusion (7 to 15 mL/100 g/min) leads to the suppression of the EEG activity. Below 12 to 15 mL/100 g/min, neural damage begins to occur, making the EEG a useful monitor for cortical ischemia.

In addition to ischemia caused by CCC, EEG changes may be seen with shunt malfunction, hypotension, contralateral carotid stenosis, or cerebral emboli. EEG also has the advantages of being very sensitive for large areas of cortical ischemia without the need for averaging, and it is relatively simple, noninvasive, practical, and inexpensive. However, as

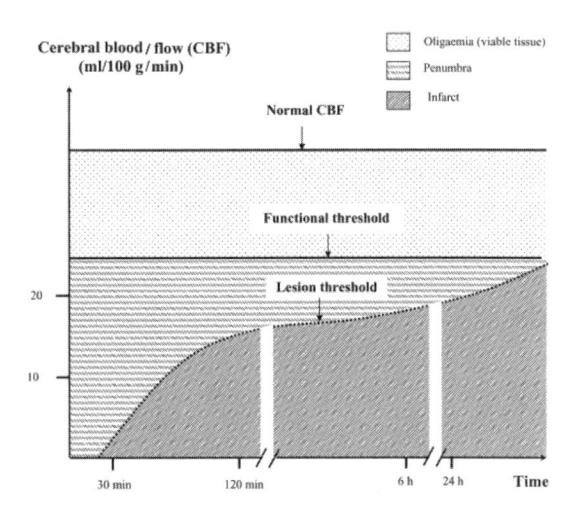

FIGURE 16.7 Brain perfusion thresholds as a function of time. [Reproduced with permission from Florence et al. (8).]

noted above, it is limited by an inability to detect subcortical injury, a high false-positive rate (lower specificity, mainly due to sensitivity to anesthesia and drugs), and a diminished sensitivity in patients who have a history of stroke. EEG is perhaps most significantly limited by the fact that the majority of intraoperative strokes are thought to be embolic and therefore unlikely to improve with shunting. Additionally, most strokes occur postoperatively. Therefore monitoring may be able to prevent only a minority of perioperative strokes in patients undergoing CEA.

To improve the ability to detect deep brain and brainstem ischemia, SEPs can be used in combination with EEG. Unlike EEG, SEPs are able to evaluate deep brain and brainstem structures, not just the cerebral cortex. Ischemic damage to cortical or subcortical neurons produces a characteristic, detectable pattern: a decrease in signal amplitude and concomitant increase in signal latency. Electrical stimulation of a peripheral nerve passes through first- and second-order neurons to synapses in the brainstem and then on to target neurons in the somatosensory cortex. There are many studies showing SEPs to be a valuable monitor of cerebral ischemia. SEPs are particularly useful for patients who have an abnormal EEG as a result of prior stroke.

Studies performed in anesthesized baboons have shown that SEP amplitude decreases for CBF values ranging from 16 to 20 mL/100 g/min. In humans, a 50% reduction in SEP amplitude is observed when flow decreases below 14 mL/100 g/min. Similarly, an increase in the central conduction time (CCT) occurs for CBF values lower than 15 mL/100 g/min. The CBF value resulting in a loss of spontaneous neuronal activities is extremely variable (6 to 22 mL/100 g/min). This large variability can be explained by the differences among individual neurons in energy metabolism and local features of blood supply. Cortical SEPs disappear for CBF values between 12 to 15 mL/100 g/min (8).

EEG Monitoring Technique

Scalp EEG is primarily used to monitor for cortical ischemia. Both unprocessed or raw EEG (REEG) and quantitative EEG (QEEG) may be assessed and provide similar information. REEG refers to unmodified signals in the range of 0.3 to 70 Hz recorded from scalp channels, similar to those recorded in most diagnostic EEG laboratories. QEEG analyzes brief epochs of REEG using a mathematical process called fast Fourier transformation (FFT). This process dissects signals into sine waves, which, if added together, would recreate the original REEG. The amplitudes of sine waves within any designated frequency range are squared and summed, resulting in a measure of power for that range. Once quantified in this manner, many additional measures of the EEG can be assessed, such as the power of any given frequency range, the total power of the EEG, or the frequency with a predetermined proportion of power above or below it [i.e., spectral-edge frequency (SEF), median power frequency].

There is some controversy on the number of channels used and the use of QEEG versus REEG. A 16-channel REEG recording viewed in an anterior-posterior, longitudinal, bipolar montage is typically considered the "gold standard" for EEG monitoring alone. This should be used whenever enough channels are available. Most centers use more than one modality of monitoring (REEG, QEEG, and SEP), so more restricted montages can be used for the EEG if only 8 channels are available. Reports suggest that significantly fewer channels of EEG are needed, providing high degrees of sensitivity and specificity if the appropriate montage is used. This particular montage selectively records EEG from the area of cerebral hemisphere where blood supply is most compromised by CEA surgery, specifically the middle cerebral artery distribution. Channels that provide a frontoparietal and frontotemporal coverage correlate with the distribution of the blood supply of the superior and inferior M2 branches of the middle cerebral artery, respectively. For four-channel recordings F3-C3, F7-T3 / T3-T5 and F4-C4, F8-T4 / T4-T6 or C3-P3, F7-T3 / T3-T5 and C4-P4, F8-T4 / T4-T6 should be used (9). With the newer 16-channel NIOM machines (and recently even 32-channels have become available), one can record F3-C3, C3-P3, F7-T3 / T3-T5 and F4-C4, C4-P4, F8-T4 / T4-T6 as a minimum. If more channels are available, recording can be modified to include the classic 16-channel EEG montage.

The inclusion of QEEG as a part of monitoring is less controversial. QEEG has the advantage of easier interpretation for nonexpert electroencephalographers. In some instances, QEEG may provide additional information, but expert electroencephalographers gain little and may consider it an annoyance rather than an additional tool. QEEG should always be used in conjunction with REEG because only REEG reliably identifies noise, seizure activity, and burst-suppression patterns.

Strategies for Optimizing Detection of Cerebral Ischemia

The sensitivity of the EEG recording is set at 3 to 5 μV/mm for better assessment of low-voltage anterior beta activity. Longitudinal bipolar montages are most appropriate for analysis, as mentioned above. Compressing the EEG with a slow time base (5 or 15 mm/second as opposed to 30 mm/second) enhances assessment of change over time and allows easier detection of slow activity. Having a preoperative EEG is an advantage as it allows comparison to a baseline. At least a preinduction and premedication baseline should be recorded in order to assess any pre-existing asymmetries or abnormalities. It is recommended that at least 10 minutes of preclamp baseline EEG be recorded while the patient is anesthetized to appreciate any clamp-associated changes (10). Similarly, monitoring for a 10-minute period following restoration of blood flow upon clamp release is important to ensure that any intraoperative changes have resolved.

SEP recordings should be obtained preoperatively if possible. Certainly operative baselines should be obtained prior to CCC. Displaying cortical, subcortical, and peripheral waveforms is optimal if enough channels are available. This allows more precise localization of ischemia and helps with troubleshooting. The signal-to-noise ratio of the SEP waveforms should be maximized so that reproducible waveforms can be obtained with the least number of repetitions. An attempt should be made to reproduce the SEP waveforms every 30 seconds during CCC to provide rapid feedback.

Anesthetic Effects on the EEG and SEPs

The EEG anesthesia pattern consists of fast anterior dominant rhythmic activity [FAR; also known as widespread, anteriorly maximum rhythmic activity (WAR)], anterior intermittent slow waves (AIS), and widespread persistant slow waves (WPS). Compressing the EEG with a slow time base enhances assessment of change over time. Adjusting gain until the FAR pattern produces a deflection of about 1 cm helps detect the signs of ischemia. The proportion of the three anesthesia patterns varies between patients and within a given patient. The preclamp EEG is classified as stable or unstable depending on the persistence of these components and as symmetric or asymmetric. Fluctuations of the anesthesia pattern are usually generalized and relate to anesthesia, analgesia, and systemic factors such as mean arterial pressure (MAP), and they can confound interpretation. The anesthesiologist should seek a stable level of anesthesia prior to CCC. Otherwise confusion at the time of clamping may arise from suboptimal patterns, such as frontal intermittent rhythmic delta activity (FIRDA), a burst-suppression pattern, etc.

An asymmetric EEG usually occurs with antecedent cerebral lesions. Usually over the abnormal hemisphere there is less FAR and more WPS patterns. Unluckily anesthesia may affect preoperative focal EEG abnormalities by either activating or obscuring them (which is one of the reasons SEPs are useful in this scenario).

Clamp-related EEG changes usually occur within 1 minute. Mild to moderate ischemia produces a reduction in the FAR pattern with or without an increase in the WPS pattern. Severe ischemia produces EEG suppression; usually changes are ipsilateral, but they may be bilateral when the clamped vessel provides flow to the contralateral hemisphere as well.

Various anesthetic agents have different effects on the EEG. Agents considered inhibitory are nitrous oxide, halogenated agents, propofol, and barbiturates. Agents causing augmentation are ketamine and etomidate. Neutral or near neutral agents include narcotics and benzodiazepines. Neuromuscular blocking agents are considered neutral, but they help reduce muscle artifact in EEGs and increase signal-to-noise ratios for SEPs. Propofol and barbiturates suppress EEGs as mentioned, with less effect on SEPs, which can still be recorded when the EEG is isoelectric (11) (Figure 16.8).

Anesthetic effects on SEPs are described in detail elsewhere in this book. Briefly, inhalation agents will cause suppression of the cortical waveforms, especially of the tibial SEPs. Intravenous anesthetics, such as propofol, have little effect on SEPs. However, high doses of even these agents can cause suppression of the cortical waveforms. Neuromuscular blocking agents reduce electromyographic (EMG) artifact and make SEP acquisition quicker owing to an improved signal-to-noise ratio. Intravenous narcotics and benzodiazepines have little effect on SEPs.

Alarm Criteria

Alerting the surgeon when changes in REEGs, QEEGs, or SEPs are seen is important. The criteria used most often are presented in Table 16.1. Ischemia-related changes are seen on the EEG within one minute of CCC. If changes are not seen in this period of time, there is adequate collateral circulation to perfuse the ipsilateral hemisphere. The most typical criteria for alerting the surgeon based on REEG are when the amplitude drops by 50%, when then there is 50% decrease of FAR, or when there is doubling of WPS. A minor change is when there is a visually uncertain, less than 20% reduction of FAR with or without an increase of WPS. The CBF with such a change is about 23 mL/100 g/min. A mild change of REEG is when there is a clear but less than 50% reduction of FAR with or without an increase of WPS. This corresponds to a CBF of about 18 to 23 mL/100 g/min. A moderate change is when a greater than 50% reduction of FAR is noted with or without an increase of WPS (Figure 16.9A and B). This occurs with a CBF of about 17 to 22 mL/100 g/min. Finally, a major change is when there is suppression of the REEG, which is consistent with a CBF of less than 17 mL/100 g/min. A moderate or major change should prompt the surgeon to insert a shunt. Patients with preexisting focal EEG abnormalities are more likely to have a major change during CEA. Once a shunt is in place, there is resolution of the EEG changes.

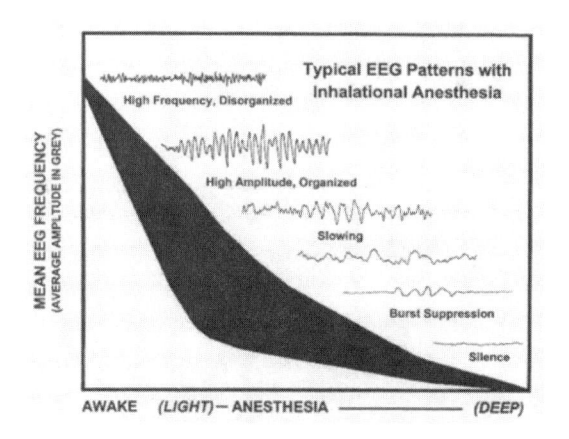

FIGURE 16.8 Typical changes in the EEG at different levels of anesthesia. [Reproduced with permission from Sloan (11)].

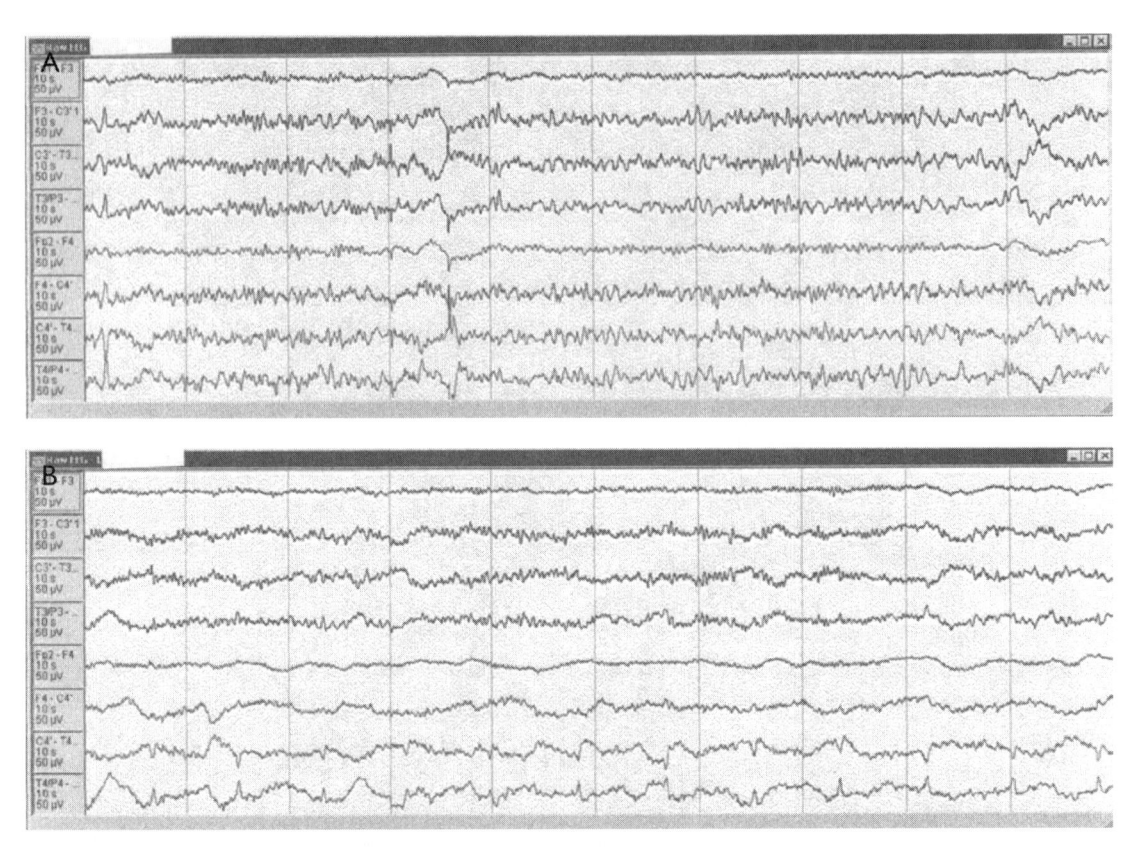

FIGURE 16.9 A. Normal raw EEG recording at baseline in a CEA case. B. A change in the raw EEG recording in a CEA case, showing bilateral, right more than left (last two channels) centrotemporal slowing.

QEEG-based warning criteria have also been used (12). When there is a 75% loss of total power, an alarm should be sounded (Figure 16.10). In general, a decrement of the alpha + beta / theta + delta ratio correlates well with reduced perfusion. When propofol anesthesia is used, the delta power is the best parameter to use to gauge cerebral perfusion. The best montage for this type of monitoring is F3-Cz, P4-Cz, C4-Cz, F7-Cz. For isoflurane anesthesia, SEF of 90% is the most commonly used marker for cerebral perfusion; the best montage for monitoring this is F8-Cz, T4-Cz, C4-Cz, F4-Cz. Knowing the anesthetic agent to be used along with the number of channels available should dictate the use of the specific QEEG method and modification of derivations used for EEG. It is important to keep the surgeon informed of the degree of change seen in both the REEG and QEEG.

SEP changes can also occur with CCC if adequate collateral circulation does not exist (Table 16.1). CCC related SEP changes occur within a few minutes. SEP changes are significant when they occur unilaterally; bilateral changes most often indicate systemic changes such as anesthesia or blood pressure fluctuations. The most sensitive SEP marker of ischemia is cortical waveforms. A minor change is a 50% reduction of amplitude or 5% latency prolongation of the cortical waveforms. A major change is near complete loss of the cortical waveforms. This occurs when CBF falls to 15 to 20 mL/100 g/min. Subcortical waveforms may not be affected when cortical waveforms are nearly completely lost. When the CBF falls to 10 to 15

TABLE 16.1 EEG and SEP Alarm Criteria Used in CEA

Significant change	Raw EEG: 50% ↓ overall amplitude 50% ↓ loss FAR Doubling of WPS	
EEG	REEG changes	CBF (mL/100 g/min)
Minor	20% ↓ FAR, ± ↑ WPS	23
Mild	< 50% ↓ FAR, ± ↑ WPS	18–23
Moderate	> 50% ↓ FAR, ± ↑ WPS	17–22
Severe	Suppression	< 17
Quantitative EEG		
Significant change	75% loss of total power	
Propofol anesthesia	↑ relative delta power	
Isoflurane anesthesia	SEF 90%	
SEP		
Significant change	50% ↓ amplitude of cortical waveforms 5% ↑ latency of cortical waveforms	
	SEP changes	CBF (mL/100 g/min)
Minor	< 50% ↓ amplitude of cortical waveforms	15–20
Major	> 50% ↓ amplitude of cortical waveforms, 5% ↑ latency of cortical waveforms	< 14
Severe	Loss of cortical waveforms, ↓ amplitude of subcortical waveforms	12–15

FAR = fast anterior dominant rhythmic activity; WPS = widespread persistant slow waves, CBF = cerebral blood flow; SEF = spectral edge frequency.

mL/100 g/min, significant loss of subcortical waveform amplitude may be seen. A major change should prompt the surgeon to insert a shunt. As with EEG, SEP changes resolve once the shunt is in place.

Occasionally focal EEG and unilateral SEP changes can occur randomly during CEA—i.e., not related to CCC. Often these changes are transient and related to fluctuations in blood pressure or anesthetics. If they resolve spontaneously, they are not likely to be associated with postoperative morbidity. If presurgical focal EEG abnormalities are present, they may be accentuated with anesthesia, thus appearing to be new focal changes. These, too, are not associated with new postoperative deficits. Emboli may arise from the site of surgery and lodge in a distal vessel ipsilaterally. This can result in focal EEG and unilateral SEP changes. These changes will be persistent; increasing the blood pressure may help resolve them. But if they persist, they will likely be associated with new postoperative deficits.

Sample CEA NIOM Case

A 43-year-old man with an asymptomatic 80% left internal carotid artery stenosis and diffuse vascular disease underwent a left CEA with EEG and SEP NIOM. Upon initial clamping of the carotid artery, a marked loss of left more than right hemispheric QEEG total power was seen (Figure 16.11A). A Pruitt shunt was placed and all signals recovered (Figure 16.11B). The same pattern of signal loss and recovery was seen later in the procedure when the vessel was clamped again for

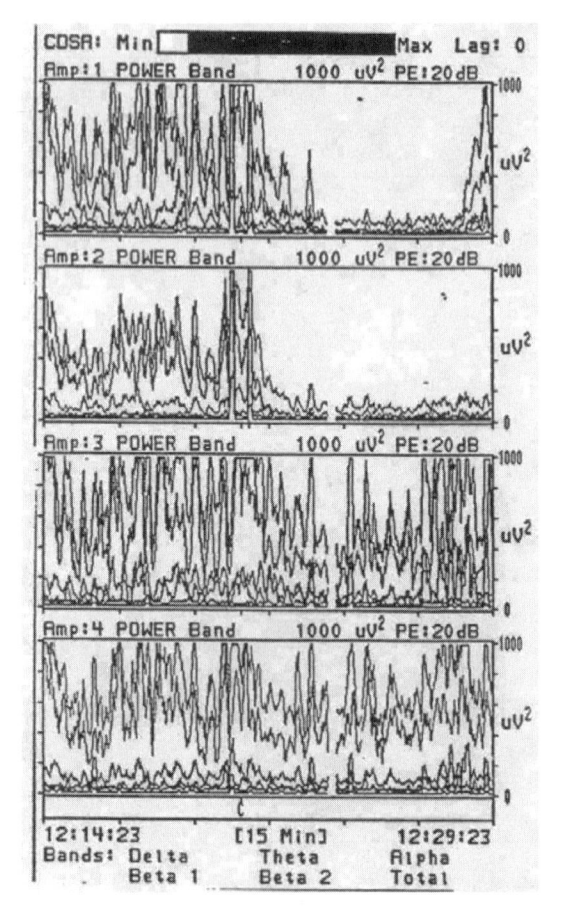

FIGURE 16.10 Example of a left-sided change (upper two channels) of QEEG during CCC.

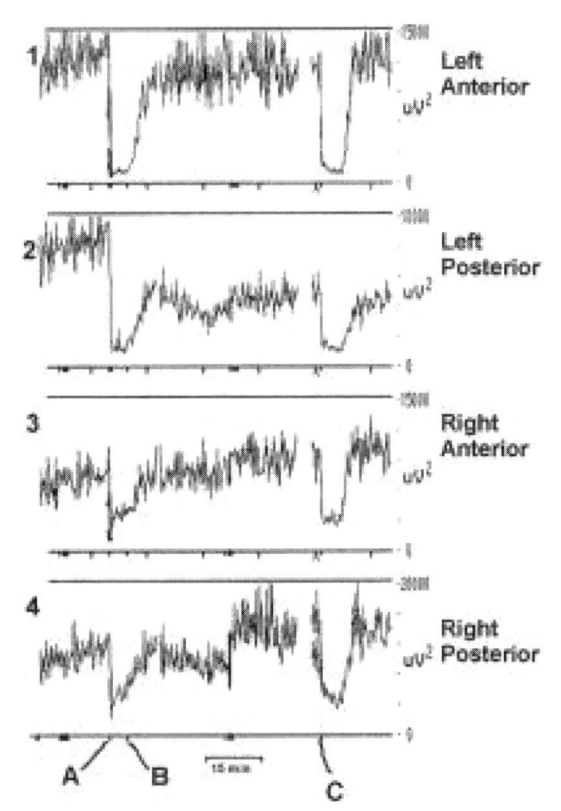

FIGURE 16.11 QEEG total power changes during a CEA case. Left more than right total power dropped upon clamping, followed by a recovery after shunting. At point "A," the left carotid artery was clamped. A sudden drop in power was seen bilaterally, left worse than right. Point "B" marks institution of a shunt; notice prompt return of the waveforms to near normal levels. Toward the end of the case, at point "C," the carotid artery is clamped again for shunt removal. There is sudden loss of total power, which returns after releasing the clamp.

shunt removal (Figure 16.11C). The amplitude of the right median nerve SEP cortical response was also dramatically reduced in association with the initial carotid artery clamping, as was the amplitude of the right tibial nerve SEP cortical response(Figure 16.12). All signals recovered and the patient remained neurologically intact after surgery (7).

Other Vascular Surgeries

Surgeries involving distal branches of the internal carotid artery (anterior and middle cerebral and anterior and posterior communicating arteries) as well as arteries of the vertebrobasilar system require more complicated NIOM. This is not discussed in detail as monitoring for these surgeries is uncommonly performed. An overview of the modalities used most often is presented below. REEG, QEEG, and SEPs are used for most vascular surgeries, and brainstem auditory evoked potentials (BAEPs) are used for surgeries on the vertebrobasilar system.

When vascular surgery involves the middle or posterior cerebral or posterior communicating arteries, contralateral tibial nerve SEPs are more sensitive than median nerve

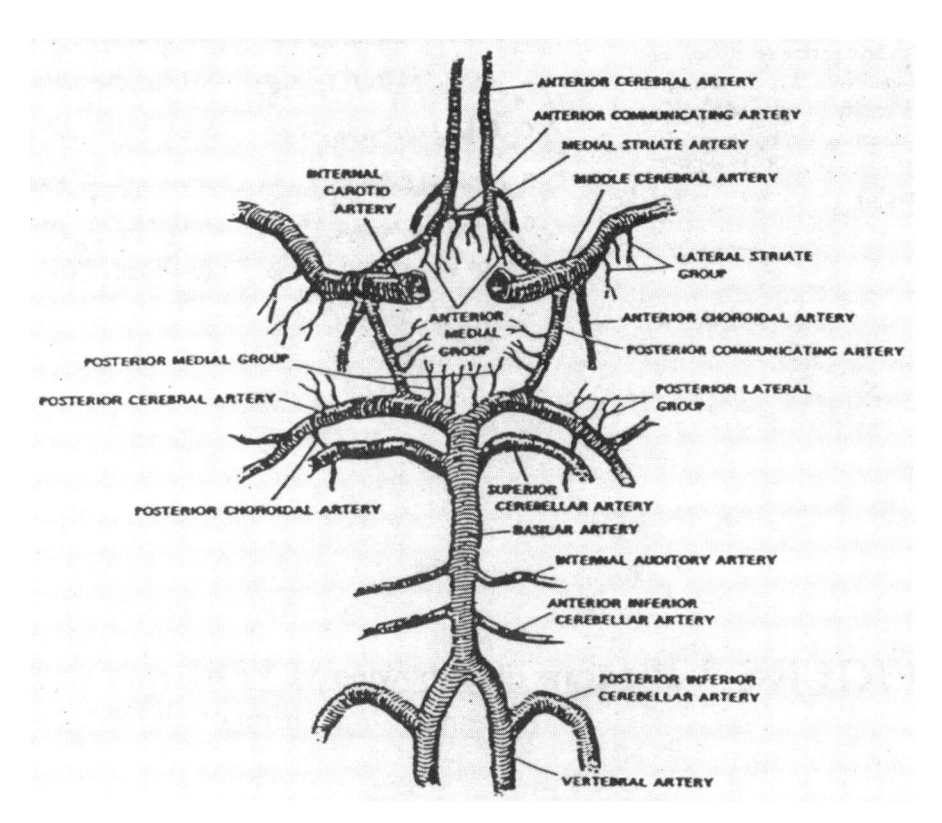

FIGURE 16.12 Median nerve SEP changes during a right CEA. Right median nerve SEP response deteriorates after clamping with improvement after shunting without left median nerve SEP change.

SEPs. For surgeries on the A1 segment of the anterior cerebral and anterior communicating arteries, the contralateral tibial nerve SEP is most sensitive, followed by the ipsilateral tibial nerve SEPs, followed by the contralateral median nerve SEPs. Surgery on the A2 segment of the anterior cerebral artery is best monitored by contralateral tibial and median nerve SEPs. When the basilar or vertebral arteries are involved, both tibial and median nerve SEPs are useful, as are BAEPs. REEG and QEEG are used during surgery on all cerebral vessels.

Evidence Supporting Use of NIOM in Carotid Endarterectomy

It is difficult to determine whether NIOM with EEG or SEP helps decrease the morbidity of CEA, as most surgeons shunt the carotid artery if neurophysiologic changes are noted. However, a report from a center where none of the patients receive shunts regardless of EEG findings noted that 55 of 176 (31%) patients undergoing CEA had significant clamp-associated REEG changes (10). These changes resolved after the clamp was released in 36 (65%) patients. Five (9%) developed new neurologic deficits, and in two (1%) of these patients the deficits were permanent. Similarly, in a study of 312 CEA procedures, 28 (8%) had significant alterations of SEPs (13). In 24 of these patients, the abnormalities were completely reversed with shunting, and in another 2 patients the abnormalities were partially reversed. None of these patients had any postoperative deficits. In 2 patients in whom there was persistent absence of SEPs, contralateral hemiparesis was noted after surgery.

Another way to evaluate the efficacy of EEG and SEP monitoring is to evaluate their sensitivity and specificity in identifying cerebral ischemia. In a recent review, the sensitivity and specificity of REEG was noted to be 0.27 and 0.87. QEEG was slightly better, with sensitivity and specificity of 0.58 and 0.99. SEPs also seemed to be better than REEG, with a sensitivity and specificity of 0.52 and 0.98 (8). Multimodality monitoring may be more effective than any single modality alone.

TECHNICAL CONSIDERATIONS

Preparation

In preparing for CEA or other surgery involving the carotid arteries, it is best to review the anatomy of the cerebral vasculature. A handy reference demonstrating the vascular anatomy around the circle of Willis is useful to have available.

There are many patient-related conditions that may affect NIOM; it behooves the NIOM team to recognize these so that monitoring can be adequately adapted. Prior hemispheric stroke or demyelinating diseases may result in slowing of EEG frequencies at baseline. This must be kept in mind in interpreting focal slowing after CCC. The presence of peripheral neuropathy, neuromuscular disorders, myelopathy, and cerebral palsy may affect SEPs. Preoperative EEG and SEP studies done at least a day in advance of the surgery have the advantage of alerting the NIOIM team of preexisting abnormalities in neurophysiologic tests.

An adequate number of electrodes should be available. The exact number and types of electrodes needed will depend on which modalities are monitored. Sterile, disposable, subdermal, stainless steel needle electrodes can be used for all standard procedures. They are optimal due to low impedances and easy application. If special techniques such as BAEPs are to be used, appropriate electrodes for these modalities should also be made available. Details of obtaining BAEPs are discussed elsewhere in this book.

The surgical team is responsible for informing the patient about the procedure and risks prior to the surgery. It is a good idea to include the remote risk of needle burn in the list of possible complications. If possible, the NIOM team should meet the patient prior to the administration of anesthesia and explain their roles in the procedure.

Procedure

Setup for a CEA or other carotid surgery will depend not only on the modalities to be monitored but also on how many channels are available on the NIOM machine. Older machines had 8 channels, greatly restricting the number of EEG and SEP channels that could be recorded. Now 32-channel machines are available; however, most machines used currently have 16 channels.

At least four EEG channels are used; the most useful montage has been described earlier (F8 Cz, T4-Cz, C4-Cz, F4-Cz or F3-Cz, P4-Cz, C4-Cz, F7-Cz). A slightly different montage is used for aneurysm surgery (F1–C3, C3–O1, F2–C4, C4–O2). If extra channels are available or if separate machines are used for monitoring EEG and SEPs, a 16-channel, anterior-posterior longitudinal montage should be used. For SEP monitoring, electrodes on the scalp (C3, Cz, C4), cervical spine (C5S), Erb's point, and popliteal fossa are used. Stimulating electrodes for the median and tibial nerves are placed at the wrists and medial aspect of the ankles. The recording and stimulating electrodes for SEPs can be either of the needle or surface type.

Anesthesia can affect both EEG and SEP NIOM. A discussion with the anesthesia team about the modalities being monitored and the best anesthetic regimen is important. Generally for CEA and other types of carotid surgeries, complete neuromuscular blockade is acceptable. Inhalation agents are also acceptable in these cases. The NIOM team must keep in mind the effects of these agents on the EEG, as discussed earlier. If the minimum alveolar concentration (MAC) is increased much above 1, there may be suppression of the cortical waveforms of the SEPs. Propofol and barbiturates may also be used by the anesthesia team to induce burst-suppression (for cerebral protection). This makes interpretation of the EEG more difficult; however, it may be needed for cerebral protection. The NIOM team can help the anesthesia team by keeping them informed of the duration of the suppression; usually 7 to 10 seconds of suppression are required between "bursts" to protect the cortex. Propofol and barbiturates have minimal effect on the SEPs. Etomidate can induce burst suppression but causes a marked increase in amplitude of the EEG; this should be avoided because comparisons to baseline will no longer be valid. Whenever possible, it is best that a constant level of anesthesia be used, as bolus doses of any agent can produce sudden changes in both the EEG and SEPs, making interpretation difficult.

Baseline NIOM data should always be obtained once the anesthetic regimen has been stabilized. It may be useful to print a sample of the EEG baseline prior to CCC for comparison to later tracings. Similarly, an SEP baseline should be obtained for later comparison. At least the cortical response (and preferably the subcortical and peripheral responses as well) should be displayed, as it is usually the highest in amplitude and therefore has the best signal-to-noise ratio. If a change in noted in the cortical responses, other responses will also have to be viewed for localization of the change. Most new NIOM machines allow display of multiple panels, so that REEG, QEEG, and SEPs can be viewed simultaneously.

REEGs and QEEGs are acquired in a free-running mode during the surgery. SEPs are obtained as frequently as possible, particularly during the riskiest segment of the procedures (CCC, coiling, embolization, etc).

Changes unrelated to surgical injury must be identified as such to avoid raising a false alarm. These changes can be induced by anesthesia, a drop in blood pressure, blood loss, peripheral nerve compression (positioning, blood pressure cuff), electrical noise, mechanical noise (drilling, suctioning), and physiologic artifacts [electrocardiogram (ECG), electromyogram (EMG), breathing]. It is the role of the NIOM team to recognize and troubleshoot the confounding factors in collaboration with the anesthesia team.

Technical problems often occur in the operating room. The technologist, with the help of the neurophysiologist, should attempt to resolve these as quickly as possible. Problems with stimulation (for SEPs) may occur if the stimulating needles are pulled out during positioning. The stimulator itself may be malfunctioning. If the needles are pulled out, the NIOM machine will often alert the operator that an impedance limit has been reached. Changes in the SEPs will consist of signal loss, including loss of peripheral responses.

Problems can also occur with the recording system. This results in excessive artifact seen in the EEG and very noisy traces or excessive input rejection of the amplifier for SEPs. The first step is to check impedances. If impedances are high, the corresponding electrodes should be checked to make sure they are making adequate contact. The connection of the electrode leads to the amplifier must also be checked. The head box connection holes must also be checked, as they may be defective; other holes can be tried. Finally, the electrode itself may need to be replaced, as the connection between the electrode and its lead may be broken. If impedances are acceptable, all previous problems are ruled out. The technologist must then concentrate on identifying and eliminating noise sources if possible. Devices that may be causing artifact and may be disconnected include the surgical bed, body warmers, blood warmers, and electrical islands. Prior to unplugging any device in the operating room, the circulating nurse must be consulted to ensure that the device can be safely unplugged. The NIOM machine should not be plugged in islands or where multiple devices are plugged. If possible the EEG and SEP electrode wires should be braided, as this reduces artifact as well. Filtering specific electrical noise frequencies can also be attempted if other methods to reduce this artifact fail (i.e., 60 Hz filter). Excessive EMG contamination of the EEG or SEPs can be reduced by asking the anesthesia team to administer neuromuscular blocking agents.

When the NIOM technologist sees certain changes, they should be discussed with the neurophysiologist and anesthesia team before raising an alarm for the surgeon. This includes any global change affecting either EEG or SEPs and is not correlated with critical steps of the procedure. It must be determined as soon as possible if there have been changes in anesthetic parameters, blood pressure, temperature, etc. If the cause of these changes cannot be attributed to a nonsurgical cause or one of the alarm criteria described earlier is met, the surgeon must be notified immediately.

Communication between the NIOM, surgery, and anesthesia teams is critical for optimal monitoring. Surgeons should announce every step of the surgery or any ongoing adverse event. The anesthesia team must inform of any parameter change or fluctuation in vital signs. The NIOM team must immediately inform the surgeon about any change that may imply ischemia or injury or discuss with the anesthesia team any nonsurgical change. Documentation of all events is extremely important.

Postprocedure

Needle electrodes must be removed cautiously, avoiding injury to both the patient and others working in the operating room. The needle electrodes must be discarded in an appropriate container. In case of accidental needle-stick injury, hospital protocols for such injuries should be followed. All tape fragments must be removed carefully as well. Surface electrodes, if reuseable, should be appropriately cleaned and disinfected for future use. Burn injuries are very rare, but when they occur, they should be reported and documented. Equipment should undergo scheduled maintenance by the biomedical department of the hospital. Technical malfunctions should be reported immediately and will require an immediate assessment by the engineers.

After surgery, a report of the NIOM procedure should be written providing relevant data and sequence of events for accuracy. This report is also of important medicolegal value: whatever is not reported is considered not to have been done. Lack of thorough reporting may be interpreted as "sloppy" and unprofessional monitoring. Documentation must include patient demographics, diagnosis, relevant clinical or complementary data, and any adverse event or change in NIOM. Consider including baseline and closing data printouts, including SEP curve stacks and numerical data, as part of the patient's NIOM chart. This data can also be stored digitally, depending on the NIOM machine's capability.

CONCLUSIONS

NIOM during CEA and other types of carotid surgery can provide the surgeon with critical information that may modify the surgical procedure. With assistance from the NIOM team, the surgeon may elect to shunt the carotid artery during CEA or may modify the clip placed on an aneurysm. REEG and QEEG analysis during these surgeries is critical for assessment of cortical perfusion. With the addition of SEP monitoring, subcortical ischemia can also be detected. Recognizing appropriate alarm criteria is important, as instantaneous feedback to the surgeon is mandatory. A complementary working environment between the

NIOM, surgery, and anesthesia teams will ensure the best monitoring.

REFERENCES

1. Netter FH. *Nervous System: Neurologic and Neuromuscular Disorders*. West Caldwell, NJ: Ciba-Geigy, 1992.
2. Netter FH. *Atlas of Human Anatomy*, 3rd ed. Teterboro, NJ: Icon Learning Systems, 2003.
3. Yadav JS, Wholey MH, Kuntz RE, et al. Protected carotid-artery stenting versus endarterectomy in high-risk patients. *N Engl J Med* 2004;351:1493–1501.
4. Allain R, Marone LK, Meltzer J, Jeyabalan G. Carotid endarterectomy. *Int Anesthesiol Clin* 2005;43:15–38.
5. Liu AY, Lopez JR, Do HM, et al. Neurophysiological monitoring in the endovascular therapy of aneurysms. *AJNR Am J Neuroradiol* 2003;24:1520–1527.
6. Babikian VL, Cantelmo NL. Cerebrovascular monitoring during carotid endarterectomy. *Stroke* 2000;31:1799–1801.
7. Minahan RE. Intraoperative monitoring. *Neurologist* 2002;8:209–226.
8. Florence G, Guerit JM, Gueguen B. Electroencephalography (EEG) and somatosensory evoked potentials (SEP) to prevent cerebral ischaemia in the operating room. *Neurophysiol Clin* 2004;34:17–32.
9. Laman DM, van der Reijden CS, Wieneke GH, et al. EEG evidence for shunt requirement during carotid endarterectomy: optimal EEG derivations with respect to frequency bands and anesthetic regimen. *J Clin Neurophysiol* 2001;18:353–363.
10. Blume WT, Sharbrough FW. EEG monitoring during carotid endarterectomy and open heart surgery. In: Niedermeyer E, Da Silva FL, eds. *Electroencephalography: Basic Principles, Clinical Applications, and Related Fields*. Baltimore: Williams & Wilkins, 1999:797–805.
11. Sloan TB. Anesthetic effects on electrophysiologic recordings. *J Clin Neurophysiol* 1998; 15:217–226.
12. Laman DM, Wieneke GH, van Duijn H, et al. QEEG changes during carotid clamping in carotid endarterectomy: spectral edge frequency parameters and relative band power parameters. *J Clin Neurophysiol* 2005;22:244–252.
13. Amantini A, Bartelli M, de Scisciolo G, et al. Monitoring of somatosensory evoked potentials during carotid endarterectomy. *J Neurol* 1992;239:241–247.

17 Epilepsy Surgery

William O. Tatum, IV
Fernando L. Vale
Kumar U. Anthony

More than 3 million people in North America have epilepsy, and 20% to 40% have seizures that remain uncontrolled with antiepileptic drugs (AEDs). Most adults with seizures refractory to AEDs have localization-related epilepsy (LRE) and recurrent complex partial seizures. Up to 50% of these patients may be candidates for neurosurgical intervention. Surgical candidates must have a definitive diagnosis of LRE, fail at least two or three adequate trials of an appropriate AED, be impaired by their seizures, and be motivated to undergo epilepsy surgery. The role of the neurophysiologist in epilepsy surgery is to localize the epileptogenic zone, elucidate the functional anatomy of the neurophysiologic generator, and predict the outcome after epilepsy surgery.

Localization of the epileptogenic zone is based upon concordance of the preoperative evaluation, which includes interictal and ictal electroencephalograms (EEGs) recording from the scalp and various types of neuroimaging. However, scalp EEG localization may be difficult when the epileptogenic zone is in a deep-seated location, small in size, associated with rapid low-amplitude rhythmic ictal discharges, or limited by movement artifact that obscures the recording. In these situations, invasive recordings may be necessary to clarify the site of ictal origin.

Once the site of ictal onset has been identified, neurophysiologic intraoperative monitoring (NIOM) is often necessary during the resective surgery. NIOM in these cases includes electrocorticography (ECOG) and functional brain mapping. ECOG is a neurophysiologic technique that records cortical electrical potentials directly from the surface of the brain. It was pioneered during brief exposures of the brain in the operating room in an effort to determine the site and borders of epileptogenicity and offer predictive information about postsurgical outcome. Functional brain mapping using electrical stimulation is helpful in defining and confining the excision to noneloquent cortex. These two techniques are further discussed in this chapter.

ANATOMY AND PHYSIOLOGY

The brain is compartmentalized into the frontal, parietal, occipital, and temporal lobes. Much of the cerebral cortex has surface area that is "buried" beneath the skull and is therefore inaccessible to scalp EEG recording. Additionally, individual variations in skull thickness create differences in scalp EEG potentials from patient to patient and between the left and right hemicranium. Brain functional compartmentalization also varies from patient to patient. This is especially important in defining a cortical map of functional neuroanatomy. Cortical representation of a body region is illustrated best by an individualized homunculus. The homunculus is a functional, three-dimensional, disproportionate human caricature with regional accentuations (i.e., face and hand enlargements) superimposed on the surface of the brain. In the homunculus, the head and hands are positioned inferolaterally and the legs superomedially upon the midsurface of the brain. The amount of cortical representation depends upon individualized development or previous injury restricting regions of involvement.

The central sulcus is a critical landmark that helps to identify the principal sites of motor and sensory function. The primary motor cortex is demarcated by the precentral gyrus residing at the posterior margin of the frontal lobe. The primary somatosensory cortex is represented by the postcentral gyrus located in the anteriormost parietal lobe; it integrates sensory functions, although it also has representation from the corticospinal tracts to impart motor function as well.

The location of language function is dependent on cerebral dominance. The principal functions of the temporal lobe are the functional integration of language within the dominant hemisphere and mediating functions responsible for memory and learning. Language function is processed by reception of written or spoken words through cortex located at the supramarginal and angular gyrus of the anterior parietal lobe. Expression of language is effected through the Broca area in the posterior-inferior frontal lobe. The more posterior temporal-occipital lobe connections and occipital lobe serve visual functions mediated by the primary visual cortex.

The temporal lobe is frequently the site of epilepsy onset (temporal lobe epilepsy, or TLE); consequently it is a common site for surgical intervention. The borders of the temporal lobe are the Sylvian fissure superiorly, the middle cranial fossa inferiorly, and the sphenoid bone anteriorly, with an approximate border from the parietal and occipital lobes posteriorly. The hippocampal formation is oriented in the inferomesial portion of the temporal lobe along its anteroposterior extent and consists of the parahippocampal gyrus, subiculum, hippocampal sulcus, dentate gyrus, alveus, and fimbriae, creating convolutions of the brain that mimic the appearance of a seahorse.

Scalp EEG measurement of the epileptogenic zone represents a two-dimensional projection from a three-dimensional source. A single interictal epileptiform discharge (IED) detected at the scalp electrodes reflects large synchronous electrical discharges of several million neurons. Therefore the cortical potentials produced at the scalp are often not representative of small interictal or ictal sources. Furthermore, dipole localization using scalp EEG to infer the origins of an IED creates the inverse problem of source localization due to volume conduction inherent in scalp EEGs, which "scatters" the electrical activity from the intrinsic sources, preventing accurate source prediction. In addition, most of the human cortex is buried deep beneath the scalp surface and is far removed from the detection of scalp EEGs (Figure 17.1). Hence, intracranial EEGs may clarify neurophysiologic localization when noninvasive investigations are discordant or nonlocalizing on scalp EEGs (Figure 17.2).

PATHOLOGY

Resection of the epileptogenic zone that represents the anatomic site of epileptogenesis is essential to a favorable surgical outcome for patients with intractable seizures. While the pathology of TLE is most often hippocampal sclerosis, the pathology of extratemporal epilepsy is much more varied. Slow-growing tumors such as low-grade astrocytomas, oligodendrogliomas, gangliogliomas, and

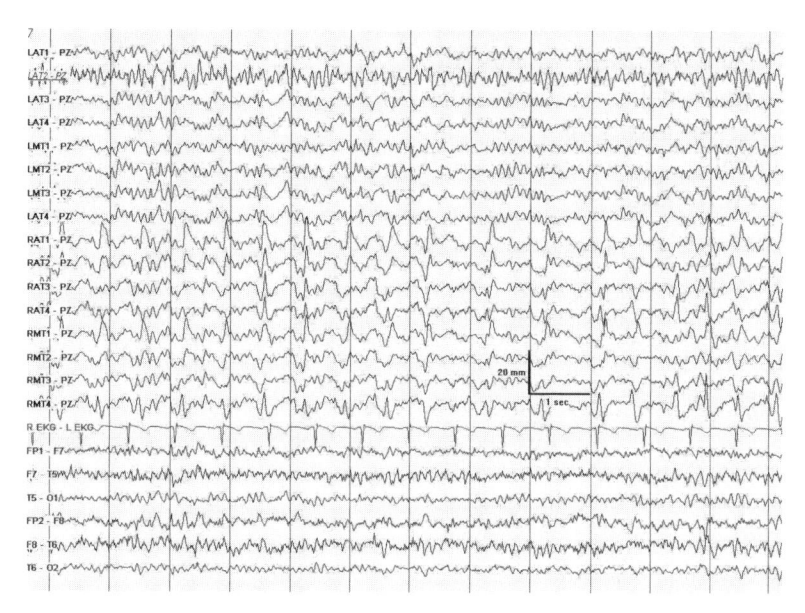

FIGURE 17.1 Concomitant scalp and intracranial EEG demonstrating repetitive right temporal IEDs, which are seen on the intracranial channels but not on the scalp channels in a patient with temporal lobe epilepsy. LAT = left anterior temporal; LMT = left midtemporal; RAT = right anterior temporal; RMT = right midtemporal; lower channels = scalp EEG. [Reproduced with permission from Tatum WO, Benbadis SR (14).]

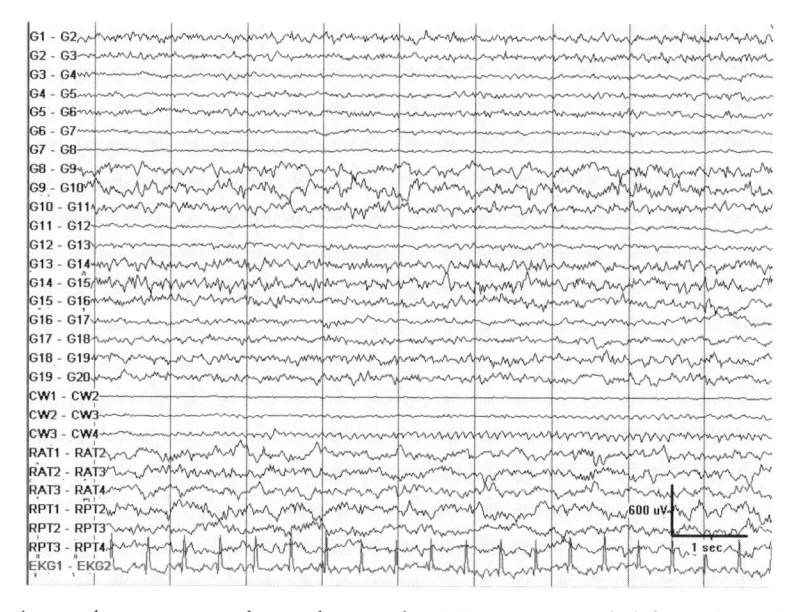

FIGURE 17.2 Auras that were not detected on scalp EEG were recorded from the wall of an area of encephalomalacia in a patient with symptomatic extratemporal epilepsy. An array of two right temporal strips, a strip within the cyst wall, and a grid were implanted unilaterally. G = grid; CW = cyst wall; RAT = right anterior temporal; RPT = right posterior temporal.

dysembryoplastic neuroepithelial tumors are frequently discovered. Malformations of the brain due to abnormal cortical development are common pathologic substrates and are being visualized with increasing frequency owing to advancements in neuroimaging. Cortical dysplasia represents a wide range of neuronal migration disorders that create a structural and neurophysiologic disturbance. Vascular malformations such as cavernous vascular malformations and arteriovenous malformations may lead to intractable epilepsy. Encephalomalacia of various etiologies—including trauma, infection, and cerebral infarction in addition to other causes—may also produce seizures.

ECOG

Background

Hans Berger initially performed ECOG in the late 1920s, when he recorded human EEGs through craniotomy sites with intracortical needle electrodes (1). In the mid-1930s, EEG was introduced into the operating room (2). ECOG is best appreciated as a technique that is used in the operating room to record EEGs from surgically exposed brain.

ECOG is composed of the same combination of cortical rhythms found on scalp recording. However, the amplitudes of ECOG are 10-fold greater than at the level of the scalp. Faster frequencies enhanced by medications may appear similar to pathologic polyspike discharges when compared with the scalp EEG owing to the absence of the skull and scalp, which normally attenuates the voltage of the low-amplitude fast frequencies. Regional differences in cortical representation of the different frequencies are more discrete and therefore more apparent with ECOG. In addition, normal variations and variants, such as the mu rhythm, are more precisely demarcated and restricted on ECOG, mimicking abnormal IEDs.

Intraoperative Recording

Intraoperative ECOG refers to the recording of neurophysiologic potentials directly from the brain within the confines of the operating room. When used as a presurgical tool, intraoperative ECOG is limited because of the brief opportunity for recording during surgery, and preoperative localization information creates a bias toward exposure. However, there are benefits to intraoperative ECOG, with the potential to avert risks from the initial surgical procedure, move and direct electrode locations within the surgical field, and perform intraoperative ECOG with cortical stimulation for mapping.

ECOG is recorded with standard EEG equipment brought to the operating room. Electrodes of various types and styles may be used. Seizures are seldom recorded in utilizing ECOG; the IED provide the bulk of the information obtained within the operating room. Intraoperative ECOG has been used in an effort to localize the site of epileptogenicity through the demonstration of IED persistence, frequency, and distribution.

Because neural tissue is complex, pitfalls in utilizing IED as a marker for seizure onset lie in the fact that the functional relationships between IED and seizure onset are not always commensurate. Additionally, the epileptogenic zone and the sites of IED formation may be of dissimilar sizes; widespread discharges may be noted despite a smaller zone of epileptogenesis. Furthermore, spikes and sharp waves that are propagated or even volume-conducted are not readily distinguishable from spikes and sharp waves involved in the primary generator. Hence, seizures may arise from sites outside the ECOG sites of interictal epileptiform abnormalities.

Extraoperative Recording

Interest in intraoperative ECOG in guiding resection of dysfunctional cortex has now evolved to include advances made within neuroradiology as well as digital instruments available for long-term video–EEG monitoring. With the need for invasive recordings of seizures and functional mapping of eloquent cortex, extraoperative ECOG has become the foundation for excisional epilepsy surgery when intracranial electrodes are necessary. While anesthesia is not utilized outside the operating room, analgesia is typically required. Extraoperative ECOG allows clarification of briefer intraoperative recordings by increasing the length of recording and obtaining information from intracranial ictal EEGs. It also allows more prolonged cortical mapping time when necessary.

Intraparenchymal (intracortical or depth) or extraparenchymal (subdural strip/grid) recordings are used during the intracranial phase of epilepsy monitoring. Deep-seated anatomic structures—including the hippocampus, amygdala, and subcortical abnormalities within the brain—may serve as generators for seizures. As such, volume conduction of these electrical fields from deep generators may interfere with precise localization at the level of the scalp. New frameless systems for the placement of depth electrodes near these generators allow for more accurate localization.

Electrodes

The initial intraoperative ECOG pioneered in Montreal, Canada, by Jasper and Penfield used a series of eight insulated silver wires with chloride ball tips as recording electrodes. They were capable of being redirected to different sites of the exposed brain. Artifact-contaminated reference recordings quickly gave rise to bipolar montages. Today, subdural electrodes constitute the main method of recording ECOG and are available from several electrode-dedicated vendors. Subdural electrodes are available in various configurations that comprise grid and strip electrodes involving multiple contacts and sizes that can be tailored for individual implantation (Figures 17.3 and 17.4). Stainless steel and

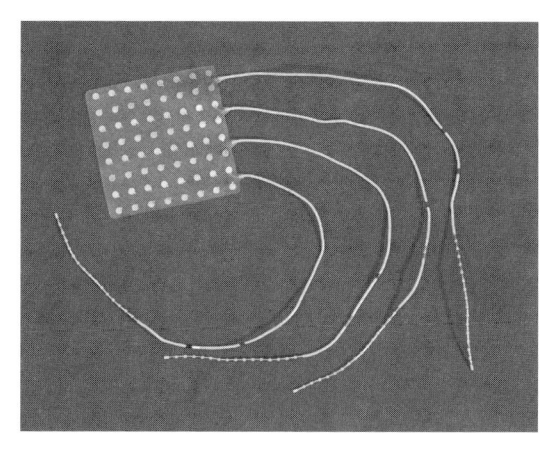

FIGURE 17.3 Photograph of an 8 by 8 contact subdural grid electrode.

platinum alloys are the principal compounds composing the electrodes; they are embedded in a clear malleable silicone or polyurethane array to permit visualization of underlying cortical structures during placement (Figure 17.5). A variety of electrode styles is available; these typically include strips with 2 to 8 contacts and grids that contain 4 to 64 contacts. Each contact may vary in diameter but commonly is 5 mm wide, and they are spaced 1 cm apart. Individual sizes and spacing depend upon clinical requirement as well as manufacturing capabilities.

Subdural electrodes are placed over the site of cortex that is potentially epileptogenic or eloquent for an essential function (i.e., primary

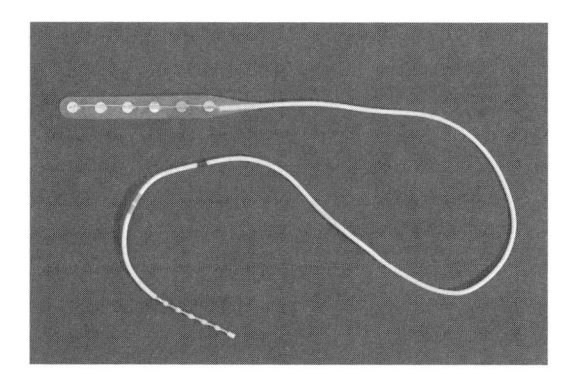

FIGURE 17.4 Photograph of a six-contact subdural strip electrode. Each contact is separated by 1 cm.

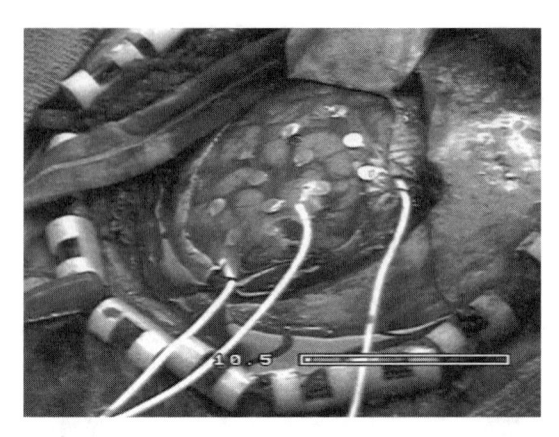

FIGURE 17.5 Operative placement of a 4 by 5 contact subdural grid in a patient with medically intractable epilepsy. Note the retracted dura mater at the top and the cables connecting to the EEG at the bottom.

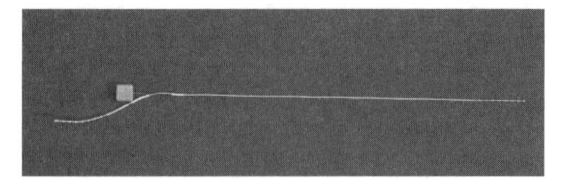

FIGURE 17.6 Photograph of a depth electrode. This electrode has eight contacts.

sensory, motor, visual, or language cortex). The advantages of subdural electrodes over depth electrodes are that they are less likely to create morbidity, are easier to implant, and can cover a larger cortical surface.

Depth electrodes are intraparenchymal electrodes that sample a small surrounding area of brain at the site of placement (Figure 17.6). This form of stereo–EEG recording provides a limited sampling and represents the most invasive of all the commonly used electrodes for direct recording from the brain. Depth electrodes have the advantage of allowing more precise localization from the mesial temporal structures when seizures arise from the amygdala and hippocampus. Other less invasive electrodes include foramen ovale and epidural electrodes for localizing the epileptogenic zone to one mesial temporal region.

Technique

After the patient is taken to the operating room and has undergone general anesthesia, the head is secured using Mayfield pin holders, shaved, prepped, and draped in a sterile fashion. The site or sites of operation, positioning, and incisions are individualized for placement of electrodes, cortical stimulation, or resection. A craniotomy (or craniectomies) is preformed to expose the dura mater, which is then opened to expose the cortical surface for placement of electrodes or for intraoperative cortical stimulation. The placement of subdural grid electrodes requires a craniotomy, while strip electrodes may be placed through individual burr holes.

After the neurophysiologic evaluation is completed, resection of brain tissue is performed using deep retractors, and adequate visualization is obtained using the operating microscope. Corticectomy and resection of the targeted regions are then performed. Tissue cultures are taken from the surgical wound site and antibiotics used to reduce the risk of unexpected infection. Thereafter, Surgicel is applied to the brain surface, retractors and the operating microscope are removed, the dura mater is reapproximated with sutures, and the bone flap is secured in place. Surrounding soft tissues are also reapproximated with sutures, and the skin is stapled. Perioperative antibiotics and steroids are administered and the patient is released to the anesthesia service for recovery.

Recording ECOG inside and outside the operating room uses the same technique. A preoperative plan is developed prior to surgery. Selection of electrode type(s) to be used and plans for an implanted electrode array are required. Electrode placement occurs under aseptic conditions. The leads from the individual electrodes connect to the EEG machine for direct recording in the operating room and reconnected to cable (or radio) telemetry for further extraoperative recording. For extraoperative recording, the electrode leads are tunneled under the skin and exit through a stab wound a short distance away from the craniotomy site. This helps minimize the risk of cerebrospinal fluid leakage and infection. Following completion of epilepsy monitoring with or without extraoperative functional mapping, the electrodes are removed during a second surgery.

Sterile technique during placement and throughout the time of ECOG is essential. The risk of infection and hemorrhage with insertion of subdural strip electrodes is less than 1%, while subdural grid electrodes carry a higher risk of complications. Besides infection, transient neurologic deficits, hematoma, increased intracranial pressure, cerebral infarction, and herniation can occur due to the mass effect, which may be created by placement of the electrodes. The greater the number of electrodes implanted, the longer the recording time, the older the patient, the greater the number of skull breaches, or dominant hemispheric implantation, the greater the risk of complications.

Unlike subdural electrodes, depth electrodes penetrate brain parenchyma and may cause intracerebral hemorrhage when placed near vascular structures. Examination of resected tissue has demonstrated gliosis and cystic degeneration around the trajectory of the depth electrode. Typically, however, the risk of intracranial bleeding or infection is only 0.5% to 4% (3).

In the localization of seizure foci, intraoperative surgical navigation systems have been utilized to coregister subdural electrodes to regions of known radiographic pathology. This provides a link between noninvasive and invasive data to further develop the relationship between brain function and anatomic variability.

Interpretation

Epileptiform Abnormalities

Spikes are more evident on ECOG than the scalp EEG (Figure 17.1). About 25% of patients with TLE have IEDs on ECOG that are not noted on the scalp EEG (2). Additionally, the area containing IEDs with ECOG is frequently larger than that obtained with scalp recordings. Compared to scalp-recorded IEDs, ECOG-recorded IEDs have greater amplitude (500 to 1000 µV) and are shorter in duration, sometimes even less than 20 ms. Furthermore, ECOG IEDs may appear in several regions distant to the site of epileptogenicity.

When patients have few or rare IEDs on ECOG, activation techniques are used to augment interictal abnormalities. Unlike scalp recordings that use hyperventilation, photic stimulation, and sleep as activating techniques, pharmacologic activation is used during ECOG. Methohexital and thiopental are used most frequently. Abnormalities that can be induced include focal reduction of fast frequencies, induction of focal slow activity, and an increase in the number, extent, and frequency of IEDs. However, IEDs noted with activation may extend beyond the proposed site of resection and region of neuroanatomic abnormality. Consequently the clinical usefulness of drug-induced IED in guiding resective surgery is limited.

Information obtained from ECOG has been used to tailor resections of epileptogenic tissue. However, resection of the entire region with IEDs is not essential to render patients seizure-free. This is because the IEDs arise not only from the epileptogenic zone (which is resected) but also from adjacent regions of secondary cortical neurophysiologic involvement (which do not need to be resected). Therefore some investigators have found no additional information using ECOG beyond that obtained from the preoperative scalp video–EEG monitoring (3,4). On the other hand, areas of high density computer-detected spike discharges on ECOG have been suspected to be areas in the primary epileptogenic zone, with resection resulting in a more favorable surgical outcome (5).

Dysplastic cortex often produces a unique pattern of epileptiform abnormalities on

ECOG. Prominent, widespread IEDs that may be very complex, repetitive, and have polyspike morphology are typically seen. Nearly continuous spikes and periodic spikes can also occur in long runs. It has been suggested that beyond localizing dysfunctional cortex, the morphology and topography of the IEDs may be predictive of pathology in cortical dysplasia.

Nonepileptiform Abnormalities

Nonepileptiform abnormalities identified by ECOG include abnormalities of a variety of frequencies. A reduction of certain frequencies (i.e., beta activity) during spontaneous or pharmacologic activation identifies dysfunctional cortex. However, regions of low amplitudes on ECOG may reflect the technical limitations from bipolar recording of similar generators. Additionally, low-amplitude activity may signify proximity to vascular or noncerebral materials (Gelfoam, pledglets, saline irrigation, etc.) rather than pathology.

Focal slow activity may be recorded on ECOG. This activity usually reflects dysfunctional cortex and may be helpful when IEDs are not present on the preexcision ECOG, although its lack of specificity limits its usefulness. With spectral analysis of ECOG in 40 patients, the area of maximal delta slowing coincided with the site of maximal spike activity in approximately 50% of patients in one study (5). However, given the difficulty in separating the surgical effects from underlying pathology after the start of operation, interpretation of intraoperative focal slowing merits suspicion of a nonepileptogenic source.

Event related desynchronization of the normal alpha and beta frequencies has been used to detect differences during functional activation of sensorimotor cortex. Broad somatotopic networks demonstrate functional overlap of different body parts for alpha and beta frequencies. Comparatively, the topographic patterns of gamma activity (30 to 100 Hz) in the lower or upper limits of the bandwidth appear more discrete with respect to somatotopic specificity, appearing over the contralateral somatosensory cortex during limb movement. In addition, coherence patterns identified with ECOG have suggested characteristic patterns that may help define the anatomy of individual brain regions. In defining the central sulcus, low phase coherence may decrease, while high phase-shift coherences increase.

Importantly, pathologic alterations of brain function may be suggested by certain abnormalities. High-frequency oscillations ranging from 100 to 250 Hz (ripples) or 250 to 500 Hz (fast ripples) have been recorded using intracranial electrodes. Electrographic seizure onset has been associated with ripples; thus they have localizing value. Fast ripples occur preferentially in the hippocampus ipsilateral to the seizure onset, and their generators may be important in identification and mapping of the epileptogenic process.

Evidence of Usefulness

Preexcision ECOG

The evidence to suggest that the preexcision ECOG helps to determine the degree of resection for temporal, extratemporal, lesional, and nonlesional surgeries to provide a favorable clinical outcome has been limited (5,6). Early reports in adults and children with ECOG-guided resection of slow-growing glial lesions noted more favorable results with younger patients (7). A small series of patients with symptomatic intractable epilepsy caused by gangliogliomas reported improved outcome when ECOG-guided resection was performed compared with those who simply underwent a lesionectomy (5). ECOG often reveals widespread abnormalities beyond the site seen on neuroimaging. However, cortical dysplasias and glioneuronal tumors often cause localized or regional continuous spiking, bursts, and recruiting discharges (8). ECOG often reveals widespread abnormalities beyond the site seen on neuroimaging. A complete resection of the epileptiform abnormalities correlates with a favorable surgical outcome in some series (8).

Other investigators, however, report that more than one independent spike focus noted on preexcision ECOG predicts a poor postoperative outcome. Studies of nonlesional TLEs have not been able to identify favorable predictors for successful postoperative outcome (3–6). The correlation between underlying pathology and the location of IEDs on ECOG has not been reliable (3). This is likely due to frontal, parasagittal, and occipital foci having a more widespread neuronal network, leading to the propagation of IEDs widely over the hemisphere (or even the contralateral hemisphere).

Postexcision ECOG

As with the preexcision ECOG, evidence for a beneficial role of the postexcision ECOG to predict surgical outcome has been inconsistent. Early reports suggested that the postexcision ECOG had predictive outcome potential when preexcision IEDs were no longer present after resection. One early study with 5-year follow-up demonstrated a significant difference when the postexcision ECOG did not have IEDs. When postexcision IEDs were present, only 36% of 104 patients had a good outcome (5).

Other studies have demonstrated that residual postexcision spikes have no predictive value. This may be especially true of hippocampal or deep-seated lesions. One case series of pure lesionectomy (normal tissue at the edge of resection) patients reported seizure freedom to be independent of spike distribution or even spike presence on ECOG before or after resection (9). Additionally, another study found no difference with the use of ECOG in patients with TLE, though resection margins may have encompassed the majority of the IEDs (5). Some locations, such as the posterior parahippocampal gyrus and insular cortex, appear to lack prognostic significance when persistent spiking is encountered on the postexcision ECOG (2).

IEDs may appear on the ECOG following initial resection when none were present prior to resection. Postexcision activation of spikes is more benign than the presence of residual spikes unaltered by the resection and may indicate injury potentials from surgical manipulation. Discharges that remain unaltered after resection may carry a poorer prognosis for a seizure-free outcome, especially in frontal lobe epilepsy when three or more gyri contain IEDs. However, in a recent study, 80 patients with mesial TLE underwent a resection tailored to remove up to 7 cm of tissue, depending upon the presence of neocortical spikes and eloquent cortex. Interestingly, the presence of neocortical spikes was found to be associated with a more favorable prognosis for postoperative cognitive outcome (10).

FUNCTIONAL BRAIN MAPPING

Electrical Stimulation

Electrical stimulation of the brain has been primarily used for diagnostic purposes, although therapeutic uses also exist. The latter are beyond the scope of this chapter. Intracranial electrodes that are surgically implanted in the form of either strips or grids are capable of performing not only ECOG but also electrical stimulation of the cortex for functional brain mapping. Electrical stimulation can be useful for providing an individualized functional map that identifies areas of eloquent cortex. However, if a site on the map involved with a particular function is accidentally sacrificed during surgery, it does not necessarily imply that there will be a permanent deficit of that function. Often other neural networks are available to compensate for the lost function. Young children are able to demonstrate such plasticity better than adults. Stimulation of brain structures has been performed by direct application of electrical current to both cortical and subcortical structures.

Utility

Electrical stimulation has been performed in every lobe of the brain. It may be performed extraoperatively at the bedside through implanted electrode arrays or intraoperatively using handheld probes directed to specific cortical areas of interest by the neurosurgeon. Low-frequency stimulation (i.e., 1 Hz) is less likely to induce seizures than high-frequency (50 Hz) stimulation. However, even with low-frequency stimulation, seizure induction has been noted with stimulation of temporal lobe white matter as well as the neocortical gray matter (11). Low-frequency electrical stimulation of the temporal lobe with simultaneous ECOG results in a gradual increase in spikes with or without the occurrence of low-voltage fast activity. This has been reported to help define the epileptogenic zone (11).

Electrical stimulation to define the cortical representation of sensorimotor or language function of the dominant hemisphere has been a principal goal of brain mapping. Individual variations of the classic human homunculus are common, especially when lesions are present. One study found variation in the organization of primary motor cortex in 19.4% of 36 patients (12). In addition, functional overlap between two different areas was found in 11.1% of patients. The responses obtained from electrical stimulation of eloquent and "silent" regions of the brain allow the neurophysiologist to design a pictorial map of individualized cortical function that is task-specific. Thus this type of mapping is critical for optimizing postoperative outcomes.

Localization for Reproduction of Symptoms and Signs

Various symptoms and signs can be reproduced by electrical stimulation. Negative and positive clinical correlates may be noted during functional brain mapping through electrical stimulation of the brain. Stimulation of negative motor areas within the frontal lobe, such as the supplementary motor area, may cause interruption fine motor movements, focal negative myoclonus, or bilateral atonia. Interruption of tongue, finger, or toe movement may be induced without loss of muscle tone when the patient is asked to perform continuous movement tasks during testing. Numbness or scotomata can occur with stimulation of somatosensory and visual cortices. Stimulation of language areas may result in naming difficulties (as noted during the picture identification task), speech arrest, or difficulties in comprehension during reading.

Positive motor phenomena include tonic or clonic contraction of a group of muscles and may be subjectively detected through an increase in tone or objectively noted on direct visualization. Tingling or phosphenes reflect positive involvement of the somatosensory or visual systems. In the low postcentral region, cortical landmarks determined by localizing tongue and face sensation are more reliable than stereotactic coordinates of the same area. Experiential or psychic symptomatology, visual imagery, and memory recall have been demonstrated during electrical stimulation of the mesial temporal lobe.

If negative or positive phenomena are produced with stimulation, a second trial should be conducted for validation. This allows development of a functional map of the cortex. Additionally, by reproducing symptoms characteristic of the patient's spontaneous events, the site of seizure onset can be better localized.

Beyond defining the clinical function of neural tissue, electrical stimulation using depth electrodes for the purpose of triggering partial seizures has been performed. Identifying the epileptogenic zone from the irritative zone is done by reproducing the entire habitual seizure semiology. This technique has been inconsistent for specifically reproducing the habitual seizure. Additionally, more than one site from the ipsilateral and contralateral hemispheres may be capable of reproducing the same aura (11). Therefore electrical reproduction of the habitual aura lacks localizing and lateralizing specificity. However, when a typical aura is elicited by brain stimulation, the lobe of origin of the seizure can be established with some accuracy.

Localization of Afterdischarges

Afterdischarges (ADs) are electrical events that represent elicited epileptiform activity similar to a restricted focal electrographic seizure. ECOG is used in conjunction with cortical stimulation to elicit and detect ADs. ADs have a threshold that reflects the degree of ease of seizure generation. They may arise from normal and pathologic brain tissue. Although the morphology remains stable in a given region of the brain, there is prominent variability from region to region and from patient to patient (12). The ADs may appear either as repetitive IEDs or brief rhythmic discharges. They serve as an electrographic warning sign that a seizure may be impending. No specific morphology predicts an underlying pathology, and a wide range of patterns with different frequencies may occur.

If symptoms are produced with the ADs, it does not confirm proximity to functional cortex, as symptoms may be produced from propagated electrical discharges (11,12). Symptoms produced with and without ADs spreading beyond the site of stimulation have included not only sensory and motor responses but also visceral sensory, autonomic, thermoregulatory, experiential, and vocalization symptoms. Furthermore, specific clinical responses can often be elicited from more than one site, frequently from noncontiguous areas in the same or both hemispheres (11).

AD thresholds reflect the degree of electrical current that is required to generate an AD. Thresholds do not appear to be AED concentration-dependent. The ADs vary in morphology, duration, and location and demonstrate greater excitability and lower thresholds at the site of seizure onset. Thresholds evoking ADs that are lower or more prolonged may carry a greater likelihood of corresponding to the site of spontaneous seizure onset, while morphology is probably less predictive (2). Thresholds will vary from patient to patient, and even the same site in the same patient may vary from day to day. Furthermore, AD thresholds may tend to increase with subsequent stimulations or following prolonged ADs (2). Thresholds also depend on the location of the brain that is stimulated, with the mesial temporal lobe typically having the lowest threshold (13). Extratemporal neocortex has a higher threshold, and the motor cortex has the highest. Depth electrodes are amenable to cortical stimulation and have also been used to demonstrate sites of low current thresholds to electrical stimulation.

However, AD thresholds have not held a consistent relationship with the ability to identify the site of spontaneous seizure onset (13). Also, they may demonstrate variability, with some thresholds being higher and some lower in the region of the epileptogenic zone. Because ADs probably require a certain neuronal density, in areas of significant neuronal loss (i.e., hippocampal sclerosis), thresholds may be higher in the region of epileptogenicity owing to the greater stimuli needed to recruit a smaller cellular population. Similarly, the presence of a foreign tissue lesion also makes the determination of the site of epileptogenicity using AD thresholds unreliable. Hence, AD thresholds have not been able to consistently identify epileptogenic and nonepiletpogenic tissue.

Technique

Like ECOG, electrical stimulation for functional brain mapping can be performed in and out of the operating room. Electrical stimulation studies are usually performed in patients with indwelling electrodes following epilepsy monitoring. Sessions usually last anywhere from 30 minutes to several hours and may require more than one day to complete a functional map (Figure 17.7). Testing usually requires patients to be awake in order to obtain sensory, motor, visual, and language information. This may be tiring for the patient, although it is usually not painful.

Stimulations are performed sequentially through pairs of adjacent subdural grid or strip contacts, with EEGs recorded simultane-

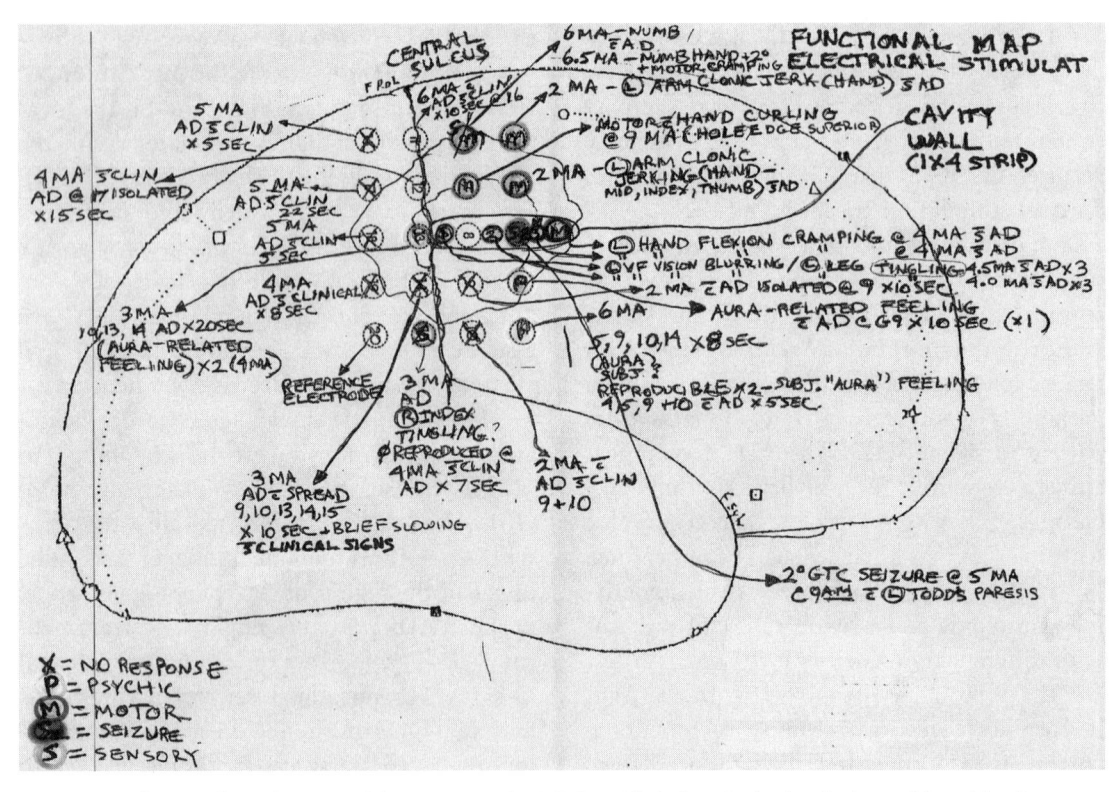

FIGURE 17.7 Working functional brain map of ECOG-guided electrical stimulation with a 4 by 5 contact subdural grid and a cavity wall 1 by 4 subdural strip placed over the central sulcus and inside an cystic cavity. Stimulation is repeated at each site and the duration and spread of the ADs as well as the clinical correlate is noted. Note the variability of stimulation, with the second inferior grid contact not reproducing sensory function and the third superior grid contact with sensory and motor function demonstrated during the second trial of stimulation.

ously from other contacts. Stimulation is with constant-current bipolar square-wave pulses delivered at 50 Hz for a duration of 0.5 ms. Initial stimulation intensity is 1 to 2 mA and is increased by 0.5 to 1 mA up to maximal settings allowable for the individual stimulator utilized (i.e., 10–15 mAs) and depending on the surrounding AD thresholds. Stimulation is continued for 4 to 5 seconds, with an AD defined as periodic epileptiform discharges or rhythmic epileptiform activity lasting at least 1 second in at least one contact. Two trials are performed to verify function, AD threshold without clinical symptoms, or no response at the maximum of 10 mA. When one trial results in an AD and another not, the tissue is regarded as noneloquent as long as no symptoms are registered during the trial with the AD. Repeat attempts to electrically stimulate sites of the cortex in gradually increasing intensities will often elicit an AD. During stimulation, stimulus artifact obscures the ECOG at the site of stimulation as well as adjacent electrodes (Figure 17.8).

ADs are similar to restricted focal seizures and often consist of a sudden onset of recurrent rhythmic or epileptiform discharges that last for seconds to several minutes or more and can involve neighboring contacts. They may cease abruptly, have postictal suppression in the affected contacts, or evolve into a clinical seizure. Different locations within the brain have variable stimulus thresholds. Typically, mesial temporal stimulation has the

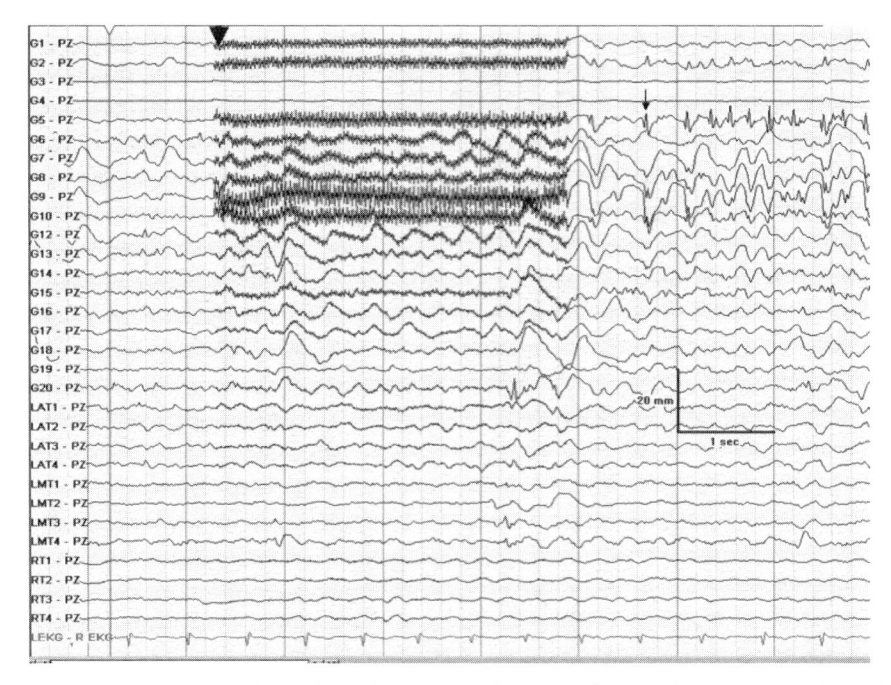

FIGURE 17.8 AD present at G5 electrode with some involvement of G8 and G9 on an implanted 20 contact subdural grid following 3.5 seconds of stimulation. Note the thick arrow at the onset of stimulus artifact and the thin arrow during the AD. LAT = left anterior temporal; LMT = left midtemporal; RT = right temporal.

lowest threshold for inducing ADs. However, there is a wide threshold range for eliciting ADs within the same cortical location of the same patient. In one study, up to a 9-mA difference was found within the temporal lobe and up to a 5.5-mA difference between adjacent electrodes on the temporal lobe (13). Furthermore, AD thresholds do not necessarily parallel a functional threshold, although this may vary from one site to another in an individual patient. Differences may even be seen from trial to trial or from day to day, making precise mapping even more complicated for precise demarcation of functions. A delay in responses to a single pulsed stimulation may reflect a higher risk of epileptogenicity than those appearing within 100 ms.

The ECOG should always be monitored during electrical stimulation to assess the presence of ADs (Figure 17.8). If a seizure occurs with stimulation, the stimulus intensity is reduced and slowly retitrated up. In some cases this allows the current to be advanced to higher or even maximal threshold intensity. Alternatively, the use of benzodiazepines may reduce the likelihood of an AD. When an AD occurs with postictal slowing, return of the EEG to baseline is required before continuing functional mapping. If a clinical seizure is precipitated by the stimulation, notation as to the habitual nature is documented and return of the EEG and the patient to baseline is required prior to continuing mapping. If lorazepam is required for a seizure lasting longer than 5 minutes, the session is usually aborted until a later time. Fortunately, seizures occur rarely during mapping sessions.

Other Forms of Functional Brain Mapping

ECOG and electrical stimulation of the brain for functional mapping may be performed in conjunction with other techniques that help localize areas of eloquent cortex. Intraoperative median nerve somatosensory evoked potentials (SEPs) are commonly obtained when identification of motor cortex is necessary. To record these potentials, a subdural grid or strip electrode is placed on the exposed cortex. The contralateral median nerve is stimulated. Cortical waveforms of the SEPs are obtained from the various electrode contacts referenced to a distal electrode, such as one on the contralateral mastoid. The N20 waveform is seen over the somatosensory cortex while a P22 (sometimes called the P20) waveform is seen over the motor cortex. The central sulcus lies between the electrodes generating the highest amplitude N20 to P22 complex and is easily delineated by the phase reversal that is generated (14) (Figure 17.9). This is not a true phase reversal, since the negative and positive waveforms do not represent two ends of a single dipole; rather, they represent two different dipoles. Hence this is often called a pseudo–phase reversal.

Several other nonneurophysiologic techniques are also used for brain mapping. The intracarotid amobarbital (Wada) test is used to lateralize language and memory; it is used most often in surgeries of the mesial temporal lobe. Functional magnetic resonance imaging (MRI) and positron emission tomography (PET) have shown utility in localizing motor, sensory, and language functions. Optical imaging is being used to map the spatiotemporal relationship between excitatory and inhibitory neuronal activity during epilepsy surgery. Neurophysiologic mapping with source and frequency analyses with magnetoencephalography (MEG) dipole analysis provides unique information not obtainable with anatomic or functional neuroimaging. Specialized surgical navigational systems are being developed that will coregister anatomic, functional, and neurophysiologic data to allow more precise delineation of the anatomic–functional boundaries of lesions.

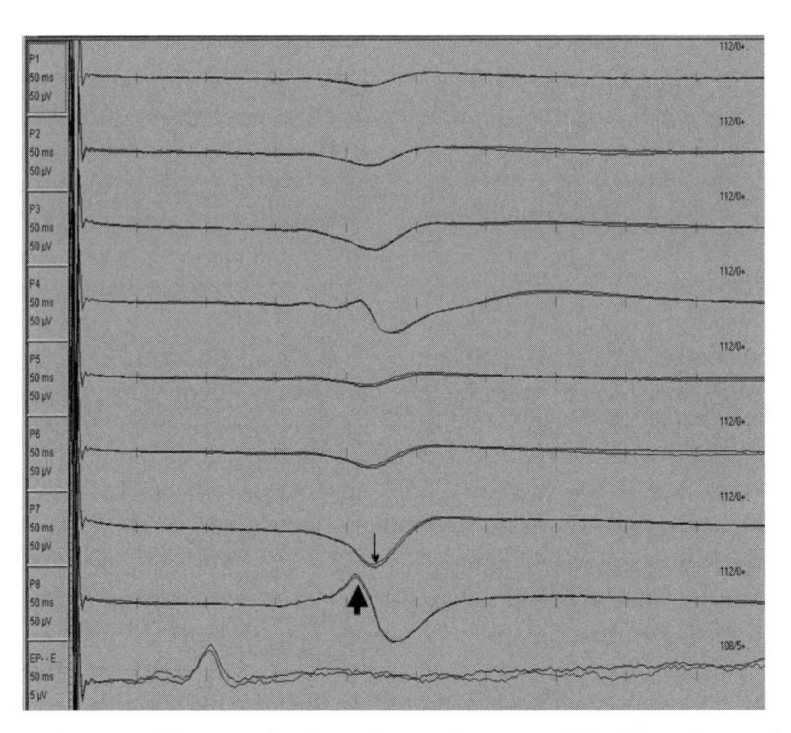

FIGURE 17.9 Localization of the central sulcus using median nerve SEPs. Note the pseudophase reversal of the N20 (thick arrow) and P22 (thin arrow) waveforms at contacts 7 and 8 of the grid. The last channel demonstrates Erb's point's potential, verifying adequacy of stimulation. [Reproduced with permission from Husain (14).]

ANESTHESIA

General anesthesia may produce significant alteration of the EEG background activity as well as the provoking epileptiform activity on the ECO General anesthesics are minimized or discontinued prior to intraoperative ECOG. However, they are a common choice during the induction phase of anesthesia for epilepsy surgery. Opioid analgesics such as fentanyl and remifentanil may activate IEDs and produce behavioral seizures. As noted previously, spike discharges may also be augmented or activated with methohexital. On the other hand, the use of benzodiazepines may accentuate both faster and slower frequencies on ECOG but act as suppressants for IEDs and seizures. Intravenous benzodiazepines remain the principal agents for aborting seizures both in and outside of the operating room.

Propofol, etomidate, and barbiturates are general anesthetics that have dose-dependent effects upon ECOG, initially accentuating faster frequencies and then augmenting slower frequencies at higher doses. Inhalation halogenated anesthetics such as halothane, enflurane, and sevoflurane can influence or suppress background activity and alter epileptiform discharges. At higher concentrations, generalized delta frequencies become apparent and even a burst-suppression pattern may be noted. Enflurane may produce IEDs in nonepileptic patients or broaden the field of spread in those with seizures (2). Nitrous oxide can also suppress IEDs, and in addition, because of slowing introduced into ECOG, it is often discontinued prior to recording (6). Substituting nitrous oxide with intravenous anesthesia in concert with paralytic agents may minimize the effects on the recording.

Local anesthesia is utilized when intact cognition is desirable for functional mapping. This is especially useful when regions close to eloquent cortex are to be excised. However, local anesthesia requires stable head position, cooperation from the patient, is more time consuming, and is difficult in the cognitively challenged and younger age group. Even when local anesthesia is used for functional mapping, general anesthetics are used during the remainder of the surgery. Patients are awakened (transitioned to local anesthetic) when mapping is to be performed. Once mapping is complete, they are transitioned back to general anesthesia.

SAFETY

Electrical safety of the brain is dependent on the charge density delivered to cortical tissue. Charge density [in microcoulombs (µC) of charge per square centimeter of tissue per phase of stimulation] is a measure of the amount of current applied during electrical stimulation. At the routine extraoperative settings utilized for functional mapping, no alteration in parenchymal architecture has been found with light microscopy at the sites of subdural electrode stimulation (15). Furthermore, no evidence of cumulative histologic injury at the electrode sites has been shown in any clinical trial using cortical or deep brain stimulation. Extraoperative stimulation using subdural electrodes may produce a charge density of 50 to 60 µC per square centimeter per phase (15). However, intraoperative stimulation can produce a much higher charge density (15,16).

Repeated trials of stimulation have not demonstrated evidence of secondary epileptogenesis (i.e., kindling) in humans. Animal models, however, have demonstrated this phenomenon. It is thought that the human neocortex is much more difficult to kindle, and the irregular and limited electrical stimulation used for mapping is insufficient to produce this phenomenon.

Morbidity may be associated with placement of depth and subdural electrodes. Cerebral edema with shifting of midline structures and infection are the primary concerns. Postoperative computed tomography (CT) of the brain and perioperative antibiotics are routinely used to detect and prevent these complications. Presence of purulent wound drainage, unrelenting fever, disproportional change in mental status, or a notable increase in seizure frequency or status epilepticus should raise suspicion for complications.

TECHNICAL ISSUES

Preparation

Epilepsy surgery is different than other types of surgeries where NIOM is used. Rather than a standard procedure, in epilepsy surgery the procedure is individualized for the patient based on preoperative and intraoperative neurophysiologic findings. Prior to surgery, the NIOM team must be aware of the preoperative workup and the type of surgery planned. A discussion between the surgeon and neurophysiologist should establish whether ECOG, brain mapping, or both are to be performed. This must also be communicated to the anesthesiologist so that appropriate anesthetics are used.

The NIOM team should discuss the monitoring that will be done during the procedure with the patient. The site of the incision and the amount of hair that will need to be shaved should be reviewed. During this time any potential issues that may hamper full patient cooperation are brought to the attention of the surgeon. An example of such an issue may be the need for the patient to have his or her glasses available during language mapping. Potential complications, especially in cases in which electrodes will be implanted for extraoperative recording, should be discussed with the patient.

The NIOM technologist must make certain that appropriate equipment is available for the surgery. If ECOG is to be performed in the operating room, an EEG machine with the capacity to record 16 to 128 channels must be available. Newer portable digital EEG machines usually have this capability. If functional mapping is to be performed, an electrical stimulator should also be available. A common type of stimulator is the Ojemann electrical stimulator which has a ball-tipped, handheld stimulating probe.

A discussion between the surgeon and the NIOM team should establish the type of electrodes that will be used during the procedure and where they will be placed. This may include subdural grid or strip or other types of electrode. The size of these electrodes should also be determined. A few extra electrodes should be available in case the electrodes malfunction or are accidentally contaminated during surgery. All electrodes and stimulating probe should be sterilized prior to surgery.

Procedure

Unlike other types of NIOM, a lot of patient preparation for monitoring is not needed after induction of anesthesia. If necessary, a scalp electrode contralateral to the side of surgery should be glued on with collodion for use a reference electrode. If median nerve SEPs are to be obtained, stimulating electrodes along the median nerve in the forearm and recording electrodes at Erb's point should be placed. The rest of the electrodes will be placed by the surgeon after exposure. The electrodes to be used should be handed to the scrub nurse using sterile technique.

Once surgical exposure is complete, the surgeon places the electrodes in predetermined locations. Once the electrodes are in position, the neurophysiologist with the help of the surgeon maps the location of the electrodes on a cartoon of the brain. This helps with identifying the location of abnormal discharges on the ECOG and mapping. Leads from the electrodes are passed to the NIOM technologist who inserts the pins into the jack box. Care must be taken to ensure that leads are inserted into the correct positions. A mistake in this can cause misinterpretation of the site of abnormal discharges. ECOG is recorded for several minutes and feedback regarding the presence of spikes is given the by the neurophysiologist to the surgeon. The electrodes are then removed from the surgical field and resective surgery begins. In some situations the surgeon may request ECOG again after partial or complete resection. The virtues of postexcision ECOG have been discussed previously.

After the initial ECOG, the surgeon may stimulate various cortical regions to determine AD thresholds. As noted previously, the surgeon stimulates initially with low intensity and then gradually increases the intensity. When an AD is noted, the NIOM team alerts the surgeon. When the ADs stop, the surgeon is again informed.

If brain mapping to reproduce symptoms is to be performed, the anesthesiologist is informed and anesthesia is altered to awaken the patient. Motor and sensory mapping is performed by observing and talking with the patient during electrical stimulation of various parts of the cortex. Language mapping involves presenting pictures to the patient and asking him or her to name objects while different brain regions are stimulated by the surgeon. During this mapping, ECOG is monitored to note for ADs. If they occur, the surgeon is immediately notified.

Median nerve SEPs are obtained if localization of the motor cortex is to be performed. Parameters for stimulation of the median nerve are the same as for other types of median nerve SEPs. The Erb's point response is recorded as a measure of adequacy of stimulation. Cortical responses are recorded from the grid or strip electrodes placed on the surface of the brain. Usually a referential montage is used, with each subdural contact referenced to a distal electrode, usually on the contralateral mastoid. The grid or strip electrode is moved to different locations, and the site where the N20/P22 complex is of highest amplitude is noted.

When subdural or depth electrodes are implanted for extraoperative recording, the NIOM team's primary role in the operating room is to clearly identify which electrode is in which location. This enables correct labeling of channels once the electrodes are connected to the EEG machine. After surgery, the patient undergoes x-ray andCT of the head to determine the sites of the electrodes. As soon as possible thereafter, the patient should be connected to the EEG machine and data acquisition started.

Postprocedure

After surgery the electrodes are disposed in an appropriate container. If median nerve stimulation electrodes were used, they are removed and disposed of. A report documenting the findings is created as part of the patient's permanent medical record.

If extraoperative ECOG monitoring will be performed, the NIOM technologist places the head wrap as soon as the sterile dressings are placed. This is also done under the direct supervision of the circulating nurse or anesthesia team. Intracranial electrode leads are cleaned with saline or alcohol, dried, and attached to the recording cables, which will be maintained outside the sterile field. Surgical drains that have been placed may be moved to one side so that they can be removed safely at the bedside by the neurosurgeon without strain on the electrode leads. Once the patient arrives in the epilepsy monitoring or intensive care unit, the leads are connected to the jack box of the EEG machine. Monitoring is continued until an adequate number of seizures are recorded and all extraoperative functional mapping is completed. Thereafter the patient returns to the operating room for removal of the electrodes. The NIOM team is usually not needed during this procedure.

CONCLUSIONS

Epilepsy remains the prime target for using ECOG. The application of ECOG for patients with known structural lesions noted on brain MRI has been controversial, and resection of the lesion is usually performed with excellent results. Most of the ECOG-guided reports have been associated with temporal lobe resections in adults with epilepsy and have been retrospective in nature. The utility of preexcision ECOG to tailor resections has been inconsistent. Similarly, the prognostic value of postexcision ECOG has also been mixed, with outcomes contingent on the margins of the resection. Unfortunately, IEDs found on ECOG have not demonstrated consistent results, and "spike chasing" during intraoperative ECOG has not yet proven to be of value. Therefore the use of ECOG in isolation has not received validation to recommend its routine use to extend cortical resections, although questions still remain regarding its utility in an individual patient. Additionally, the potential benefits of using ECOG in patients without seizures, newly diagnosed seizures, or controlled epilepsy are still to be defined. Electrical brain stimulation for functional brain mapping is routinely used in conjunction with ECOG. It provides a map of eloquent cortex that can guide surgical resection. ECOG and electrical stimulation of the brain are potentially beneficial and have been applied toward helping patients with medically intractable seizures undergoing epilepsy surgery.

REFERENCES

1. Chatrian G-E. Intraoperative electrocorticography. In: Ebersole JS, Pedley TA, eds. *Current Practice of Clinical Electroencephalography*, 3rd ed. Philadelphia: Lippincott Williams & Wilkins, 2003:681–712.
2. Luciano D, Devinsky O, Pannizzo F. Electrocorticography during cortical stimulation. In: Devinski O, Beric A, Dogali M, eds. *Electrical and Magnetic Stimulation of the Brain and Spinal Cord*. New York: Raven Press, 1993:87–102.
3. Engel J Jr, Driver MV, Falconer MA. Electrophysiological correlates of pathology and surgical results in temporal lobe epilepsy. *Brain* 1975;98:129–156.
4. Tran TA, Spencer SS, Marks D, et al. Significance of spikes recorded on electrocorticography in nonlesional medial temporal lobe epilepsy. *Ann Neurol* 1995;38:763–770.
5. Keene DL, Whiting S, Ventureyra EC. Electrocorticography. *Epileptic Disord* 2000; 2:57–63.
6. Binnie CD, Polkey CE, Alarcon G. Electrocorticography. In: Luders HO, Comair YG, eds. *Epilepsy Surgery*. Philadelphia: Lippincott Williams & Wilkins, 2001:637–641.
7. Berger MS, Ghatan S, Haglund MM, et al. Low-grade gliomas associated with intractable epilepsy: seizure outcome utilizing electrocorticography during tumor resection. *J Neurosurg* 1993;79:62–69.
8. Ferrier CH, Aronica E, Leijten FS, et al. Electrocorticographic discharge patterns in glioneuronal tumors and focal cortical dysplasia. *Epilepsia* 2006;47:1477–1486.
9. Tran TA, Spencer SS, Javidan M, et al. Significance of spikes recorded on intraoperative electrocorticography in patients with brain tumor and epilepsy. *Epilepsia* 1997;38: 1132–1139.
10. Leijten FS, Alpherts WC, Van Huffelen AC, et al. The effects on cognitive performance of tailored resection in surgery for nonlesional mesiotemporal lobe epilepsy. *Epilepsia* 2005; 46:431–439.
11. Fish DR, Gloor P, Quesney FL, Olivier A. Clinical responses to electrical brain stimulation of the temporal and frontal lobes in patients with epilepsy. Pathophysiological implications. *Brain* 1993;116(Pt 2):397–414.
12. Branco DM, Coelho TM, Branco BM, , et al. Functional variability of the human cortical motor map: electrical stimulation findings in perirolandic epilepsy surgery. *J Clin Neurophysiol* 2003;20:17–25.
13. Lesser RP, Luders H, Klem G, et al. Cortical afterdischarge and functional response thresholds: results of extraoperative testing. *Epilepsia* 1984;25:615–621.
14. Husain AM. Neurophysiologic intraoperative monitoring. In: Tatum WO, Husain AM, Benbadis SR, Kaplan PW, eds. *Handbook of EEG Interpretation*. New York: Demos, 2007:223–260.

15. Gordon B, Lesser RP, Rance NE, et al. Parameters for direct cortical electrical stimulation in the human: histopathologic confirmation. *Electroencephalogr Clin Neurophysiol* 1990;75:371–377.

16. Pouratian N, Cannestra AF, Bookheimer SY, et al. Variability of intraoperative electrocortical stimulation mapping parameters across and within individuals. *J Neurosurg* 2004;101(3): 458–466.

Index

Note: Bold numbers indicate illustrations, italic *t* indicates a table.

access to patient, 15, 16–17
achondroplasia, 97
ACNS. *See* American College of Neurosurgeons
afferent pathway of spinal cord, 118–119
afterdischarge (AD) localization, 293
alfentanil, 130
American Board of Electroencephalographic and Evoked Potential Technologists (ABRET), 70–71
American College of Neurosurgeons (ACNS), 73, 78, 81, 100
American Medical Association (AMA), 67
amplifiers and operational amplifiers, 73, 74, 79–80, **79**, **80**, 81*t*
   common-mode rejection ratio in, 80–81, **80**
   electroencephalography (EEG), 81
   electromyography (EMG), 81
   evoked potentials (EPs), 81
   input impedance in, 81, **81**
   nerve conduction studies (NCS), 81
   operational, 79–80, **79**, **80**, 81*t*
   process of, 81–82
   voltage-divider rule in, 81, **81**
amplitude of MUPs, 26
anal sphincter function monitoring, 161–162, **161**
analog filters, 82–83
analog-to-digital conversion (ADC), 83–86, **85**
anesthesia, 15, 55–66
   agents used in, 55, 58–63, 58*t*, 59*t*
   anterior intermittent slow waves (AIS) in, 272
   barbiturates in, 60, 60*t*, 61, 130
   benzodiazepine in, 60, 60*t*, 61
   blood flow and, 57
   brainstem auditory evoked potentials (BAEPs) and, 43, 59, 64, 201
   carotid endarterectomy (CEA) and, 272–273, 278
   classification of, 119, 119*t*
   compound muscle action potentials (CMAPs) and, 205
   desflurane in, 58, 58*t*
   dexmedetomidine in, 63
   electrocorticography (ECOG) and, 297
   electroencephalography (EEG) and, 56–60, 59*t*, 239–240, 272–273, **273**, 278–279, 297
   electromyography (EMG) and, 28–29, 172, 173, 205
   enflurane in, 58, 58*t*
   epilepsy/epilepsy surgery and, 297
   etomidate in, 60, 60*t*, 62–63, 130
   equipment used for, 11, **11**
   evoked potentials (EPs) and, 58, 58*t*, 60, 60*t*
   extradural, 119–121, 119*t*
   extramedullary, 119–121, 119*t*
   fast anterior dominant rhythmic activity (FAR) in, 272, 273
   frontal intermittent rhythmic delta activity (FIRDA) in, 272
   gamma aminobutyric acid (GABA) and, 61
   general, 55
   halogenated agents in, 59
   halothane in, 58, 58*t*
   hematology and, 57
   hyper- and hypotension and, 57
   induction of, 55
   inhalation agents used for, 58, 58*t*, 59*t*, 130
   intracranial pressure and, 57–58
   intramedullary, 119–121, 119*t*
   intravenous agents in, 60–63, 60*t*
   isoflurane in, 58, 58*t*
   ketamine in, 60, 60*t*, 62, 130
   local, 55
   mean/minimal alveolar concentration (MAC) and, 55–56, 58, 59, 62, 63, 64, 130, 239, 272
   motor evoked potentials (MEPs) and, 37–38, 38*t*, 59, 60, 129–130, 239
   nerve action potentials (NAPs) and, 204
   neuromuscular blockade type, 130, 147–148, **148**, **149**

anesthesia *(continued)*
  nitrous oxide in, 58, 58t, 60, 130
  nonpharmacologic factors and, NIOM and, 56–58
  opioids in, 60, 60t, 61–62, 130
  paralytics in, 63, 64
  potassium/sodium/calcium balance in, 58
  principles of, 55–56
  propofol in, 60, 60t, 61, 130
  regional, 55
  relative insensitivity of NIOM to, 64
  sedation as, 55
  selective dorsal rhizotomy (SDR) and, 172, 173
  sensitivity to, 64–65
  sevoflurane in, 58, 58t
  somatosensory evoked potentials (SEPs) and, 33, 57, 59, 60, 64, 128–130, 239–240, 244, 272–273, 278–279
  spinal cord surgery and, 128–130
  techniques for, 63–65
  temperature and, 56–57
  thoracic aortic surgery and, 239–240, 243–244, 246
  total intravenous (TIVA), 60, 61, 62, 64, 128, 130, 243–244, 246
  train-of-four (TOF) blockade and, 63, 147–148, **148, 149**
  ventilation and, 57
  vertebral column surgery and, 112–113
  widespread anteriorly maximum rhythmic activity (WAR) in, 272
  widespread persistent slow waves (WPS) in, 272, 273
anesthesia team/technician/resident, 7
anesthesiologist, 7
aneurysmal bone cyst, 119–121, 119t
aneurysms, 41, 229–231, **229, 230**
anterior cervical discotomy and fusion, 98
anterior intermittent slow waves (AIS), 272
anterior spinal release surgery, 98
antiepileptic drugs (AEDs), 283
aorta/aortic diseases. *See* thoracic aortic surgery
aortic dissection, 231–232, **231**
arachnoid cysts, 215t. *See also* tumors of the cerebellopontine angle
Arnold-Chiari malformation, 97
arteries of spinal cord, 119
arteriovenous malformations (AVM), 41, 117
artifacts, 74
  automated rejection of, 83, **84**
  electroencephalography (EEG) and, 40
  free-running EMG and, 142–143, **143**
  operating table, **13**
ascending aorta and aortic arch, 232–233, **232, 233,** 238–241, 249–254, 256. *See also* thoracic aortic surgery
aseptic technique, 3–6
aspirator, Cavitron ultrasonic surgical (CUSA), 11
astrocytoma, 119–121, 119t
asynchronous EMG pattern, 25–26
atherosclerosis formations, 263–264, **265**

atracurium, 130
attendants, OR, 8
attending anesthesiologist, 7
attending surgeon, 6
attire for the operating room, 5, 17
auditory pathways, for brainstem auditory evoked potentials (BAEPs) and, 41–42
auditory stimulation, 77–79
  piezoelectric transducers for, 78–79
  sound and decibel scale in, 77–79
  sound pressure level (SPL) and, 78
  sound reference and decibel scale in, 78
  types of, 78–79
autoclaves, 4
automatic artifact rejection, 83, **84**
Axon Systems, 106
axonal injury and EMG activity, 26–27

bandpass filter, 82, **82**
barbiturates, 60, 60t, 61, 130, 239, 297
Bell, Alexander Graham, 77
benzodiazepine, in, 60, 60t, 61, 239, 297
Berger, Hans, 286
bilateral independent lateralized epileptiform discharges (BiPLEDs), 240
billing. *See* coding and billing
biopsy, fascicle selection for, 190
bits and vertical resolution, 85–86
blood flow and NIOM, 57, 96
BrainLab, 12, **13**
brainstem auditory evoked potentials (BAEP), 15, 21, 41–43
  anesthesia and, 43, 59, 64, 201
  auditory stimulation and, 41–42, 78, 79
  electromyography (EMG) and, 43
  factors affecting, 43
  filtration in, 82
  indications for, 43
  interpretation of, 42–43, 201–203, **201, 202, 203**
  intracranial pressure and, 58
  ketamine and, 62
  microvascular surgery (MVD) and, 199–203, **200, 201, 202, 203,** 206, 207, **209**
  operational amplifiers in, 80
  paralytics in, 63, 64
  preparation, procedure, postprocedure, 207–210, 221–226
  recording techniques for, 42
  stimulation techniques for, 42, 78, 79
  tumors of the CPA and, **214,** 216–220, **216, 221, 222**
  vascular surgeries and, 276–277
burns, 16
bursts, EMG, 23, **24**

C-arm, 11, **12**
Cadwell, 106
carbon dioxide (CO_2) lasers, 11, 122
cardiopulmonary bypass (CPB), 8, 9, **9,** 232, 233–234, **234,** 237–238

carotid cross clamping (CCC) procedure, 270, 273–275
carotid endarterectomy (CEA), 261–281
    alarm criteria during, 273–275, **275**
    anatomy and pathology in, 261–265, **262, 263, 264, 265**
    anesthesia and, 272–273, 278–279
    atherosclerosis formations in, 263–264, **265**
    brainstem auditory evoked potentials (BAEPs) and, 276–277
    carotid cross clamping (CCC) procedure in, 270, 273–275
    cerebral blood flow (CBF) assessment during, 2, 269–270, **270**, 273–275
    clinical symptoms/presentation of atherosclerotic disease and, 265–267
    collateral circulation in, 261–262, **263**
    electroencephalography (EEG) and, 39, 40, 41, 270–278, **276**
    electromyography (EMG) in, 279–280
    evidence supporting NIOM use during, 277–278
    hypoglossal nerve and, 262, **264**
    mean arterial pressure (MAP) and, 272
    other vascular surgeries and, 276–277
    quantitative EEG (QEEG) in, 271–276, **276**, 278–280
    raw EEG (REEG) in, 271–276, **274**, 277–280
    reversible ischemic neurologic deficit (RIND) in, 266
    sample NIOM case in, 275–276
    somatosensory evoked potentials (SEPs) in, 270–276, **277**, 277–278
    surgical procedure for, 267–269, **268**
    technical considerations in, preparation, procedure, postprocedure, 278–280
    transcranial Doppler (TCD) in, 270
    transient ischemic attack (TIA)/stroke and, 263, 266–267, **266**
    utility of NIOM during, 269–270
    vagus nerve and, 262, **264**
carotid surgery. *See* carotid endarterectomy
carpal tunnel syndrome, 188, 189
Cavitron ultrasonic surgical aspirator (CUSA), 11, 122, 135
CD storage media, 88
cell savers, 12
cerebellopontine angle surgery, tumor. *See* tumors of the cerebellopontine angle
cerebral blood flow (CBF) assessment, 269–270, **270**, 273–275
cerebral palsy, 97, 169–170. *See also* selective dorsal rhizotomy
cerebrospinal fluid (CSF) tests, 121, 242
cervical spondylosis, 97, 98
chaining of stimulators, 74. *See also* interleaving
channels for EP machines, 73–74
chemical sterilization, 4
chondroblastoma, 119–121, 119*t*
chondrosarcoma, 119–121, 119*t*
chordoma, 119–121, 119*t*

circulating nurse, 8
clean-up of OR, 17
client-server systems, in remote monitoring, 51–52
clinical registered nurse anesthetist (CRNA), 7
CMAPs. *See* compound muscle action potentials
Cobb angle, 96
Code 95829, 69
Code 95920, 68–69, 68*t*, 68
Code 95955, 69
Codes 95961/95962, 69
Codes 95970–95979, 69, 70*t*, 69
coding and billing, 67–69, 70*t*
    cortical and subcortical localization (Codes 95961/95962) in, 69
    Current Procedural Coding (CPT) for billing, 67
    electrocorticography (ECoG; Code 95829) in, 69
    intraoperative neurophysiology CPT, 67, 68*t*
    intraoperative neurophysiology testing (Code 95920) in, 68–69, 68*t*
    neurostimulator programming and analysis (Codes 95970–95979) in, 69, 70*t*
    nonintracranial EEG (Code 95955 in, 69
    Relative Value Units (RVU) in, 67
    Resource Based Relative Value System (RBRVS) in, 67
collateral circulation in carotid artery, 261–262, **263**
common peroneal neuropathy at the knee, 189
common-mode rejection ratio, op amps, 80–81
compound muscle action potential (CMAPs), **29**, 125, 129–131, 133–135
    anesthesia and, 205
    interpretation of, 205–206
    lumbosacral surgery and, 148, **149**, 150, 152
    microvascular surgery (MVD) and, 205–206
    neuromuscular blockade and, 148, **149**
    peripheral nerve surgery and, 182, 183–188, 190–191
    tethered cord syndrome (TCS) and, 158–159, **159**
    trigeminal nerve monitoring using, 220
    tumors of the CPA and, 219, 224
compressed spectral array (CSA) EEG, 89
compression, spinal, 97
computed tomography (CT), 121, 158
computer system for NIOM machines, 83–89
    in remote monitoring, 45–48
connecting to a network, for remote monitoring, 47–50
constant voltage vs. constant current, in stimulators, 76–77, **76**
contradictions to NIOM, 14
conversion, analog-to-digital (ADC), 83–86, **85**
cords and cables, safety, 15–16
cortical and subcortical localization (Codes 95961/95962), 69
cortical potentials, SEP, 100–104
corticospinal tracts, 96
Crawford classification of aortic aneurysms, 230, **230**

credentialing of staff, 70–71
Current Procedural Coding (CPT) for billing, 67
cutoff frequency, filter, 83, **83**

data displays, 88–89
data packet, in remote monitoring, 47–48, **48**
data transmission, for remote monitoring, 50–54
DeBakey and Stanford classification of aortic dissection, 231, **231**
decibel scale, 77–79
decompression, microvascular. *See* microvascular decompression
decompression, posterior, 99
decussation (SEPs), 100–104, **101**
deep hypothermic circulatory arrest (DHCA), 232–241, **234, 240, 241,** 241*t*, 249–250
  electroencephalography (EEG) and, 240–241, **240, 241,** 241*t*
  somatosensory evoked potentials (SEPs) and, 241
default gateways for remote monitoring computers, 47
density spectral array (DSA) EEG, 89
dermatomal somatosensory evoked potentials (DSEP), 139, 140
descending thoracic and thoracoabdominal aorta, 233–235, **235,** 241–245, 250–252, 254–257. *See also* thoracic aortic surgery
desflurane, 58, 58*t*, 59
dexmedetomidine, 63
diastematomyelia (split-cord malformation), 97, 157. *See also* tethered cord syndrome
diazepam, 170
digital filters, 87–88
Digitimer, 106
disinfection, 17
display software, in remote monitoring, 50–51
displays, 88
distal nerve disturbances, 110
documentation, 17–18, 71
dorsal column, 118
dorsal nerve rootlet, selective dorsal rhizotomy (SDR) and, 174–177, **175, 176**
dorsal rhizotomy. *See* selective dorsal rhizotomy, 169
drapes for sterile field, 5–6
drill, surgical, 13
dural sinus thromboses, 215*t*. *See also* tumors of the cerebellopontine angle
duration of stimulus, 75–76, **75**
DVD storage media, 88
dwell time, 84–85
dysplasia, vertebral, 96

ECG. *See* electrocardiograph
ECOG. *See* electrocorticography
EEG. *See* electroencephalography
efferent pathway of spinal cord, 118–119, **118**
EKG. *See* electrocardiograph
elbow, ulnar neuropathy at (UNE), 188
electrical safety, 15–16

electrocardiography (ECG/EKG)
  peripheral potentials in, 105
  signal-to-noise ratio (SNR) and, 86
  thoracic aortic surgery and, 251
electrocautery unit, 9, **9**
electroconvulsive therapy (ECT), 61, 62
electrocorticography (ECOG), 69, 283, 286–291
  anesthesia and, 297
  background of, 286
  electroencephalography (EEG) used with, 286, 287, 289
  electrodes used in, 287–288, **287, 288**
  epilepsy/epilepsy surgery and, 283, 286–291
  epileptiform abnormalities in, 289–290
  evidence of usefulness of, 290–291
  extraoperative recording using, 286–287
  functional brain mapping and, 291–296
  interictal epileptiform discharges (IEDs) and, 286, 289
  interpretation of, 289–290
  nonepileptiform abnormalities in, 290
  postexcision, 291
  preexcision, 290–291
  preparation, procedure, postprocedure, 298–299
  technique for, 288–289
  temporal lobe epilepsy (TLE) and, 291
  video-EEG and, 287, 289
electroencephalography (EEG), 9, 15, 21, 38–41, **39,** 74, 249–250
  amplification in, 81
  anesthesia and, 56, 58, 59, 59*t*, 60, 239–240, 272–273, **273,** 278–279, 297
  aneurysms and, 41
  anterior intermittent slow waves (AIS) in, 272
  applications for, 41
  arteriovenous malformations (AVMs) and, 41
  artifacts in, 40, 83
  benzodiazepines in, 61
  bilateral independent lateralized epileptiform discharges (BiPLEDs) in, 240
  carotid endarterectomies (CEAs) and, 39, 40, 41, 270–278, **276**
  changes of significance in, 41
  coding and billing for, 67, 69
  compressed spectral array (CSA), 89
  data analysis of, 88
  data displays for, 89
  deep hypothermic circulatory arrest (DHCA) in, 240–241, **240, 241,** 241*t*
  density spectral array (DSA), 89
  digital signals in, 84
  electrocorticography (ECOG) and, 286, 287, 289
  epilepsy/epilepsy surgery and, 283–300, **285**
  etomidate in, 62–63
  fast anterior dominant rhythmic activity (FAR) in, 272, 273
  filtration in, 82
  frequency classification of, 39
  frontal intermittent rhythmic delta activity (FIRDA) in, 272

functional brain mapping and, 295
generalized periodic epileptiform discharges (GPEDs) and, 240, **240**
generators for, 38–39
montages of recording in, 39, **39**, **40**
motor evoked potentials (MEPs) and, 40, **40**
opioids in, 61–62
paralytics in, 63, 64
patterns seen in, 39–40
periodic lateralized epileptiform discharges (PLEDs), 240
preparation, procedure, postprocedure for, 251–257, 278–280, 298–299
processing methods for, 40–41
propofol in, 61
quantitative (QEEG), 271–276, **276**, 278–280
raw (REEG), 271–276, **274**, 277–280
signal-to-noise ratio (SNR) and, 86
somatosensory evoked potentials (SEPs) and, 41
temperature effects on, 56
tethered cord syndrome (TCS) and, 158
thoracic aortic surgery and, 239–240
tumors of the CPA and, 222
vertebral column surgery and, 101
video-, 287, 289
widespread anteriorly maximum rhythmic activity (WAR) in, 272
widespread persistent slow waves (WPS) in, 272, 273
electromagnetic interference (EMI), 177
electromyography (EMG), 15, 21, 74
amplification in, 81
amplitude of MUPs in, 26
anatomy, physiology and, 21, 23
anesthesia and, 28–29, 172, 173, 205
asynchronous pattern in, 25–26
brainstem auditory evoked potentials (BAEPs) and, 43
bursts and trains in, 23, **24**
carotid endarterectomy (CEA) and, 279–280
characterization of, 23
compound muscle action potentials (CMAPs) and, 150, 152
data analysis of, 88
data displays for, 88–89
digital signals in, 84
facial nerve monitoring using, 219
filtration in, 82
firing rate of MUPs in, 25–26
free-running, 21–29, 139–143, **140**
hemifacial spasm (HFS) and, 196
interpretation of, 23, 205–206
ischemia and, 27
lumbosacral surgery and, 139–154, **140**
microvascular surgery (MVD) and, 199, 205–207
motor nerve conduction studies (triggered) using, 27–29
motor unit potential (MUP) in, 21, 23, 25–26
muscle selection for, 21, 23t, 152–153
myotomes and, 21
needle electrodes for, 186, **186**
nerve dysfunction vs. activity on, relation of, 26–27
neuromuscular blockade monitoring using, 147–148, **148**, **149**, 153
parameters for, 150t
patient safety and, 153
pedicle holes and screws evaluation by, 27–28, 28t, **29**, 144–147, **144**, **145**, 146t
peripheral nerve surgery and, 186–187
preparation, procedure, postprocedure, 177–180, 190–191, 207–210, 221–226
radiculopathy in, 110
recording and stimulating parameters used in, 21, 22t
recording electrodes for, 150, 150t, **151**
reflexive activity and, 25
sampling frequency for, 85
selective dorsal rhizotomy (SDR) and, 171–172, 173
shape of MUPs in, 26
signal-to-noise ratio (SNR) and, 86
"significant" activity on, communicating with the surgeon, 27
sphincter function monitoring using, 161–162, **161**
spinal cord surgery and, 136
stimulating electrodes and parameters for, 75, **151**, 152, **152**
subdermal needle electrodes used in, **173**
surgical events and, relationship between, 24–25, **26**
tethered cord syndrome (TCS) and, 158–163, **160**
threshold ratios (TR) and, 173–174, 175t
trigeminal nerve monitoring using, 219–220
tumors of the CPA and, 217–220, **221**, 225
EMG. *See* electromyography
endovascular stent grafts (EVSG), 235–237, **236**, **237**, 246–251
endovascular thoracic aortic repair, 235–237, **236**, **237**, 246–251. *See also* thoracic aortic surgery
enflurane, 58, 58t, 59, 297
EPs. *See* evoked potentials
ependymoma, 119–121, 119t
epidermoids, 215t. *See also* tumors of the cerebellopontine angle
epilepsy/epilepsy surgery, 283–301
afterdischarge (AD) localization in, 293–295, **295**
anatomy and physiology in, 283–284
anesthesia and, 297
antiepileptic drugs (AEDs) and, 283
bilateral independent lateralized epileptiform discharges (BiPLEDs) in, 240
electroencephalography (EEG) and, 283–300, **285**, 295
electrocorticography (ECOG) and, 283, 286–291
functional brain mapping and, 283, 291–296

epilepsy/epilepsy surgery (continued)
  generalized periodic epileptiform discharges
      (GPEDs), 240, **240**
  interictal epileptiform discharge (IED) in, 284,
      285
  intracarotid amobarbital (Wada) test and, 296
  localization-related (LRE), 283
  magnetic resonance imaging (MRI) and, 296
  magnetoencephalography (MEG) and, 296
  pathology in, 284–286
  periodic lateralized epileptiform discharges
      (PLEDs), 240
  positron emission tomography (PET) and, 296
  safety precautions for, 297–298
  somatosensory evoked potentials (SEPs) in, 299
  technical considerations in, preparation,
      procedure, postprocedure, 298–299
  temporal lobe (TLE), 284, **285**, 291
  video-EEG and, 287, 289
equipment for NIOM, 73–92
equipment for the OR, 8–13
Erb's point, 104
errors in medical care, 71
Ethernet connector, 47, **47**
ethical responsibility of staff, 70–71
etiquette of the OR, 16–17
etomidate in, 60, 60t, 62–63, 130, 297
evoked potentials (EPs), 73
  amplification in, 81
  anesthesia and, 58, 58t, 60, 60t
  artifact rejection in, 83
  auditory stimulation for, 78
  data displays for, 88–89
  digital signals in, 84
  distal nerve disturbances in, 110
  interpretation of, 108–111
  ketamine and, 62
  opioids in, 61–62
  pathologic decrements in, 110, 113, **114**
  peripheral potentials in, 105
  preparation, procedure, postprocedure for,
      111–115
  proximal nerve or plexus disturbances in, 110
  radiculopathy in, 110
  signal averaging and, 86–87
  signal-to-noise ratio (SNR) and, 86, 87
  spinal cord compromise in, 110–111, **111**
  stimulators and, 75, 78
  systemic factors affecting, 109
  technical factors affecting, 109–110
  temperature effects on, 56
  tumors of the CPA and, 219
  vertebral column surgery and, 95
  warning criteria for, 108–111, **109**
  waveform of, 86–87, **87**
Ewing's sarcoma, 119–121, 119t
extradural spinal tumors, 119–121, 119t
extramedullary spinal tumors, 119–121, 119t

facial nerve monitoring, 219
Faraday cage, 73

fascicle selection for nerve biopsy, 190
fasciculus gracilis, 118
fasciculus cuneatus, 118
fast anterior dominant rhythmic activity (FAR),
    272, 273
feedback rapidity, in SEPs, 100
fentanyl, 297
fiber tracts of spinal cord in, 118–119
filtering data, in remote monitoring computers,
    47–48
filters, 74, 82–83, **82**, **83**
  amplitude vs. frequency in, 82–83, **82**
  analog, 82–83
  bandpass, 82, **82**
  cutoff frequency of, 83, **83**
  digital, 87–88
  high-cut, 82–83
  low-cut, 82–83
  order of, 82–83
  roll-off of, 82–83
firewalls, in remote monitoring computers, 47, **48**,
    50, 51 53, **53**
firing rate of MUPs, 25–26
fluoroscopy, 11, 16
follow-up, 17
fractures, spinal, 97, 98
Free Software Foundation, 52
free-running EMG, 21, 139. *See also*
    electromyography
  artifacts in, 142–143, **143**
  muscles suitable for, 141, 141t
  outcome data from, postop, 141, 142t
  output from, 140–141, **141**
  precautions for, 142–143
  radiculopathy and, 142–143, 143t, **143**
  sensitivity of, 141–142, 142t
  technique for, 140–141
  tethered cord syndrome (TCS) and, 161, 162
Friedreich's ataxia, 97
frequency, electroencephalography (EEG) and, 39
frontal intermittent rhythmic delta activity
    (FIRDA), 272
fully qualified names, for remote monitoring and
    computers, 51
functional brain mapping, 283, 291–296
  afterdischarge (AD) localization using,
      293–295, **295**
  electroencephalography (EEG) and, 295
  epilepsy/epilepsy surgery and, 283,
      291–296
  intracarotid amobarbital (Wada) test and, 296
  localization using, 292–293, **296**
  magnetic resonance imaging (MRI) and, 296
  magnetoencephalography (MEG) and, 296
  positron emission tomography (PET) and, 296
  preparation, procedure, postprocedure,
      298–299
  somatosensory evoked potentials (SEPs) and,
      296–297
  technique for, 293–295, **294**, **295**
  utility of, 291–292

future directions
    tethered cord syndrome (TCS) and, 166–167
    thoracic aortic surgery and, 257

gamma aminobutyric acid (GABA), 61
ganglioglioma, 119–121, 119*t*
general anesthesia. *See* anesthesia
General Public License, 52
generalized periodic epileptiform discharges (GPEDs), 240, **240**
generators, for somatosensory evoked potentials (SEPs), 30–31, 30*t*
giant–cell tumor, 119–121, 119*t*
globus tumors, 215*t*. *See also* tumors of the cerebellopontine angle
glossopharyngeal neuralgia (GPN), 195, 197, 199. *See also* microvascular decompression
GoToMyPC, remote monitoring and, 52
gowns, masks, drapes, 5–6
grounding, 16

halogenated agents in anesthesia, 59. *See also* anesthesia
halothane in, 58, 58*t*, 59, 297
Health Insurance Portability and Accountability Act (HIPAA), 53, 88
heat sterilization, 3–4
hemangioblastoma, 119–121, 119*t*
hemangioma, 119–121, 119*t*
hematology, anesthesia and, 57
hemifacial spasm (HFS), 195, 196–199. *See also* microvascular decompression
hemivertebrae, 96
high-cut filters, 82–83
history of NIOM technology, 73–74
horizontal gaze palsy and progressive scoliosis (HGPPS), 97
horizontal resolution, 84–85
hypertension, 57
hypocarbia, 57
hypoglossal nerve, 262, **264**
hypotension, 57, 110
hypoxia, 57

image capture, for remote monitoring, 53–54
image-guided surgery systems, 12, **13**
infection control, 16
infratentorial lateral supracerebellar approach (ILSA), 197, 198
inhalation agents used for anesthesia, 58, 58*t*, 59*t*
injectors, fluoroscopy, 12
Inomed, 106
input impedance, amplifiers, 81, **81**
Institute of Medicine, 71
Institutional Review Board (IRB), 77
intensity of stimulus, 75, **75**
interictal epileptiform discharge (IED), 284, **285**, 286, 289, 291
interleaving, 74
internal carotid artery (ICA). *See* carotid endarterectomy (CEA)

Internet and remote monitoring, 45–48
interpeak latency (IPL), 217
interpreting
    BAEP, 42–43, 201–203, **201**, **202**, **203**
    compound muscle action potentials (CMAPs), 205–206
    electrocorticograph (ECOG), 289–290
    electromyography (EMG), 23, 205–206
    muscle evoked potential (MEP), transcranial, 35–36
    nerve action potentials (NAPs), 204–205
    somatosensory evoked potentials (SEPs), 31–33
intracarotid amobarbital (Wada) test, 296
intracranial pressure, anesthesia and, 57–58
intramedullary spinal tumors, 119–121, 119*t*
intraoperative neurophysiology CPT codes, 67, 68*t*
intraoperative neurophysiology testing (Code 95920) in, 68–69, 68*t*
intraoperative ultrasound, 10
intrathecal pumps, spasticity and, 170
intravenous agents for anesthesia, 60–63, 60*t*
inverting op amp, 79–80, **79**, **80**, 81*t*
IP (Internet Protocol) addresses, in remote monitoring computers, 45, 48, 51
ipconfig command, in remote monitoring computer systems, 45, 47
ischemia, electromyography (EMG) and, 27
isoflurane in, 58, 58*t*, 59

keep-alive signals, in remote monitoring, 52–53, **53**
ketamine, 60, 60*t*, 62, 130
knee, common peroneal neuropathy at, 189

laptop NIOM machines, 74
lasers, 11, 122
lateral suboccipital infrafloccular approach (LSIA), 197
legal issues, 71
leiomyosarcoma, 119–121, 119*t*
liability for errors, 71
lipoma, 119–121, 119*t*, 215*t*. *See also* tumors of the cerebellopontine angle
local anesthesia. *See* anesthesia
localization, somatosensory evoked potentials (SEPs) and, 30–31, 31*t*
localization-related epilepsy (LRE), 283
lorazepam, 170
Louisiana State University, 188
low-cut filters, 82–83
lower limb derivations (SEP), 101–104, **102**, **103**, 104*t*
lumbosacral surgery, 139–154
    compound muscle action potentials (CMAPs) in, 148, **149**, 150, 152
    dermatomal somatosensory evoked potentials (DSEP) in, 139, 140
    free-running EMG in, 139–143, **140**
        artifacts in, 142–143, **143**
        muscles suitable for, 141, 141*t*
        outcome data from, postop, 141, 142*t*
        output from, 140–141, **141**

lumbosacral surgery *(continued)*
    precautions for, 142–143
    radiculopathy and, 142–143, 143*t*, **143**
    sensitivity of, 141–142, 142*t*
    technique for, 140–141
  MEPs in, 139
  muscle selection for EMG in, 152–153
  neuromuscular blockade monitoring in, using EMG, 147–148, **148, 149,** 153
  patient safety and, 153
  pedicle hole/screw evaluation in, using EMG, 144–147, **144, 145,** 146*t*
  preoperative studies for, 150
  recording electrodes and parameters for, 150, 150*t*, **151**
  somatosensory evoked potentials (SEPs) in, 139, 140
  stimulating electrodes and parameters for, **151,** 152, **152**

magnetic resonance imaging (MRI), 12, 121
  epilepsy/epilepsy surgery and, 296
  hemifacial spasm (HFS) and, 197
  peripheral nerve surgery and, 190
  tethered cord syndrome (TCS) and, **157**
  trigeminal neuralgia (TN) and, 196
  tumors of the CPA and, 215
magnetoencephalography (MEG), 296
masks, 5–6
mean/minimum alveolar concentration (MAC), 55–56, 58, 59, 62–64, 130, 239
mean arterial pressure (MAP), 243, 272
median neuropathy at the wrist (carpal tunnel syndrome) and, 188, 189
medical students, 6–7
medical-legal issues, 71
meningioma, 119–121, 119*t*. *See also* tumors of the cerebellopontine angle
MEPs. *See* motor evoked potentials
methohexital, 297
microscope, 9–10, **10**
microvascular decompression (MVD), 195–210
  brainstem auditory evoked potentials (BAEPs) in, 199–203, **200, 201, 202, 203,** 206, 207, **209**
  compound muscle action potentials (CMAPs) in, 205–206
  electromyography (EMG) in, 199, 205–207
  in glossopharyngeal neuralgia (GPN), 195, 197, 199
  in hemifacial spasm (HFS), 195, 196–199
  infratentorial lateral supracerebellar approach (ILSA) in, 197, 198
  lateral suboccipital infrafloccular approach (LSIA) in, 197
  microvascular decompression; MVD. *See* microvascular decompression (MVD), 195
  monitoring techniques used in, 199–206
  nerve action potential (NAPs), vestibulocochlear nerve in, 204–205, **204,** 206
  nerve conduction studies (NCS) in, 207
  somatosensory evoked potentials (SEPs) in, 199, 206
  surgical technique for, 197–199
  technical considerations in, preparation, procedure, postprocedure, 207–210
  transcondylar fossa approach (TFA) in, 197
  in trigeminal neuralgia (TN), 195–196, 198
  tumors of the CPA and, 197
  utility of NIOM in, 206
minimal alveolar concentration (MAC). *See* mean/minimum alveolar concentration
monitoring equipment, 9–12, **10, 12,** 15, 71, 73. *See also* NIOM machines; remote monitoring
montages, electroencephalographic (EEG) and, 39, **39,** 40
morphine, 130
motor evoked potentials (MEPs), 9, 10–11, 14, 15, 17, 21, 29, 97, **128**
  anesthesia and, 37–38, 38*t*, 59, 60, 129–130, 239
  barbiturates in, 61
  benzodiazepines in, 61
  compound muscle action potentials (CMAPs) in, 125, 129–131, 133, 134, 135, 148, **149**
  data displays for, 88–89
  electroencephalography (EEG) and, 40, **40**
  etomidate in, 62–63
  interpretation of, 108–111
  intracranial pressure and, 58
  ketamine and, 62
  lumbosacral surgery and, 139
  muscle potentials in, 106–107, **107,** 108
  nerve action potentials (NAPs) in, 125, **126**
  neuromuscular blockade and, 130
  opioids in, 61–62
  paralytics in, 63, 64
  preparation, procedure, postprocedure for, 111–115, 134–136, 163–166, 251–257
  propofol in, 61
  radiculopathy in, 110
  right-body, during scoliosis correction, 36
  spinal cord compromise in, 110–111, **111**
  spinal cord stimulation in, recording from muscles/nerves, 125
  spinal cord surgery and, 117, 124–137, **128**
  stimulators and, 75–77
  systemic factors affecting, 109
  technical factors affecting, 109–110
  thoracic aortic surgery and, 239, 242–251, 244*t*, **247, 248**
  transcranial (tceMEP), 33–38, 77
    anesthesia and, 37–38, 38*t*
    complications of, 37
    contraindications of, 37
    degraded signals in, 35, **35**
    indications for, 37
    interpretation of, 35–37
    recording of, 34
    signal optimization in, 34
    stimulation for, 34
    techniques for, 34

transcranial electric stimulation (TES) and, 106–107, **107**, **108**, 125, **125**, 129, 133
tumors of the CPA and, 218–220
vertebral column surgery and, 96–115
warning criteria for, 108–111, 130–133, **132**, **133**
motor nerve conduction studies (triggered EMG), 21–29. *See also* electromyography
motor unit action potentials (MUAPs)
    peripheral nerve surgery and, 186–187
    selective dorsal rhizotomy (SDR) and, 171
motor unit potential (MUP), 21, 23, 25–26
multichannel EP machines, 73–74
multiple myeloma, 119–121, 119*t*
muscle potentials, SEP, 106–107, **107**, **108**
muscles commonly monitored by EMG, 21, 23*t*
muscular dystrophy, 97
MVD. *See* microvascular decompression
myotomes, 21

NAPs. *See* nerve action potentials
NCS. *See* nerve conduction studies
needle electrodes, 16, **173**, 186, **186**
nerve action potentials (NAPs), 125, **126**
    anesthesia and, 204
    biopsy and fascicle selection using, 190
    interpretation of, 204–205
    knee neuropathy and, 189
    microvascular surgery (MVD) and, 204–207
    peripheral nerve surgery and, 182–191, **185**
    preparation, procedure, postprocedure, 207–210
    tumors of the CPA and, 219
    tumors of the peripheral nerves and, 189
nerve conduction studies (NCS), 74
    amplification in, 81
    data displays for, 88–89
    microvascular surgery (MVD) and, 207
    peripheral nerve surgery and, 183–186
    stimulators and, 75
    tumors of the CPA and, 219
nerve dysfunction vs. EMG activity, 26–27
networked computers, remote monitoring and, 45–48
neural tube defects, 97, 156. *See also* tethered cord syndrome
neuroblastoma, 119–121, 119*t*
neurofibroma, 119–121, 119*t*
neurofibromatosis, 96
neuromuscular blockade, 130
    electromyography (EMG) monitoring of, 147–148, **148**, **149**, 153
neuromuscular disease, 97
neurophysiologic intraoperative monitoring (NIOM), 3, 21–44
neurostimulator programming and analysis (Codes 95970–95979), 69, 70*t*
Nicolet Endeavor stimulator, 106
NIOM machines, 73–92
    amplifiers for, 79–83
    analog-to-digital conversion (ADC) in, 83–86, **85**
    bits and vertical resolution in, 85–86
    CD or DVD storage in, 88
    comparison of, 89, 90–91*t*
    data displays in, 88–89
    dwell time in, 84–85
    filtering and smoothing in, 87–88
    filters in, 82–83, **82**, **83**
    horizontal resolution in, 84–85
    operational amplifiers in, 79–80
    sampling frequency in, 84–85, **85**
    signal averaging and, 86–87
    signal-to-noise ratio (SNR) and, 86, 87
    stimulators in, 74–79
    storage in, 88
    trending in, 88
NIOM. *See* neurophysiologic intraoperative monitoring
nitrous oxide, 58, 58*t*, 60, 130, 297
nonintracranial EEG (Code 95955), 69
noninverting op amp, 79–80, **79**, **80**, 81*t*
nurse practitioner (NP), 7
nursing team, 7–8
Nyquist theorem, 85

Ohm's law, 76
Ojemann stimulator, 298
oligodendroglioma, 119–121, 119*t*
operating room, 3–19
    access to patient in, 15, 16–17
    aseptic technique and sterilization in, 3–6
    attire for, 5, 17
    clean-up of, 17
    documentation of procedures in, 17–18
    equipment of, 8–13
    etiquette and protocol of, 16–17
    personnel for, 6–8
    preparing for surgery in, 13–15
    safety in, 15–16
operational amplifiers, 79–80, **79**, **80**, 81
    common-mode rejection ratio in, 80–81
    input impedance in, 81, **81**
    polarity and inverting/noninverting, 79–80, **79**, **80**, 81*t*
    voltage-divider rule in, 81, **81**
opioids in, 60, 60*t*, 61–62, 130
oscilloscope, 73
ossification of the posterior longitudinal ligament (OPLL), 97, 98
osteoblastoma, 119–121, 119*t*
osteochondroma, 119–121, 119*t*
osteoid sarcoma, 119–121, 119*t*
osteosarcoma, 119–121, 119*t*

pancuronium, 130
paragangliomas, 215*t*. *See also* tumors of the cerebellopontine angle
paralytics, and anesthesia, 63, 64
pathologic EP decrements, 110, 113, **114**
patient access, 15, 16–17
pcAnywhere, 52
pedicle holes and screws, EMG evaluation of, 27–28, 28*t*, **29**, 144–147, **144**, **145**, 146*t*

perfusionist, 8
periodic lateralized epileptiform discharges (PLEDs), 240
peripheral nerve stimulation, recording from spinal cord, 122, **123**
peripheral nerve surgery, 181–193
    common peroneal neuropathy at the knee and, 189
    compound muscle action potential (CMAPs) in, 182, 187, 188
    compound muscle action potential (CMAPs) in, 183–186, 190–191
    electromyography (EMG), needle electromyography in, 186–187, **186**
    fascicle selection for nerve biopsy and, 190
    localizing lesions for, 182
    magnetic resonance imaging (MRI) in, 190
    median neuropathy at the wrist (carpal tunnel syndrome) and, 189
    motor unit action potentials (MUAPs) in, 186–187
    nerve action potentials (NAPs) in, 182–191, **185**
    nerve conduction studies in, 183–186
    stimulator placement in, mono- and bipolar, 183–184, **184**
    technical considerations in, preparation, procedure, postprocedure, 190–191
    technical problems encountered in, 187–188
    tumors of the peripheral nerves and, 189
    ulnar neuropathy at elbow (UNE) and, 188
peripheral neuropathies, 97
peripheral potentials, SEP, 105
personal firewalls, remote monitoring and, 51
personal protective equipment, 16
personnel of the operating room, 6–8
physician assistant (PA), 7
piezoelectric transducers, stimulators and, 78–79
pinging a network connection, 46, **47**
plasmacytoma, 119–121, 119*t*
plexus disturbances, 110
plotters, 73
polarity of operational amplifiers, 79–80, **79**, **80**, 81*t*
polio, 97
port numbers, in remote monitoring computers, 47
portable NIOM machines, 74
positron emission tomography (PET), 296
posterior decompression, 99
posterior spinal fusion (SPF), 98
postoperative documentation, 18
postsurgical testing, 17
potassium/sodium/calcium balance, anesthesia and, 58
potential fade, 109, **109**
preoperative documentation, 17
preoperative studies, 13–14
preparing for surgery, 13–15
processing methods, electroencephalography (EEG) and, 40–41

propofol, 60, 60*t*, 61, 130, 239, 297
protocol in the OR, 16–17
proximal nerve or plexus disturbances, 110

quantitative EEG (QEEG), 271–280, **276**

radiation sterilization, 4–5
radiculopathy, 110
    free-running EMG and, 142–143, 143*t*, **143**
radiology technician, 8
raw EEG (REEG), 271–280, **274**
recording electrodes and parameters, EMG, 150, 150*t*, **151**
reflexive activity, on EMG, 25
regional anesthesia. *See* anesthesia
registered EEG technologist (R EEG T), 70, 71
registered evoked potential technologist (R EP T), 70, 71
registered nurse (RN), 8
Relative Value Units (RVU), in billing/coding, 67
remifentanil, 130, 297
remote application servers, 49–50, **50**
remote monitoring, 15, 45–54
    client-server systems in, 51–52
    computer systems for, 45–48
    connecting to the network for, 47, 48–50
    data packet used in, 47–48, **48**
    data transmission in, 50–54
    default gateways for computers used in, 47
    display software used in, vendor-specific, 50–51
    Ethernet connector for, 47, **47**
    filtering of data in, 47–48
    firewalls in network computers used in, 47, **48**, 50, 51, 53, **53**
    fully qualified names of computers in, 51
    HIPAA policies and, 53, 88
    image capture in, 53–54
    in-hospital vs. remote display systems in, 51
    Internet and, 45–48
    IP (Internet Protocol) address of computers in, 45, 48, 51
    keep-alive signals and, 52–53, **53**
    pcAnywhere and, 52
    personal firewalls in, 51
    pining a network connection for, 46, **47**
    port numbers of computers used in, 47–48
    remote application servers used in, 49–50, **50**
    reverse-connection software for, 52–53, **53**
    screen capture software for, 51–52
    security of signal in, 52, 53, 88
    servers for, 53–54
    virtual network computing (VNC) in, 52
    virtual private networks (VPNs) for, 48–49, **49**, 51, 52
    Web servers for, 53–54
    Windows-based systems for, 45–46, **46**, **47**
repetitive microtrauma of nerve, EMG activity, 26–27, **26**
resident, anesthesia, 7
resident, surgical, 6

resolution, horizontal, 84–85
resolution, vertical, 85–86
Resource Based Relative Value System (RBRVS), in billing/coding, 67
responsibility of staff, 70–71, 70
reverse-connection software, in remote monitoring, 52–53, **53**
reversible ischemic neurologic deficit (RIND), 266
rhizotomy. *See* selective dorsal rhizotomy
roll-off, in filtration, 82–83
room attendant, 8

safety in the OR, 15–16
sampling frequency, 84–85, **85**
schwannoma, 119–121, 119*t*, 215*t*. *See also* tumors of the cerebellopontine angle
scoliosis, 96–97. *See also* vertebral column surgery
 Cobb angle and, 96–97
 surgical treatment of, 98
 vertebral column surgery and, 96–97
Scoliosis Research Society, 33
screen capture software, for remote monitoring, 51–52, 51
screws, EMG evaluation of, 27–28, 28*t*, **29**, 144–147, **144, 145**, 146*t*
scrub nurse, 8
security of data, 52, 53, 88
sedation. *See* anesthesia
selective dorsal rhizotomy (SDR), 169–180
 anesthesia and, 172
 anesthetic/nerve root verification in, 173
 dorsal nerve rootlet selection in, 174–176, **175, 176**
 dorsal nerve rootlet sparing in, 176–177
 electromyography (EMG) and, 171–173
 exposure/anatomic identification in, 172
 indications for, 170
 motor unit action potentials (MUAPs) and, 171
 muscle monitoring in, 171, 171*t*
 NIOM techniques for, 170
 preoperative preparation for, 171–172, **173**
 somatosensory evoked potentials (SEPs) and, 171
 standard montage used for, 173–174, 174*t*
 stimulation and recording parameters in, 172–173
 subdermal needle electrodes used in, **173**
 technical considerations in, preparation, procedure, postprocedure, 177–180
 threshold ratios (TR) and, 173–174, 175*t*
sensitivity of NIOM to anesthesia, 64–65
SEPs. *See* somatosensory evoked potentials
servers, remote application/remote monitoring, 49–50, **50**, 53–54
setup for NIOM, 14–15
sevoflurane in, 58, 58*t*, 59, 297
shape of MUPs, 26
shock hazards, 15–16
signal averagers, 73, 86–87
signal optimization, MEP, transcranial and, 34

signal rejection, 74
signal-to-noise ratio (SNR), 86, 87, 99–101, **101**
smoothing of digital signals, 87–88
somatosensory evoked potentials (SEPs), 9, 15, 21, 29–33, **32**, **127**, 127*t*, **132, 133**
 anesthesia and, 33, 57, 59, 60, 64, 128–130, 239–240, 244, 272–273, 278–279
 barbiturates in, 61
 blood flow and, 57
 carotid endarterectomy (CEA) and, 270–278, **277**
 cortical potentials in, 100–104
 decussation and, 100–104, **101**
 deep hypothermic circulatory arrest (DHCA) and, 241
 distal nerve disturbances in, 110
 electroencephalography (EEG) and, 41
 epidural spinal cord stimulation in, 124
 epilepsy/epilepsy surgery and, 299
 feedback rapidity in, 100
 filtration in, 82
 functional brain mapping and, 296–297
 generators of, 30–31, 30*t*
 hematologic status and, 57
 importance of, 29–30
 indications for, 33
 interpretation of, 31–33, 108–111
 intracranial pressure and, 58
 ketamine and, 62
 localization of, 30–31, 31*t*
 lower limb derivations for, 101–104, **102, 103**, 104*t*
 lumbosacral surgery and, 139, 140
 microvascular surgery (MVD) and, 199, 206
 muscle potentials in, 106–107, **107, 108**
 neuromuscular blockade and, 130, 147–148, **148, 149**
 paralytics in, 63, 64
 peripheral nerve stimulation in, recording from spinal cord, 122, **123**
 peripheral potentials in, 105
 preparation, procedure, postprocedure for, 111–115, 134–136, 163–166, 207–210, 221–226, 251–257, 278–280
 propofol in, 61
 proximal nerve or plexus disturbances in, 110
 radiculopathy in, 110
 sampling frequency for, 85
 selective dorsal rhizotomy (SDR) and, 171
 signal-to-noise ratio (SNR) in, 99–101, **101**
 "significant" degradation in, 31, **32**, 33
 spinal cord compromise in, 110–111, **111**
 spinal cord stimulation in
  epidural, 124
  recording from scalp, 123–124, **124**
  recording from spinal cord, 122–123
 spinal cord surgery and, 117, 122–137, **127**, 127*t*, **132, 133**
 spinal potentials in, 105
 stimulators and, 75
 subcortical potentials in, 104–105

somatosensory evoked potentials (SEPs) *(continued)*
  systemic factors affecting, 109
  technical factors affecting, 109–110
  tethered cord syndrome (TCS) and, 160–162
  thoracic aortic surgery and, 239–251, 239, 244t, **248**, **249**
  thoracic decompression and fusion shown on, **32**, 32
  total intravenous anesthesia (TIVA) in, 128, 130
  transcranial electric stimulation (TES) and, 106–107, **107**, **108**
  trigeminal nerve monitoring using, 220
  tumors of the CPA and, 217–220, **218**, **221**
  upper limb derivations for, 100–101, **101**
  ventilatory status and, 57
  vertebral column surgery and, 96–115
  warning criteria for, 108–111, 130–133, **132**, **133**
sound and the decibel scale, 77–79
sound pressure level (SPL), 78
sound reference and decibel scale, 78
spasticity, selective dorsal rhizotomy (SDR) for, 169–170. *See also* selective dorsal rhizotomy
sphincter function monitoring, 161–162, **161**
spinal cord
  afferent and efferent pathways of, 118–119
  anatomy of, 96, 117–119
  arteries of, 119
  blood supply of, 96
  compromise of, 110–**111**
  fiber tracts of, 118–119
  spinal cord stimulation
    epidural, 124
    recording from muscles/nerves, 125
    recording from scalp, 123–124, **124**
    recording from spinal cord, 122–123
spinal cord surgery, 117–137
  anesthesia and, 128, 129–130
  arteries of spinal cord in, 119
  carbon dioxide (CO_2) laser in, 122
  Cavitron ultrasound surgical aspirator (CUSA) in, 122, 135
  cerebrospinal fluid (CSF) tests for, 121
  clinical presentation in, 121
  compound muscle action potentials (CMAPs) in, 125, 129–131, 133, 134, 135
  CT and MRI in, 121
  diagnostic evaluation for, 121
  electromyography (EMG) in, 136
  fiber tracts of spinal cord in, 118–119
  MEPs in, 117, 124–137, **128**
  nerve action potentials (NAPs) in, 125, **126**
  paradigms common to, 125–126
  peripheral nerve stimulation in, recording from spinal cord, 122, **123**
  somatosensory evoked potentials (SEPs) in, 117, 122–137, **127**, 127t, **132**, **133**
  spinal cord anatomy in, 117–119
  spinal cord stimulation in
    epidural, 124
    recording from muscles/nerves, 125
    recording from scalp, 123–124, **124**
    recording from spinal cord, 122–123
  surgical procedure for, 121–122
  technical considerations in, preparation, procedure, postprocedure, 134–136, 163–166
  total intravenous anesthesia (TIVA) in, 128, 130
  transcranial electrical stimulation (TES) in, 125, **125**, 129, 133
  tumors of spine and, 119–122, 119t
  utility of NIOM in, 133–134
  warning criteria in, 130–133, **132**, **133**
spinal dysraphism. *See* tethered cord syndrome
spinal potentials, SEP, 105
spinothalamic tract, 118
split-cord malformation, 157. *See also* tethered cord syndrome
spondylosis, cervical, 97, 98
staffing, training and responsibilities of, 70–71
sterile field, 5–6
sterilization methods, 3–6, 17
stimulating electrodes and parameters, EMG, **151**, 152, **152**
stimulators, 73, 74–79
  for auditory stimulation, 77–79
    brainstem auditory evoked potentials (BAEPs) and, 78, 79
    piezoelectric transducers for, 78–79
    sound and decibel scale in, 77–79
    sound pressure level (SPL) and, 78
    sound reference and decibel scale in, 78
    types of, 78–79
  bipolar, 183–184, **184**
  brainstem auditory evoked potentials (BAEPs) and, 78, 79
  constant voltage vs. constant current in, 76–77, **76**
  duration of stimulus and, 75–76, **75**
  electrical, 75
  evoked potentials (EPs) and, 78
  intensity of stimulus and, 75, **75**
  monopolar, 183–184
  transcranial MEPs (tceMEP) and, 77
storage for NIOM data, 88
stroke, 263, 266–267, **266**. *See also* transient ischemic attack
subcortical potentials, SEP, 104–105
subdermal needle electrodes, **173**
sufentanil, 130
supplies for NIOM, 14, 14t
surgical documentation, 18
surgical events and the EMG recording, 24–25, **26**
surgical resident, 6
surgical tables, 12
surgical team, 6
syringomyelia, 97
systemic factors affecting EPs, 109

tables, surgical, 12
tceMEP. *See* motor evoked potential, transcranial
technical factors affecting EP, 109–110
technologists, training and responsibilities of, 70–71
temperature and NIOM, 56
temporal lobe epilepsy (TLE), 284, **285**, 291
tethered cord syndrome (TCS), 97, 155–167
    anatomy of, 155–156
    compound muscle action potentials (CMAPs) in, 158–159, **159**
    diagnosis of, 157–158
    electroencephalography (EEG) in, 158
    electromyography (EMG) motor system monitoring during, 158–163, **160**
    future directions in treatment of, 166–167
    paradigm for, 163
    pathophysiology of, 156–157, 157*t*
    sensory system (SEP) monitoring during, 160–162
    sphincter function monitoring during, 161–162, **161**
    surgical considerations for, 158
    symptoms of, 157–158, **157**
    utility of NIOM in, 162
thermal sterilization, 3–4
thoracic aortic surgery, 227–259
    anatomy and, 227–229
    anesthesia and, 239–240, 243–244, 246
    aneurysmal disease and, 229–231, **229**, **230**
    aortic diseases amenable to, 229–232
    aortic dissection and, 231–232, **231**
    in ascending aortic and aortic arch, 232–233, **232**, **233**, 238–241, 249–256
    bilateral independent lateralized epileptiform discharges (BiPLEDs) in, 240
    cardiopulmonary bypass (CPB) in, 232–234, **234**, 237–238
    cerebrospinal fluid (CSF) pressures in, 242
    deep hypothermic circulatory arrest (DHCA) in, 232–250, **234**, **240**, **241**, 241*t*
    in descending thoracic and thoracoabdominal aorta, 233–252, **234**, **235**, 254–257
    ECG in, 251
    electroencephalography (EEG) in, 239–240, 249–250
    endovascular stent grafts (EVSG) in, 235–237, **236**, **237**, 246–249, 251
    endovascular thoracic aortic repair in, 235–237, **236**, **237**, 246–249, 251
    future directions in, 257
    generalized periodic epileptiform discharges (GPEDs) and, 240, **240**
    mean arterial pressure (MAP) and, 243
    MEPs in, 239, 242–251, 244*t* **247**, **248**
    NIOM paradigms for, 238–249
    periodic lateralized epileptiform discharges (PLEDs), 240
    somatosensory evoked potentials (SEPs) in, **32**, 239–251, 244*t*, **248**, **249**
    technical considerations in, preparation, procedure, postprocedure, 251–257

    total intravenous anesthesia (TIVA) and, 243–244, 246
    utility of NIOM in, 249–251
thoracic decompression and fusion, somatosensory evoked potentials (SEPs) and, **32**
threshold ratios (TR), EMG, 173–174, 175*t*
total intravenous anesthesia (TIVA), 7, 15, 60, 61, 62, 64, 128, 130, 243–246
train-of-four (TOF) blockade, 63, 147–148, **148**, **149**
training, 70–71
trains, EMG, 23, **24**
transcondylar fossa approach (TFA), 197
transcranial Doppler (TCD), carotid endarterectomy (CEA) and, 270
transcranial electric stimulation (TES), 106–107, **107**, **108**, 109–112, 125, **125**, 129, 133
transcranial electrical motor evoked potentials, 33–38
transesophageal echocardiography (TEE), 10–11, **10**
transient ischemic attack (TIA)/stroke, 263, 266–267, **266**
trauma, spinal, 97
trending, 88
trigeminal nerve monitoring, 219–220
trigeminal neuralgia (TN), 195–196, 198. *See also* microvascular decompression
tumors of the cerebellopontine angle (CPA), 197, 213–226
    anatomy and, 213–215
    brainstem auditory evoked potentials (BAEPs) and, **214**, 216–220, **216**, **221**, **222**
    compound muscle action potentials (CMAPs) and, 219, 224
    electroencephalography (EEG) in, 222
    electromyography (EMG) and, 217–220, **221**, **225**
    evoked potentials (EPs) and, 219
    facial nerve monitoring in, 219
    magnetic resonance imaging (MRI) and, 215
    MEPs and, 218–220
    nerve action potentials (NAPs) and, 219
    nerve conduction studies (NCS) and, 219
    NIOM techniques in, 217–220, 220*t*
    pathology of, 215, 215*t*
    somatosensory evoked potentials (SEPs) and, 217–220, **218**, **221**
    surgical procedures for, 215–216
    technical considerations in, preparation, procedure, postprocedure, 221–226
    timing of neural injury in surgeries of, 216–217
    trigeminal nerve monitoring in, 219–220
tumors of the peripheral nerves, 189
tumors of the spine, 97, 117, 119–122, 119*t*
Turner's syndrome, 97

ulnar neuropathy at elbow (UNE), 188
ultrasound, 10–11, **10**
    Cavitron aspirator (CUSA), 122, 135

ultraviolet (UV) protection, 16
upper limb derivations (SEP), 100–101, **101**
urethral sphincter function monitoring, 161–162, **161**

vagus nerve, 262, **264**
vascular surgeries, 276–277
vascular tumors, 215*t*. *See also* tumors of the cerebellopontine angle
vecuronium, 130
ventilation during anesthesia, 57
ventral posterolateral (VPL) nucleus, 118
vertebral column surgery, 95–116
    anatomy of vertebral column in, 95
    anesthesia for, 112–113
    anterior cervical discotomy and fusion as, 98
    anterior spinal release as, 98
    baseline readings for, 113
    clinical features of disorders in, 97
    cortical potentials for, 100–104
    decussation and, 100–104, **101**
    distal nerve disturbances in, 110
    electroencephalography (EEG) in, 101
    evoked potentials (EP) in, 95
    feedback rapidity in, 100
    interpretation and warning criteria in, 108–111, **109**
    lower limb derivations (SEP) for, 101–104, **102**, **103**, 104*t*
    monitoring techniques in, 99
    motor evoked potentials (MEPs) in, 96–115,
    muscle potentials in, 106–107, **107**, **108**
    pathologic EP decrements in, 110, 113, **114**
    peripheral potentials in, 105
    posterior decompression as, 99
    posterior spinal fusion (SPF) as, 98
    preparation, procedure, postprocedure for, 111–115
    proximal nerve or plexus disturbances in, 110
    radiculopathy in, 110
    scoliosis in, 96–98
    signal-to-noise ratio (SNR), 99–101, **101**
    somatosensory evoked potentials (SEPs) in, 96–115
    spinal cord anatomy in, 96
    spinal cord blood supply in, 96
    spinal cord compromise in, 110–111, **111**
    spinal potentials in, 105
    subcortical potentials in, 104–105
    surgical feedback tracing, **113**
    systemic factors affecting, 109
    technical factors affecting, 109–110
    transcranial electric stimulation (TES) and, 106–107, **107**, **108**
    upper limb derivations (SEP) for, 100–101, **101**
vertical resolution, 85–86
video-EEG, 287, 289
Viking NIOM stimulator, 106
virtual network computing (VNC), 52
virtual private networks (VPNs), for remote monitoring, 48–49, **49**, 51, 52
voltage-divider rule, amplification, 81, **81**

Wada test, 296
Web servers, remote monitoring and, 53–54
widespread anteriorly maximum rhythmic activity (WAR) in, 272
widespread persistent slow waves (WPS), 272, 273
Windows-based remote monitoring systems, 45–46, **46**, **47**
wrist, median neuropathy (carpal tunnel syndrome) at, 188, 189

X-ray machines, 11, 16

Z-meters, 177